To catch the mind and keep it still,
Is no small problem for my porous will;
As many times as I shut it down,
Unceasing thoughts on me rebound

In youth I tried through alcohol,
To ease my stress and cool my gall;
In later years I turned to grass,
The effects were good—but did not last.

At last with failing hopes I turned,
To Eastern paths, and my soul yearned
To scale the mystic heights of bliss.
Alas, no easy method this.

And now with age and turmoil weary,
All that's left me is this query:
Will heart break or mind implode,
Before my vrittis do nirode.*

*Swami Shankarananda*

*Patanjah's second sutra: *Yogash chitta vritti-nirodhah,* "Yoga is the stilling of the modifications of the mind."

# YOGA PHILOSOPHY OF PATAÑJALI

CONTAINING HIS YOGA APHORISMS WITH VYĀSA'S COMMENTARY
IN SANSKRIT AND A TRANSLATION WITH ANNOTATIONS
INCLUDING MANY SUGGESTIONS FOR THE PRACTICE OF YOGA

*BY*

Sāṁkhya-yogāchārya

SWĀMI HARIHARĀNANDA ĀRAṆYA

RENDERED INTO ENGLISH
BY

P. N. MUKERJI, C.B.E., R.B., M.A.

FOREWORD
BY

SWĀMI GOPALANANDA
*Gurudev Siddha Peeth*

STATE UNIVERSITY OF NEW YORK PRESS

ALBANY

This book was first published in English by Calcutta University Press in 1963. Revised editions were published by them in 1977 and 1981.

Published by State University of New York Press, Albany

Printed in the United States of America

For information, address State University of New York Press, State University Plaza, Albany, N.Y., 12246

**Library of Congress Cataloging in Publication Data**

Library of Congress Cataloging in Publication Data

Patanjali.
Yoga philosophy of Patañjali.

Includes index.
1. Yoga. I. Hariharānanda Āraṇya, Swami. II. Mukerji, Paresh Nath, 1882- . III. Vyāsa. Yogabhāṣya. English & Sanskrit. 1983. IV. Title.
B132.Y6P267 1983 181'.45 83-4944
ISBN 0-87395-728-8
ISBN 0-87395-729-6 (pbk.)

## CONTENTS

# FOREWORD

Patanjali's Yoga Sutras are a classical text of Eastern psychology with firm philosophical underpinnings. They give an extremely clear, precise and detailed description of the function of the mind and its relation to the different levels of consciousness. But the Sutras also go beyond the mind to the core of being, the Self, and so provide a spiritual dimension which is lacking in modern psychology and psychoanalysis. Modern psychology works toward integration of the psyche at the level of the mind and personality, but yoga aims for that central core. We can never integrate something unless we go to the heart of it, and so yoga completes the process by which all of the levels of consciousness are realized and harmonized.

There are many similarities between the Yoga Philosophy and the modern psychological model of the subconscious, affecting our lives without our being aware of it. Millenia before Freud, yoga psychology recognized a four-fold division of the psyche into the mind, ego, intellect and subconscious, all arising out of and encompassed by the inner Self. While modern psychology tries to get in touch with the subconscious material, raise it to the level of the conscious mind and deal with it there, yoga actually makes assimilation of the dark and alien contents of the subconscious easier by showing us the perfect Self from which it springs. The essence of the Yoga Philosophy's approach is stated in Patanjali's second sutra, Yogaś citta-vṛtti-nirodhaḥ: Yoga is the stilling of the modifications of the mind," and the third, "Tadā draṣṭuḥ svarūpe 'vasthānam: Then the Self is revealed."

Nothing else is needed. "If you inhibit thought and persevere," social scientist Edward Carpenter has written, "you come at length to a region of consciousness behind thought, and a realization of an altogether vaster Self than that to which we are accustomed." If this does not happen then you are in a sense deluded by your own mind. Thus, the fourth sutra declares, "Vṛtti-sārūpyam-itaratra: Otherwise the seer, or the individual appears to assume the form of the modifications and thoughts of the mind." The clear message of the Sutras is that a human being is not his mind, that he exists far beyond the level of the mind, and most of the text is simply an expansion of this basic point.

Patanjali meets the issue raised by many critics that yoga is a withdrawal or unrealistic pulling away from reality. Our true state of being, he says, is covered by all sorts of wrong ideas and concepts. It is a state of ignorance, prey to the distorting pressures of attachment and aversion, greed, anger and lust. So the first step toward recognition of the Self is withdrawal from those things that delude us. The purpose of this initial separation from the objects of sense and thought is to get in touch with ourselves completely. After we do that, we achieve perfect alignment of our inner being and our external reality, and live involved and in perfect harmony with all.

There are eight steps leading to this direct experience of the Self, according to Patanjali (his Yoga Philosophy is often called Asthanga or Eight-limbed Yoga), beginning with certain behavioral restraints. By following the "yamas" and "niyamas" as these preparatory disciplines are called, one does not actually attain a yogic state of consciousness, but rather a very purified human one. Next is asana, or the practice of physical postures helpful to meditation; pranayama, focussing and stilling the mind through breathing techniques; pratyahara, withdrawal of the senses; dharana, concentration of the mind upon a single object; dhyana, uninterrupted absorption in the object of meditation; and finally, samadhi, or merging with the object of meditation.

Looking at these eight stages, we can see a progressive movement from merely external practices leading inward toward the direct experience of the Self. Unknowingly, in the West, we have dismembered Ashtanga Yoga. Many people, for example, perform asanas independently of meditation as Hatha Yoga, while various self-awareness and mind-control methods use the techniques of pratyahara, dharana and dhyana. Most of these methods involve concentration on a particular object. But the aim of Patanjali's system of yoga is to go beyond even concentration and meditation to the state of samadhi, a state of complete absorption without even the awareness, "I am meditating on something." It is a state of pure being and pure awareness, a nondual state of total freedom and self-knowledge beyond the body, mind and senses.

The value of studying the yoga sutras is that they begin, in a very practical way, to open us to this vastly larger possibility of human functioning. Patanjali's analytical and scientific approach is, moreover, extremely palatable to the western mind. His section on supernormal powers, for example, called in this edition "Explanation of Siddhis," explains brilliantly the normally mystical and airy subject of extrasensory perception, levitation and other supernormal powers. In remarkable detail, Patanjali explains how these siddhis or powers arise. Anticipating the finding of modern science that energy is the underlying "stuff" of our universe, Patanjali implies that through the mind's power, one can manipulate that energy, and that very specific techniques exist for doing so. If the mind penetrates to the core of a particular element, then we perceive its fundamental nature and gain control of it. The Siddhis can also be viewed as feedback techniques or exercises to get control of the mind, but Patanjali does not favor the cultivation of powers, and he makes it very clear that siddhis are not necessary to yogic attainment.

Interestingly, Patanjali seems to have included this section on the occult aspects of yoga not because he is enamoured of them but simply because they actually exist. One can always find yogis with these powers, and so, to make his overview of the yoga system complete, they must be included. But basically, they are distractions and obstacles, and Patanjali cautions us to beware of powers if we really want the true goal of meditation.

With that same pragmatism, Patanjali discusses the concept of God, or Ishwara and our relationship to Him through devotion and surrender. Because God and divine grace are realities for yogis, Patanjali introduces this discussion despite his obviously strong preference for internal and psychological aspects of the yogic process. So, in the 23rd sutra of section One he tells us, "Īśvara-praṇidhānād vā: By self-surrender to God," implying that with grace one may even skip many of the stages outlined by the Yoga Philosophy and attain samadhi directly.

This practical side of Patanjali is also reflected in his literary style. Unlike most classical Indian scriptures, the Yoga Sutras do not have a notable style, and they have no particular rhythm or meter. Neither does Patanjali give lofty and romantic descriptions of exalted states. The Yoga Sutras are written more like a cookbook than like poetry; they say, do this and we will get such and such an experience: put this and this together and we get that.

Indian philosophy differs fundamentally from western philosophy in that its ultimate purpose is the direct experience of liberation. Since the means for attaining liberation is yoga, yoga penetrates and pervades every philosophical system of the East. The dharanas of Tantric works such as the **Vijnana Bhairava** are nothing but yogic practices. The ancient Vedantic and Upanishadic systems speak of stilling the mind and going to the center of the heart. There are certain yogic texts in Buddhism which give methods and techniques of meditation, and we also find yoga referred to in Jainism.

Of course there are western mystics who refer to meditation and yogic experience, but the tendency of religion in the west is to remain largely in what yogis would consider to be the stages of preparation for higher states. In these initial stages of the yamas and niyamas we become a good human being, we attain righteousness, but we don't attain yoga.

The goal of yoga is the Socratic dictum, "Know thyself." When we know ourselves, we know the universe, we know God, we know everything, since everything flows from that substratum, from that Self. For this reason, Patanjali is not really a separate path. It is a description, which we are fortunate to have, of the basic inner dynamic and ultimate stages of all paths to knowledge of the inner Self.

*Swāmi Gopalananda*
*Gurudev Siddha Peeth*
*Ganeshpuri*

# PREFACE TO THE FIRST EDITION

Yoga is one of the six systems of Indian Philosophy, and Patañjali's Yoga-sūtra is one of the earliest treatises amongst them. His Yoga aphorisms deal with the mind and its fluctuations, showing the way how they can be controlled and how complete mastery over the mind can lead to cessation of misery and attainment of peace leading to salvation. The pithy maxims were amplified by Vyāsa and this amplification has come to be regarded as an integral part of the aphorisms to ensure correct understanding of the philosophy underlying them. Various commentators in ages past gave their observations and interpretations to elucidate the complex problems relating to the human mind, but very few in recent times have attempted the task. One of these very few was Sāṁkhya-yogāchārya Śrīmat Swāmi Hariharānanda Āraṇya, Head of the Kāpila Monastery.

Under monastic convention the previous life-history of a monk is a sealed book but this much is known and can be stated that the revered Āchārya Swāmiji hailed from a well-to-do Bengali family and after a scholastic education voluntarily renounced wealth, position and comfort in search of truth in his early life. Cheerfully accepting the austerities and privations of the life of an ordained monk, he spent most of his time in solitude and a good many years in solitary caves in complete and undisturbed possession of his soul so very necessary for deep contemplation and realisation of truth as did the ancient sages of India. The first part of his monastic life was spent in the caves of Barābar hills in Bihar, hollowed out of single granite boulders bearing the inscriptions of Emperor Aśoka and very far removed from human habitation. He spent some years at Tribeni, in Bengal, at a small hermitage on the bank of the Ganges and several years at Hardwār, Rishikesh and Kurseong—all in the Himalayas. His last years were spent at Madhupur in Bihar where he lived the life of a hermit in a dwelling containing a built-up cave. The only means of contact at that time between him and his disciples was through a window opening on a big hall. He spent the last twenty-one years of his life in that solitary sequestered residence where he left his mortal abode.

While leading a hermit's life the revered Swāmiji wrote numerous philosophical treatises, the Yoga-darśana being his ***magnum opus***. Most of his books, the product of his meditation and realisation, were written in Sanskrit or in his native language, Bengali. At first most of the books were published and distributed gratis by his disciples ; nobody made his writings a commercial asset. When through the writings of other writers quoting him and his philosophical views, Western scholars came to know of his vast erudition, they started referring spiritual problems to him for solution. They also made requests for publication of his Yoga-darśana in English. This request very much perplexed him as he had retired from such undertakings long before, let alone preparation of a big book like the present one. This book has been published in Bengali by the University of Calcutta where it has been accepted as a standard work of reference in Indian Philosophy. Later, an edition of the book in Hindi was published by the University of Lucknow for the edification of the scholars of India who do not read Bengali. During the last few years of his life Swāmi Hariharānanda Āraṇya asked several scholars, both Indian and non-Indian, to take up the work of rendering his Bengali Yoga-darśana into English, but unfortunately his wish remained unfulfilled when he shuffled off his mortal coil.

I was attracted to the monastery at Madhupur when after prolonged quest in various parts of India in search of a spiritual guide I had come to this quiet little place more for rest than for search. By the merest accident I heard of the Philosophy taught at the Kāpila Monastery. The revered Āchārya Swāmiji was then fasting and would not see any visitors, I was told. But would I see the younger Swāmiji, if I really wanted to hear anything on a spiritual subject ? The monks of the monastery were very particular and as they did not like to be disturbed for nothing, were I serious in wishing to meet the Swāmiji ?

After a serious heart-searching I took courage in both hands and said 'yes'. I was informed later that I could see the younger Swāmiji the following afternoon. We met, discussed a few general spiritual points and I was directed to read a few books, published by the monastery for full answers to my questions, one of the books being the Yoga-darśana. A few months later Swāmi Hariharānanda departed from this life and Swāmi Dharmamegha Āraṇya, the younger Swāmiji referred to above, his chief disciple, was installed in his place as the Head of the Kāpila Monastery. In course of time, I was initiated into the cult of Sāṁkhya-yoga by the new Chief and I have never looked back. After years of assiduous study and as an *aide-memoire*, I compiled a little book in Bengali, primarily for the benefit of my co-disciples, giving the rudiments of the principles and practice of the Sāṁkha-yoga philosophy. While looking into this book, my master the said Swāmi Dharmamegha Āraṇya mentioned to me the unfulfilled wish of his preceptor the revered author, the great Āchārya Swāmiji as Swāmi Hariharānanda was called by all who had the good fortune to listen to his discourses. With a good deal of hesitation and full of diffidence I asked Swāmiji if I might venture upon this great task. Swāmi Dharmamegha Āraṇya gave me every encouragement, placed the library of the monastery at my disposal and passed words to all members and monks of the monastery—both lay and ordained—to give me every assistance in the preparation of the book.

In the course of the intensive study, necessary for the preparation of a faithful translation, backed by the elucidation and practical hints on Yoga from my master, I realised the vastness of the comprehension of the essential principles by the writer of Yoga-darśana before he could give such an exposition of an abstruse subject like the Yoga Philosophy, because nothing short of revelation in Samādhi could account for the wonderful insight displayed in the book. Although there is nothing new to be said about the ultimate truths which had been stated by the original teachers in ancient times, the later commentators have elucidated the methods for comprehending those truths and with their incomparable genius and uncommon insight have shed lustre of their clear intelligence in illuminating the ancient wisdom of Yoga. In Swāmi Hariharānanda's exposition will be found many things which will go to allay the doubts of ardent enquirers, to establish the appropriateness of the propositions enunciated, to elucidate many apparently unintelligible parts, as well as many new arguments which go to refute the criticism of adverse commentators. This convinced me that every word of the encomium so profusely bestowed on the Bengali edition of Yoga-darśana by the learned scholars all over India was richly deserved. Experienced readers will feel that the commentaries in this book are not the elucidation of a writer who is engaged only in a task of explaining the text without seriously following that philosophy. It is a book primarily for those whose lives have been dedicated to the principles of Sāṁkhya-yoga, who have to remove the doubts of many enquirers and who by their conduct and precept have to establish that knowledge.

Apart from its spiritual aspect, the philosophy of Yoga has a moral value and is of no small practical utility in our everyday life. The sages of old, in India, codified the rules for disciplining the mind so that better human relations could develop which are bound ultimately to bring about collective peace. It is a common error to assume that too philosophical an attitude of mind is antagonistic to social progress, but a careful perusal of the Yoga Philosophy would show that it is not tainted by sectarianism, its principles are of universal application, and that its doctrines are in harmony with human advancement all round. If the cardinal principles of human conduct enunciated in this philosophy are followed in practice, a better man will be built up, human relationship will be sweetened, a better society will come into being, and thus a better world.

I shall now explain the arrangement followed in the presentation of the subject. The aphorisms, or Sūtras as they are called in Sanskrit, have been given first in original Sanskrit with Vyāsa's introductory remarks wherever they occur. Then have bcen given Vyāsa's comments on the Sūtras in original Sanskrit. (These Sanskrit texts can be skipped over by one who does not read Sanskrit, without inferfering with the study of the subject, but these will be found highly illuminating by one who reads Sanskrit.) The English rendering of the Sūtra has been given in capital letters with numerical markings, followed by the English rendering of Vyāsa's commentary. The matters, in respect of which annotations have been given by Āchārya Swāmiji, have been denoted by numerals within brackets after them. These annotations have been given in smaller type preceded by these numerals within brackets.

The reader will find many Sanskrit words retained in the English rendering. A glossary of such words has been given as an Appendix. It has been found necessary to retain the use of such words because equivalents to denote the exact significance or import of the Sanskrit words are not available in English. Wherever possible, the English sense of the word has been given almost immediately in the text or as near to it as possible. Sanskrit words used in the book have been transliterated according to the scheme adopted by the International Congress of Orientalists. The diacritical marks used with their phonetic equivalents are given in the Appendix.

In conclusion, I wish to place on record my grateful appreciation of the valuable assistance rendered to me by my co-disciples of the Kāpila Monastery at Kurseong and the co-operation extended by the monks of the Kāpila Monastery at Madhupur, as well as my deep debt of gratitude to my most revered spiritual guide Śrīmat Swāmi Dharmamegha Āraṇya for the enlightenment given me and for looking over and correcting this book in manuscript which made my task both a pleasure and a privilege.

Kāpila Maṭha,
Madhupur,
Bihar, India.
1963

P. N. Mukerji

# INTRODUCTION

## INDIAN PHILOSOPHY OF LIBERATION

The absence of any mention of historical dates in the ancient Indian treatises makes their chronological placement extremely difficult. A careful and comparative study of the variations in linguistic idioms noticeable in the Vedas and philosophical writings of different periods may, of course, help one in determining—though not with exactitude—the age of the different works. But this method also has its limitations. For there are numerous instances of later compositions imitative of older linguistic styles and of ancient writings containing later interpolations. The Vedas contain, for example, Mantras and Brāhmaṇas composed in several varying and mutually anachronistic linguistic forms.

The names of authors of the different works do not offer any chronological clue either, as these do not refer to specific individuals. It is certain that there were more persons than one bearing the names of Vyāsa or Yājñavalkya and living in different periods of time. Similarly, there were several authors known as Patañjali which was but a family surname according to the Bṛhadāraṇyaka Upaniṣad. All these make it rather impossible to conclusively place the Sanskrit literary or philosophical works in any chronological order that will be beyond doubt. Nor is it our purpose to do so in this discussion which will be confined to a study of the Indian religious philosophies with special reference to the beginning, development and the highest fulfilment of what may be termed 'the philosophy of liberation'.

The appropriate name for the religion of the Hindus is 'Ārṣa-dharma' or the religion of the Ṛṣis. Manu, the ancient Indian law-maker and philosopher, used this name to describe the 'only true religion, not opposed to Vedic teachings'. The Buddhists also referred to this religion as Ṛṣi-mata (Isimata in Pāli) which literally meant the Doctrine of the Ṛṣis. The Vedas which formed the basis of Hinduism emanated from the Ṛṣis who were believed to be persons with extraordinary spiritual attainments. In fact, the term 'Ṛṣi' was expressive of veneration in ancient times and the Buddhists used to describe the Buddha as Maharṣi (Mahesi in Pāli) or the Great Ṛṣi. Women and non-Brāhmaṇas with superior knowledge and power were also regarded as Ṛṣis.

The Ṛṣis were broadly divided into two schools of thought. One of them preached and practised the performance of religious rites leading to worldly happiness (Pravṛtti-dharma) while the other believed in the creed or path of renunciation and liberation (Nivṛtti-dharma).* Performance of rituals advocated by the former was believed to be capable of conferring happiness on one in both the present life and the life beyond. The Ṛṣis who prescribed these rituals and 'saw' or composed their Mantras were founders of this school. The other creed of which Paramarṣi Kapila was known to be the greatest exponent owed its origin to those Ṛṣis who had discovered the way to self-realisation and evolved from their own spiritual life and experience a complete system of theory and practice for guiding others along that path. Unlike Pravṛtti-dharma (creed of worldliness) which has been prevalent in all parts of the world, Nivṛtti-dharma (creed of renunciation) originated in, and belonged exclusively to, India.

The ultimate aim of Pravṛtti-dharma is attainment of heaven and for this purpose it enjoins (i) worship of God or saints and (ii) practice of charity, benevolence, compassion and like virtues along wlth performance of good deeds. Nivṛtti-dharma points out that one's attainment of heaven through good conduct or good deeds is only temporary since this does not ensure freedom from the cycle of births. This freedom can be achieved only through perfect knowledge of one's real self. It is by proper Yoga or Samādhi (absolute mental concentration) and complete non-attachment to worldly interests that one can attain such knowledge which alone can remove Avidyā (misapprehension or imperfect knowledge of the reality), the root cause of unhappiness and the cycle of births.

The exponents or philosophers of Nivṛtti-dharma believed that true knowledge of one's Self or Ātman (soul) consisted in the realisation of its identity with an immutable reality called Puruṣa within oneself and that this realisation could be achieved only through the practice of Yoga. Differences existed, however, in their conception of the real nature of the Self or Puruṣa. The Vedantists hold, for example, that Puruṣa was Saguṇa (one having attributes) at certain stages and Nirguṇa (one beyond the attributes) at others. Sāṁkhya philosophers believed, on the other hand, that Puruṣa, whose number is many, is essentially Nirguṇa.

---

* The literal meaning of the word Pravṛtti is desire for Karma while Nivṛtti means cessation or renunciation of activity. While Pravṛtti-dharma and Nivṛtti-dharma are wide apart, all Pravṛttis need not be discarded. 'Let me be established in the path of renunciation' is also a Pravṛtti (mental activities like conation, etc. are very much a part of Karma, vide Appendix C, the Doctrine of Karma) which is highly desirable as it helps one advance on the path of Nivṛtti.

A chronological study of the genesis of different philosophical theories in India would indicate that the philosophy relating to performance of rituals and making offerings to the deities was the first to be evolved and was followed by the theory of Saguṇa Ātman or the soul with attributes. It was left to Paramarṣi Kapila to conceive and elaborate for the first time the theory of Nirguṇa Ātman. The knowledge spread gradually amongst the Ṛṣis and ultimately found its way into the Upaniṣads. This is pre-eminently noticeable in the teachings of the Kaṭha Upaniṣad.

Ṛṣi Pañchaśikha was the first to formulate the teachings of Paramarṣi Kapila into a number of aphorisms. Unfortunately, the Sāṁkhya-sūtra, as his work is called, is no longer available in its entirety, but the little that is available is sufficient to give us a coherent picture of the entire Sāṁkhya philosophy. Īśvarakṛṣṇa, a later author, compiled nearly all the Sāṁkhya doctrines in a treatise which is still available and is known as the Sāṁkhya-kārikā. The latest authoritative work on the subject is Sāṁkhya-pravachana-sūtra which is complete in six chapters.

Although in Indian thought on self-realisation and spiritual liberation the Sāṁkhya and Yoga philosophy has been traditionally divided into two distinct systems of thought, the two are inseparably related to each other. For, as has already been mentioned, no self-realisation or attainment of true knowledge of one's real self is possible without constant and unfailing practice of the disciplinal exercises of body and mind prescribed in the Yoga system. The difference between the two aforesaid systems lies, therefore, not in their acceptance or rejection of the Yoga but in the fact that while the followers of the Sāṁkhya philosophy believe in self-realisation through a correct understanding of the underlying principles of the phenomenal reality along with complete renunciation of the worldly life, the followers of the Yoga thought seek to achieve the same goal through practice of sturdy self-discipline, study of religious scriptures and repetition of Mantras and complete devotion to God. If one views the Indian philosophical thoughts on the subject of spiritual liberation as one whole system, one finds the Sāṁkhya and the Yoga to be mutually complementary, the former providing the necessary theory and the latter offering instructions on practice. This is why ancient Indian writings abound with avowals of the mutual inseparability of the Sāṁkhya and the Yoga.

According to ancient tradition, the original exponent of Yoga philosophy was Hiraṇyagarbha (the omniscient and all-pervading Creator). He was believed to have taught the system to some Ṛṣis who handed it down to others. Some consider, however, that the name Hiraṇyagarbha might have referred to Ṛṣi Kapila who was also known as Prajāpati and Hiraṇyagarbha. Followers of the Sāṁkhya thought believe that Kapila was born with superior knowledge and a spirit of non-attachment acquired in his previous birth and that he propagated his philosophy after attaining supreme spiritual heights through his own genius. Those belonging to the Yoga school hold, on the other hand, that Kapila acquired his knowledge through the grace of God (Saguṇa Īśvara or Hiraṇygarbha). This view finds mention in the Śvetāśvatara Upaniṣad which formed part of the ancient Yogic literature. Both schools admit, however, that it was Kapila who propounded the Sāṁkhya-yoga philosophy as we find it today.

Although some of the extant literature on the Sāṁkhya-yoga system are of comparatively recent origin the system itself is undoubtedly very ancient. It is profound in its wisdom, precise in its logic and is entirely free from any blind faith or bias. The code of conduct which it enjoins includes the practice of the highest human virtues like Ahiṁsā (non-injury), Satya (truth) etc. and the promotion of the noblest feelings like amity, compassion and the like. The Buddhists adopted this in its entirety. The available biographies of Buddha indicate that he had spent several years as a disciple of Arāḍa-kālāma, a noted Sāṁkhya philosopher of his time, before he left for Uruvilva in quest of further spiritual enlightenment. The practice of the Sāṁkhya-yoga consists in one's complete absorption in meditation (Dhyāna) after acquiring full mastery over one's body and mind, and culminates in Samādhi. This is what Buddha did.

The teachings of the Sāṁkhya philosophy may be summed up as follows :

(i) Mokṣa or liberation consists in the complete and permanent cessation of all sufferings. (ii) In the state of Mokṣa (*i.e.* on attainment of liberation) one abides in one's immutable and attributeless Self which is Puruṣa. (iii) In the state of Mokṣa the mind (Chitta) goes back to its original cause, Prakṛti. (iv) Cessation of the mind (Chitta) can be brought about by renunciation and supreme knowledge acquired through Samādhi. (v) Samādhi is attainable by observance of the prescribed codes of conduct and practice of meditation, concentration, etc. (vi) Mokṣa brings about cessation of the cycle of births. (vii) This cycle is without a beginning and is the result of latent impressions left by Karma (both physical and mental acts) performed in countless previous births. (viii) Prakṛti and Puruṣas (countless in number) are respectively the constituent and efficient causes of the creation. (ix) Prakṛti and Puruṣa are non-created realities with neither a beginning nor an end. (x) Īśvara is the eternally free Puruṣa.

(xi) He has nothing to do with the creation of the universe or life. (xii) Prajāpati or Hiraṇyagarbha or the Demiurge is the lord of the universe and the whole universe is being held and sustained by Him.

These teachings were accepted by all the later religious and philosophical systems of India either in their entirety or in parts.

# YOGA

## WHAT IT IS, AND WHAT IT IS NOT

The ability to stop at will the fluctuations or modifications of the mind which is acquired through constant practice in a spirit of renunciation is called Yoga. True Yoga is practised with a view to attaining salvation. The stoppage of the fluctuations of the mind or its modifications implies the art of keeping only one idea before the mind's eye and shutting out all other ideas or thoughts. In an advanced state of practice, it is possible to suspend all ideation. The two important features of Yoga to be noted are (i) that there is the suppression at will, of the modifications of the mind and (ii) that it is not casual but has been developed into a habit through constant practice, not for gaining a personal end, but in a spirit of renunciation. If without any effort, independently of any volition there is at any time a quiescence of the cognitive faculty of the mind, that is not Yoga. It has been found that some men suddenly get into a mental state of quiescence ; they imagine that at the time they were not conscious of anything. From physical symptoms, such quiescence looks like sleep. Fainting fit, catalepsy, hysteria, etc. also bring about a similar state of mental inactivity. By the conditions mentioned before, this state cannot, however, be regarded as Yoga. Again, some naturally have, or by practice acquire, the power of stopping the circulation of blood or of going without food for long or short periods, none of them is Yoga. Holding up the breath for some time in a particular physical mode or posture is not real Yoga either, because in men capable of performing such feats, the power of concentrating the mind at will on any particular object, is not found as a necessary condition.

In the Yogic concentration, where only a single item of thought is kept in the mind to the exclusion of others, there are stages. When the same item of thought can be kept constant in the mind for some length of time, the Yogic process is known as Dhyāna (meditation). When the meditation becomes so deep that forgetting everything, forgetting as it were even one's own self, the mind is fixed only on the object contemplated upon, such voluntary concentration is called Samādhi (intense concentration). This feature of Samādhi should be understood thoroughly. Ignorant people think that any form of quietness of the mind or trance or loss of consciousness of external objects is Samādhi ; but that has nothing to do with Yoga.

There are different kinds of Samādhi depending on objects concentrated upon, *viz.* Samādhi on gross objects like light, sound, etc., on faculties like Ahaṁkāra (Ego-sense) and on entities like the individual self experienced in the cognitions of 'I' and 'mine'. These are called Savīja-samādhi (*i.e.* supported or assisted by an object). The highest form of Savīja-samādhi is to be absorbed in the thought of Self, *i.e.* in concentration on pure 'I'. At first, of course, fixity of mind on an object has to be practised ; then it develops into Dhyāna. When by practice Dhyāna becomes deeper, it becomes Samādhi. For instance, to attain Samādhi on pure 'I', an idea of pure 'I' has to be formed first by ratiocination and a particular mental process ; then that idea has to be contemplated upon exclusively and developed into Dhyāna. When that deepens, it will lead to complete absorption in pure 'I'. When only the pure I-sense is present and nothing else, the Yogin is not perturbed even by serious pain. No doubt such experience depends on long and constant practice with wisdom and devotion and it is not possible without renunciation of attachment to all gross objects. When the power of Samādhi is acquired by the mind, one can be wholly absorbed in any object of the category of Grāhya (knowable, *i.e.* phenomenal objects comprehensible by the senses), Grahaṇa (internal and external organs) and Grahītā (the receiver, the empirical self). In the early stages of practice, however, devotees are instructed by experienced teachers to take up objects for meditation which would soon bring about a blissful feeling because Dhyāna on objects of the senses like light, sound, etc., does not bring about blissful feeling quickly and makes the realisation of subtle concepts like pure 'I' or individual self, more remote.

While practising devotion and in some cases spontaneously, people have been known to experience a feeling of blissfulness or an expansive feeling as if one were pervading the whole of space. When devotees get such a feeling as a result of devotional practice, it can be utilised as a support for Dhāraṇā (fixity), which in course of time can be developed into Dhyāna (meditation). If one occasionally gets such a feeling spontaneously, *i.e.* without any practice, but cannot get it when he desires it, then it is of no particular use for purposes of Yoga. Again, the coming of such a feeling does not necessarily mean that Dhāraṇā (fixity of thought), Dhyāna (meditation) and Samādhi (intense concentration) have been attained ; because even on getting such a blissful feeling or a feeling of pervading space, such minds continue to rove in many directions and are not occupied with only one idea. It cannot, therefore, come within the definition of Yoga. That feeling may be a sort of realisation and if fixity is developed on the feeling itself then it might lead to the practice of Yoga.

When success in Yogic concentration is attained, knowledge and will-power reach their fullness. One who has not got such proficiency cannot be regarded as having attained the highest perfection in Samādhi. It might be thought that a person having attained such perfection may not like to display his enlightenment or will-power. That may be true, but those who while trying to apply their knowledge and will-power are unsuccessful and still claim to be proficient in Samādhi must be labouring under a delusion.

The fruits of Yoga are the cessation of the three-fold misery. When one can control the cognitive faculty fully and rise at will above the perception of externals and attachment to the body and the senses, then only can one rise above all afflictions.

Real Yoga is of two kinds, Samprajñāta and Asamprajñāta. For Samprajñāta-yoga, one-pointedness or intentness of mind with close and undivided attention is essential. When by contemplation on divinity or on Self etc. or on a state of blissfulness, the mind can be held fixed without effort on any particular object, and no other idea intrudes itself on the mind, then the mind can be regarded as having reached a state of habitual one-pointedness. In an unsteady stage the mind can often be fixed occasionally, but oftener would it work without control. Therefore, even though temporary Samādhi might be attainable at that stage, it will not secure perpetual peace of mind for which a state of habitual one-pointedness is essential. If Samādhi is attained in such a one-pointed state of the mind and enlightenment comes in that state, then the insight gained will always remain. This process is known as Samāpatti (engrossment). If after gaining the power of acquiring knowledge in this way, one can realise the highest form of empirical self which is the Cogniser, and retain that enlightenment, then one can reach the highest stage of comprehension of the phenomenal world. Subsequently, if with discriminative knowledge, realising the phenomenal character of the empirical self, one can, by supreme renunciation, shut out even that engrossment, that would be Asamprajñāta-yoga. Then only can one attain complete quiescence of the mind and the senses, *i.e.* complete cessation of physical and psychical activity, when only the solitary existence of Puruṣa or the metempiric Self remains. That is the ultimate goal of Yoga, which is perpetual peace of mind or Kaivalya Mokṣa, *i.e.* liberation.

There can be three states of the mind, *viz.* Sāttvika or luminously calm, Rājasika or restless and Tāmasika or stupefied. Therefore, if there be reduction of Rajas or the principle of unrest, it does not necessarily follow that the mind will be Sāttvika ; it might be Tāmasika. What is commonly called 'trance' is a state of mental inactivity of that kind ; it is a Tāmasika or torpid state. Mere cessation of mental activity is, therefore, not Yoga. It would be Yoga if mental activity could be stopped at will and the mind could be fixed intently on one or other of the previously mentioned three classes of objects, *viz.* Grāhya, Grahaṇa or Grahītā. In ordinary trance, the mind is not voluntarily occupied with any of them. As a result of anaesthesia, the mind appears also to be reduced to a state of inactivity, but it is really a state of unconsciousness. Hysteria and other similar mental diseases are of the same nature. These are involuntary and torpid states, while Yoga is a voluntary and conscious state. Outwardly there is some likeness between the two states, and hence people get confused but the actual state of the mind and the ultimate result in the two conditions are as different and contrary as darkness and light.

# 卐 मंगलाचरणम् 卐

ॐ नमोऽविद्याविहीनाय ह्यस्मितारहिताय च ।
रागद्वेषप्रहीणाय निर्भयाय नमो नमः ॥ १ ॥

समाहिताय शान्ताय निःसङ्गाय निराशिषे ।
आत्मानं जानते सम्यक् स्वस्थाय च नमो नमः ॥ २ ॥

संस्थितस्त्वयि बाह्यात्मा त्वमन्तरात्मनि स्थितः ।
वितर्कविहीने हार्दे आकाशे मे महीयताम् ॥ ३ ॥

त्वयि मे सर्वम् ओम् ओम् ओम् आत्मनि मे त्वम् ओम् ओम् ओम् ।
स्मारय स्मारय ओम् ओम् ओम् चित्तं शामय शामय ओम् ॥ ४ ॥

स्मराणि सोऽहम् ओम् ओम् ओम् शान्तं चिन्मयमों माम् ओम् ।
त्वत्स्थं केवलम् ओम् ओम् ओम् स्मराणि शुद्धमों माम् ओम् ॥ ५ ॥

## INVOCATION OF THE SUPREME DEITY

My homage to that Being who is devoid of all misapprehension, free from the ME-feeling, above desire and hate, and bereft of all fear.

My homage to Him who is in perfect quiescence and peace, calm, beyond all attachments, above all cravings, who has got perfect knowledge of the metempiric Self and is self-contained.

My outer self (the body) is in Thee ; You are present in my inner self. Oh Lord, You manifest yourself in my inner heart free from all perturbations and worries.

Oh, Om ! Om ! Om ! (God), my all is in You, and You are present in my inner Self, please direct me to be mindful of Thee ; may I be led by my spirit ; may I get peace of mind.

May I have constant remembrance of Thee and of my purified Self dwelling only in Thee. Oh, Om ! Om ! Om !

# YOGA PHILOSOPHY OF PATAÑJALI

# YOGA PHILOSOPHY OF PATAÑJALI

## BOOK I

## ON CONCENTRATION

अथ योगानुशासनम् ॥ १ ॥

भाष्यम्—अथेत्ययमधिकारार्थः। योगानुशासनं शास्त्रमधिकृतं वेदितव्यम्। योगः समाधिः। स च सार्वभौमश्चित्तस्य धर्मः। क्षिप्तं मूढं विक्षिप्तम् एकाग्रं निरुद्धमिति चित्तभूमयः। तत्र विक्षिप्ते चेतसि विक्षेपोपसर्जनीभूतः समाधिर्न योगपक्षे वर्तते। यस्त्वेकाग्रे चेतसि सद्भूतमर्थं प्रद्योतयति, क्षिणोति च क्लेशान्, कर्मबन्धनानि श्लथयति, निरोधमभिमुखं करोति, स सम्प्रज्ञातो योग इत्याख्यायते। स च वितर्कानुगतो विचारानुगत आनन्दानुगतोऽस्मितानुगत इत्युपरिष्टात् प्रवेदयिष्यामः। सर्ववृत्तिनिरोधे त्वसम्प्रज्ञातः समाधिः ॥ १ ॥

**Now Then Yoga Is Being Explained. 1.**

The word 'Atha' (now then) (1) indicates the commencement of a subject which is under discussion. It is to be understood that the Śāstra dealing with the regulations relating to Yoga is now going to be explained (2). Yoga means concentration (Samādhi) (3). It is a feature of the mind in all its habitual states (4), *i.e.* concentration or Samādhi is possible in whatever state the mind may be. Such states (5) are five in number, *viz.* Kṣipta (restless), Mūḍha (stupefied), Vikṣipta (distracted), Ekāgra (one-pointed), and Niruddha (arrested). Of these, in the concentration that is attainable by a distracted mind (6) the moment of concentration is subordinated to the moments of unrest. Such concentration cannot, therefore, be regarded as pertaining properly to Yoga (7). But the concentration attained by a mind which is one-pointed (8), *i.e.* occupied with one thought, which brings enlightenment about a real entity, weakens the Kleśas (9), loosens the bonds of Karma (10) and paves the way to the arrested state (11) of the mind, is called Samprajñāta-yoga (12). Samprajñāta-yoga concerns (a) Vitarka, (b) Vichāra, (c) Ānanda and (d) Asmitā. This will be dealt with later. The concentration that is attainable when all the modifications of the mind-stuff are set at rest is called Asamprajñāta.

(1) Atha—By this word it is implied that with the first Sūtra the discourse relating to Yoga is being commenced.

(2) Anuśāsanam = discourse. The science of Yoga delineated in these Sūtras has been based on the instructions transmitted by the ancient sages. It is not a science newly evolved by the framer of the Sūtras.

Yoga is a science based not merely on logical reasoning. It was originally taught by seers who experienced the truths enunciated therein. This will be evident from the following consideration. Though the knowledge of such super-sensuous subjects as Chit, Asamprajñāta-samādhi, etc., can now-a-days be established by inferential reasoning yet for the validity of such logical process of thought an original proposition (Pratijñā) based on direct experience is necessary. Unless, therefore, something is known first hand of such super-sensuous subjects there cannot arise any occasion for applying inferential reasoning in respect of them. To us the knowledge of such things might come through tradition from generation to generation, but how could such knowledge come to the original teacher who had no instructor ? It must, therefore, be admitted that the original teacher must have acquired that knowledge through direct realisation. If that were not so, if the science of salvation were attempted to be taught by someone who had not himself been emancipated in his life-time or had not realised the ultimate principle of existence, it would be like one blind man leading another. As a blind man cannot give instructions regarding anything concerning the visual properties of objects, so the teachings of a person who has not himself realised any truth, cannot relate to any realisable principle. As stated before, matters concerning Chit, salvation, etc., on account of their being super-sensuous, are either to be taught by others or realised by oneself. To the original teacher it could not have been taught by someone else as he had no teacher ; hence he must have acquired the knowledge through direct realisation. That those matters are not imaginary or deceitful is proved by inference and reasoning. Philosophy has been promulgated to establish by reasoning the propositions enunciated by the original propounders. It has been said : "Truths are to be learnt from the Śrutis, reasoned and then contemplated upon ; these are the ways of realisation." Sāṁkhya philosophy was framed to show the way for the contemplation on the meaning of the Śrutis. Vijñāna-bhikṣu, the commentator on Sāṁkhya-pravachana-bhāṣya, has said : "These instructions have been given to aid contemplation on the meaning of the Śrutis." It is also said in the Mahābhārata : "Sāṁkhya is the philosophy of liberation."

(3) Yoga—This term has various meanings like union of Jīvātmā and Paramātmā, the union of Prāṇa and Apāna, etc., as well as other technical, derivative and conventional meanings. But in this philosophy the term 'Yoga' has been used in the sense of Samādhi or concentration which has been elaborated in the second Sūtra.

(4) The state of mind referred to here denotes the condition in which a mind habitually is.

(5) The habitual states in which a mind can be, have been indicated as five in number, *viz.* restless, stupefied or infatuated, distracted, one-pointed, and arrested. Of these, the mind which is naturally restless (Kṣipta) has not the patience or intelligence necessary for contemplation of a super-sensuous subject and consequently cannot think of or comprehend any subtle principle. Through intense envy or malice, such a mind can at times be in a state of concentration, but that is not Yogic concentration.

The second is the stupefied (Mūḍha) mind. The mind which through obsession or infatuation in a matter connected with the senses is unfit to think of subtle principles, is called a stupefied mind. People engrossed in thoughts of family or wealth generally concentrate on them. This is an example of concentration of an infatuated mind.

The third is the distracted (Vikṣipta) mind. This is different from the restless mind. Most of the spiritual devotees have this type of mind. A mind which can be calm sometimes and disturbed at other times is regarded as a distracted mind. When temporarily calm, a distracted mind can understand the real nature of subtle principles when it hears of them and can contemplate on them for a time. On account of difference in intelligence and other traits of character, there are innumerable varieties amongst men with distracted mind. There can be concentration even with a distracted mind but such concentration does not last long, because the basic trait of such a mind is calmness at one time and restlessness at another.

The fourth is the one-pointed (Ekāgra) mind. The mind which is pointed to one direction only, *i.e.* holds on to one thing only, is called a one-pointed mind. Patañjali has defined it later as a mind wherein, on the fading away of one thought, the same thought arises again in succession. In other words, when one thought vanishes from the mind and the next that arises is similar and there is a continuity of such successive states, then the mind is called one-pointed. When it becomes a habit of the mind, *i.e.* when the mind is occupied wholly with the same thought which continues even in dream, then the state of the mind can be really called one-pointed. When one-pointedness is mastered, it leads to Samprajñāta-samādhi. That Samādhi or concentration is real Yogic Samādhi leading to salvation. In the Vedas it is stated that even if a sinful thought comes unconsciously or irresistibly into the mind of such a wise person it cannot overpower him.

The fifth state is that in which the thought processes have been stopped or arrested at will by long disciplinary practice (Nirodha). This is the last state of the mind. When through practice, all thoughts can be shut out from the mind for a long time, the mind can be regarded as having reached an arrested state. When by this process the mind-stuff gradually ceases to function, then only is liberation achieved.

The minds of all beings are mainly in one or other of the above five states. The commentator has explained which state of the mind is most suitable for concentration leading to salvation.

(6) Of these, the concentration that is occasionally possible through anger, greed or infatuation, in a restless state of the mind does not lead to emancipation. For the same reason liberation cannot also be secured through concentration in a habitually distracted state of mind.

(7) The distracted mind that can be concentrated at times retains the cause of distraction in a suppressed state. In the Purāṇas we read of sages giving way to temptations. This is due to repressed passions coming into play when circumstances favourable to the fruition of suppressed desires arise.

(8) This sort of concentration is not good enough for the attainment of salvation, because when the concentration ceases, distractions arise again which interfere with the consolidation of the knowledge acquired during temporary concentration. Therefore, until the mind is freed of distraction as such and develops a lasting one-pointedness, it cannot be helpful for reaching a state of salvation.

(9-12) The Yoga by which complete and all-round knowledge of the principles, from Buddhi to the Bhūtas, is acquired so that nothing pertaining to that subject remains unknown is called Samprajñāta-yoga. It comes only from concentration in a one-pointed state of the mind. The one-pointed mind can be easily kept fixed on a desired object for any length of time. Men desire to retain the real truth about things in their minds and do not wish to have false ideas about them. In a distracted mind the subtle knowledge acquired through concentration while the mind is temporarily calm, is dispelled by later distractions. Lasting knowledge acquired through concentration is, therefore, possible only when the mind is one-pointed. The knowledge which is everlasting, *i.e.* lasts as long as Buddhi lasts, knowledge subtler than which there is none and which is not destroyed—that is the real and ultimately true knowledge. Such knowledge reveals the true nature of things, which are real and realisable. That is why the commentator has said that concentration in the one-pointed state of mind reveals the real nature of things. That is why if the forces of habit arising out of fundamental human weaknesses are allayed and the spring of our actions is sapped through renunciation based on correct knowledge, such renunciation becomes everlasting. Therefore, in that state the Kleśas are attenuated, and the bonds created by the latent impressions of previous actions are loosened. When the ultimate truth of all knowable things is realised, and by practice of supreme renunciation the process of knowing is set at rest by abandoning all acts and objects of knowing, then the mind is said to have reached a suppressed state. Since in Samprajñāta-yoga the ultimate reality or supreme knowledge is revealed, it is said to be leading to the arrested state (Nirodha).

How the work of revealing the true nature of things, real and realisable, sapping the Kleśas, loosening the bonds arising out of previous actions and leading to the arrested state is done, can be explained as follows : Concentration gives knowledge of the Bhūtas and the Tanmātras. Tanmātras are devoid of pleasure, pain or stupefaction, *i.e.* a Yogin who realises Tanmātras is not affected by the external world. In temporary concentration of a habitually distracted mind such knowledge is no doubt acquired, but when distraction sets in, the mind again feels happy, unhappy or stupefied. In the one-pointed mind, however, such a change is not possible, as the knowledge acquired in its concentration remains firmly fixed and is not obliterated by casual disturbance. It should, therefore, be noted that though knowledge of the real nature of things is possible in concentration of a distracted mind, that knowledge is not permanent as in the case of a one-pointed mind. The same is the case with human weaknesses. Suppose one is fond of wealth. In concentration of a distracted mind if one abjures love of wealth for the time being, it will reappear when the concentration is over ; but in a one-pointed mind such renunciation will become firmly established. Gradually with the elimination of feelings of attachment etc., actions which would have been dictated by such feelings cease altogether and thus the process leads on to the arrested state of the mind. It should, however, be clearly understood that Samprajñāta-yoga is not simply concentration. When the knowledge acquired by a concentrated mind becomes firmly fixed in the mind and is retained there, it is called Samprajñāta-yoga.

———

भाष्यम्—तस्य लक्षणाभिधित्सयेदं सूत्रम्प्रववृते—

योगश्चित्तवृत्तिनिरोधः ॥ २ ॥

सर्वशब्दाग्रहणात् सम्प्रज्ञातोऽपि योग इत्याख्यायते। चित्तं हि प्रख्याप्रवृत्तिस्थितिशीलत्वात् त्रिगुणम्। प्रख्यारूपं हि चित्तसत्त्वं रजस्तमोभ्यां संसृष्टमैश्वर्यविषयप्रियं भवति। तदेव तमसानुविद्धमधर्माज्ञानावैराग्यानैश्वर्योपगं भवति। तदेव प्रक्षीणमोहावरणं सर्वतः प्रद्योतमानमनुविद्धं रजोमात्रया धर्मज्ञानवैराग्यैश्वर्योपगं भवति। तदेव रजोलेशमलापेतं स्वरूपप्रतिष्ठं सत्त्वपुरुषान्यताख्यातिमात्रं धर्ममेघध्यानोपगं भवति। तत् परं प्रसंख्यानमित्याचक्षते ध्यायिनः। चितिशक्तिरपरिणामिन्यप्रतिसंक्रमा दर्शितविषया शुद्धा चानन्ता च, सत्त्वगुणात्मिका चेयमतो विपरीता विवेकख्यातिरिति। अतस्तस्यां विरक्तं चित्तं तामपि ख्यातिं निरुणद्धि, तदवस्थं संस्कारोपगं भवति, स निर्बीजः समाधिः, न तत्र किंचित्सम्प्रज्ञायत इत्यसम्प्रज्ञातः। द्विविधः स योगश्चित्तवृत्तिनिरोध इति ॥ २ ॥

This Sūtra has been enunciated to show the features of the two kinds of Yoga mentioned before.

**Yoga (1) Is The Suppression Of The Modifications Of The Mind. 2.**

In the Sūtra the word 'Sarva' or 'all' being absent (*i.e.* suppression of all modifications of the mind-stuff not having been referred to) it would appear that the word 'Yoga' is intended to include Samprajñāta-yoga as well. Since a mind has the three functions of Prakhyā, Pravṛtti and Sthiti, it must be made up of three Guṇas or constituent principles (2) *viz.* Sattva, Rajas and Tamas. When the faculty of Prakhyā (3) is influenced by the principles of Rajas and Tamas, the mind becomes inclined towards power and external objects. When it is dominated by Tamas it inclines to impious acts, false knowledge, non-detachment and weakness (4). When the veil of infatuation is completely removed and the mind becomes completely luminous, that is to say, when it has a clear conception of the cogniser, the organs of cognition, and the objects cognised, that mind being influenced by a trace of Rajas, tends towards virtue, wisdom, detachment and power (5). When the contamination of Rajas is entirely removed, the mind rests in itself (6), realises the distinction between Buddhi and the pure Self, and proceeds to that form of contemplation which is known as Dharmamegha-dhyāna. Yogins describe this form of contemplation as the highest wisdom. Chiti-śakti or Consciousness is unchangeable, untransmissible, illuminator only of things presented to it by Buddhi, pure and infinite (7). Viveka-khyāti, or the enlightenment of the distinction between the pure Puruṣa and Buddhi, is of the nature of the Sattva principle and is thus opposed to Chiti-śakti (8). As there is still a touch of impurity in Viveka-khyāti, a mind indifferent to it shuts out even that realisation. In such a state the mind retains the latent impressions alone. That is known as Nirvīja or objectless Samādhi. It is called Asamprajñāta-yoga because in this state there is no Samprajñāna (9). Thus Yoga which is cessation of the fluctuations of the mind can be of two kinds.

(1) The suppression of the fluctuations of the mind or Yoga is the highest mental power. In connection with the philosophy of salvation we find in the Mahābhārata : "There is no knowledge like that of Sāṃkhya and no power like that of Yoga." How the cessation of the fluctuations can be a source of mental strength is being explained now. The suppression of the fluctuations means keeping the mind fixed on any particular desired object, *i.e.* acquiring by practice the power of holding the mind undisturbed in the contemplation of any particular object. This is called Yoga. There are various forms of Yoga according to the

nature of the object contemplated upon and the degree of the fixation of the mind. Only external objects do not form the subject of such contemplation, mental states also come under it. When the mind acquires the power of remaining fixed, then any modification arising in the mind can also be retained to the desired extent. We should bear in mind that our mental weakness is only our inability to retain our good intentions fixed in the mind ; but if the fluctuations of the mind are overcome, we shall be able to remain fixed in our good intentions and thus be endowed with mental power. As the calmness would increase, that power shall also increase. The acme of such calmness is Samādhi (concentration) or keeping the mind fixed on any desired object, in a manner in which the awareness of one's individual self gets lost. Although on a perusal of religious and philosophical books we understand the reasons for our miseries and know the ways of escape from them, yet we cannot attain emancipation on account of our lack of mental power. The Upaniṣads teach us that one who knows the bliss of Brahman is not afraid of anything. Knowing that, and knowing fully well that death has really no horror for such persons, we cannot become fearless on account of our weakness. But one who has attained mastery over all organs through concentration and has acquired all round purity can escape from the threefold misery. One who becomes successful in concentration can be liberated even in this very life. That is why the Upaniṣads teach us to practise concentration after learning the Śāstras and meditating on them. It will thus be clear from the above that liberation cannot be attained unless one passes through the process of concentration. Liberation is the highest virtue attainable through concentration. In the Kaṭha Upaniṣad it is stated : "Neither those who have not refrained from wickedness, nor the unrestrained, nor the unmeditative, nor one with unpacified mind, can attain this only by learning." In the Śāstras it is stated that the knowledge of Self attained through concentration is the highest virtue. Happiness is the result of virtue ; knowledge of Self or the state of liberation brings about peace in the shape of cessation of misery which is the highest form of welfare. In this world, whoever is aiming at Mokṣa in whichever form it may be, is following that path in some way or other. Worship of God brings about calmness of mind ; charity and self-restraint also lead indirectly to calmness. Therefore all devotees the world over, consciously or unconsciously are practising in some form or other, the universal virtue of suppressing the fluctuations of the mind.

(2) Detailed information regarding the three faculties of Prakāśa, Kriyā and Sthiti is given in the gloss on Sūtra II.18 (Sūtra 18 of Book II). The commentator is here describing the several traits which become

dominant in the several states of mind and the things that are liked by the mind in such states.

(3-4) The Sattva Guṇa which has been transformed into Chitta, is the 'Chitta-sattva' or the pure cognizant mind. When such mind is influenced by Rajas and Tamas, *i.e.* when on account of restlessness or obstruction, the mind is not inclined to contemplate on the pure Self, then it becomes prone to love of power or to objects of the senses. That sort of disturbed mind never feels happy in meditating on the Self (Ātmā) or in being detached from the objects of the senses ; rather it feels happy in the abundant fulfilment of its desires and enjoyment of the objects of the senses. If persons with such a mind are religious devotees they hanker after supernormal powers ; if not, they aspire after the acquisition of earthly possessions. The former take delight in religious and the latter in worldly discourses. Gradually as the Sattva Guṇa develops in them and the other two Guṇas are overcome, they lose their interest in worldly objects and become happy by withdrawing into themselves. Men with distracted minds do not want real peace but only an increase of power.

Men with minds dominated by the principle of Tamas, lack the ability of discrimination between right and wrong and engage in vicious act or acts which cause great unhappiness. They are deluded and have wrong knowledge about the nature of ultimate reality. They also become greatly fond of worldly objects but through infatuation they act in a manner which brings about loss of exaltation and frustration of their desires.

(5) The principle of Rajas causes activity, *i.e.* change from one condition to another. When the state of infatuation is effectively subdued, the mind starts to have knowledge of the Self, the organs of cognition and the objects cognised. A little mental activity still persists because even then the mind is occupied with Abhyāsa and Vairāgya.

(6) When the least trace of Rajas disappears or, in other words, with the full expression of the Sattva Guṇa, the mind rests in itself. In other words, it is fully endowed with the clarity of the Sattva Guṇa, and becomes pure as gold when relieved of its dross through fire. Moreover, the mind becomes full with the realisation of Puruṣa, the pure Self, or with the knowledge thereof. This is what is called Samāpatti (*i.e.* true and balanced insight) relating to Viveka-khyāti. Such a mind remains occupied only with the realisation of the distinction between Puruṣa or the pure Self and Buddhi. When such realisation becomes permanent, and one becomes indifferent even to the attainment of powers, like

omniscience and omnipresence, then the concentration called Dharmamegha is attained (*vide* Sūtra IV.29).

The supreme knowledge means the realisation of the principle of Puruṣa or pure Self. This is also called Viveka-khyāti or enlightenment of the distinction between Puruṣa and Buddhi. Such knowledge is the effective means of preventing a relapse into empirical life. As the concentration called Dharmamegha leads to the cessation of all misery and as in that condition there arises indifference even to powers like omniscience etc., devotees call it the highest pinnacle of knowledge.

(7) Chiti-śakti or pure Consciousness has been given five adjectives, *viz.* pure, infinite, immutable, untransmissible and illuminator of things presented. The last qualification signifies that it is that to which objects are presented by Buddhi. In other words, it is that which makes Buddhi conscious and leads to the awareness of objects related to Buddhi. Although objects are revealed under its influence, pure Consciousness is neither active nor mutable. That is why it has been called untransmissible, *i.e.* inactive and detached. 'Immutable' means being without any change. It is 'pure' inasmuch as it is not liable to be influenced by the principles of inertia or action as the principle of Sattva is. Moreover, it is fully self-luminous. It is 'infinite' not in the sense of being an aggregation of an infinite number of finite units, but in the sense that the conception of finiteness is not to be applied to it in any sense.

(8) Sattva Guṇa is predominant in Viveka-buddhi or the final realisation. That manifestation which is effected with the help of a manifestor, which is more or less restless and obscured under the influence of its constant companions, Rajas and Tamas, is Sāttvika manifestation or manifestation of Buddhi. That is why things manifested by Buddhi, *e.g.* sound etc., and even the final discriminative enlightenment itself, are limited and transient. Therefore, Buddhi is opposite to self-luminant Chiti-śakti. After having realised Buddhi through concentration, when one experiences the reality of pure Consciousness in an arrested state of mind, there dawns the enlightenment of the distinction between Buddhi and pure Self and this is called Viveka-khyāti. When with the help of Viveka-khyāti and supreme renunciation the arrested state of the mind is made permanent, the state of liberation or Kaivalya ensues.

(9) When having acquired Samprajñāna or complete knowledge of all knowable things, that knowledge also is suppressed through absolute detachment, then that state of Samādhi or concentration is called Asamprajñāta. Unless Samprajñāta concentration is attained it is not possible to reach Asamprajñāta concentration.

भाष्यम्—तदवस्थे चेतसि विषयाभावाद्बुद्धिबोधात्मा पुरुषः किंस्वभाव इति—

तदा द्रष्टुः स्वरूपेऽवस्थानम् ॥ ३ ॥

स्वरूपप्रतिष्ठा तदानीं चितिशक्तिर्यथा कैवल्ये, व्युत्थानचित्ते तु सति तथापि भवन्ती न तथा ॥ ३ ॥

When the mind is in such a state, *i.e.* when Buddhi does not perceive any object, what will be the nature of Puruṣa—the knower of Buddhi (1) ?

**Then The Seer Abides In Itself. 3.**

At that time pure Consciousness—the Seer—abides in its own self, as it does in the state of liberation (2). In the empirical state, pure Consciousness does not appear to be so, though in fact it is so. (Why it is so has been explained in the next Sūtra.)

(1) Pure Consciousness is the impartial witness of Buddhi and the latter appears to it as an object. The dominant Buddhi is the sense of 'I'.

(2) Complete cessation of all fluctuations as in this state, is the state of Kaivalya. In Nirodha, suppression of the mind is for a temporary period, while in Kaivalya the mind disappears, never to appear again. The expressions the Seer's 'abiding in itself', and 'not abiding in itself' (in the sense of being identified with a mental state) are only descriptions from outside and are really verbal. (The gloss on the arrested state of mind will be found in the notes to Sūtra 18 of Book I.)

———

भाष्यम्—कथं तर्हि ? दर्शितविषयत्वात् ।

वृत्तिसारूप्यमितरत्र ॥ ४ ॥

व्युत्थाने याश्चित्तवृत्तयस्तदविशिष्टवृत्तिः पुरुषः, तथा च सूत्रम् 'एकमेव दर्शनम्, ख्यातिरेव दर्शनम्' इति । चित्तमयस्कान्तमणिकल्पं सन्निधि-

मात्रोपकारि दृश्यत्वेन स्वं भवति पुरुषस्य स्वामिनः। तस्माच्चित्तवृत्तिबोधे पुरुषस्यानादिस्सम्बन्धो हेतुः ॥ ४ ॥

Why does it appear like that? Because objects are presented to it (1).

**At Other Times The Seer Appears To Assume The Form Of The Modification Of The Mind. 4.**

The modifications of mind that take place in the empirical state appear identified with the Seer. Pañchaśikha has said on this point: "Consciousness is one; cognitive modification is Consciousness (2)." That is to say, in popular erroneous conception, a particular cognitive modification of Buddhi is taken to be the same as Consciousness. Mind is like a magnet and acts only in proximity (3), and by its character of being an object it appears to become the property of Puruṣa, its owner (4). That is how the beginningless association of the mind and Puruṣa operates as the condition of the mental modification being revealed to Puruṣa (5).

(1) That the pure Self is presented with objects has been dealt with in Sūtra I.2. On account of the close association of Buddhi and the pure Consciousness in the same cognitive process, the objects impressed on Buddhi are revealed by the Consciousness that is Puruṣa. In like manner by being the manifestor of the things taken in by Buddhi, Puruṣa appears to be indistinguishable from the functions of Buddhi.

(2) Pañchaśikha was a very ancient teacher of Sāṁkhya. It is said in the Purāṇas that Āsuri was a disciple of Kapila and Pañchaśikha was a disciple of Āsuri. Pañchaśikha was the first to compose aphorisms on the principles of Sāṁkhya philosophy. Such of his sayings as have been cited by the commentator on Yoga-sūtras in support of his observations are priceless gems. The book from which these have been extracted is now lost. About Pañchaśikha it is stated in the Mahābhārata that it was he who fully determined all the principles relating to the virtue of renunciation and had no doubts in his mind about them. The word 'Darśana' in the quotation from Pañchaśikha refers to the pure Self or pure Conscious-

ness and the word 'Khyāti' refers to the modification of Buddhi or manifestation by Buddhi.

(3) Vijñāna-bhikṣu explains the analogy as follows : "As a magnet by drawing to it a piece of iron does some service to its owner and thus becomes, as it were, a treasured possession of the owner, so does the mind serve its master, Puruṣa, by drawing to itself the objects around it and presenting them to Puruṣa and thereby become, as it were, the very self of Puruṣa."

(4) 'I shall see,' 'I shall hear,' 'I know,' 'I doubt,' etc.—amongst all these Vṛttis the common feature is 'I'. The basic knower behind all these phases of 'I' is Consciousness itself which is the Seer - the Draṣṭā. The Seer is Consciousness. Buddhi reveals things by appearing to be conscious under the influence of the Consciousness, that is, the Seer. That which is manifested or that which we come to know is the object. Colours, sounds, etc. are external objects. Knowledge relating to them is acquired through the mind. In the knowledge of objects, 'I' am the the knower, *i.e.* the subject, mind with the senses is the instrument or power of knowing, and the things known are the objects. Generally, matters relating to our mind are known to us by introspection. Therefore, when the process of knowing takes place in the mind before we come to analyse it, we first become aware of it in introspection and then, again in recollection. Though the mind acts as an instrument of the Seer in the matter of acquisition of knowledge, yet on certain occasions it itself becomes an object of knowledge to the Seer. The constituent cause of the mind is Asmitā or the cognition of 'I'. The cognitions of objects appearing in the mind are the varying modifications of the I-sense. When the power is acquired of keeping the mind calm, then we can have an intuition of this Asmitā. If we concentrate on the changing I-sense, we can realise that the knowledge of anything is a change of this Asmitā and is different from it. Then the mind perceiving the objects becomes the object and Ahaṁkāra* or the I-sense becomes the instrument of knowledge. Then when by controlling the I-sense we can remain on the pure Asmitā-level, we can realise that the Ahaṁkāra is different from the Self and is fit to be discarded. Only pure I-sense or Buddhi then becomes an instrument of knowledge. When through knowledge acquired in concentration it is realised that Buddhi is also mutable and not self-luminous, and thus one becomes aware of the existence of a Puruṣa by whom all the actions of Buddhi are manifested, then that Viveka-khyāti, or discriminative knowledge keeps on making

* Ahaṁkāra or Asmitā or Abhimāna is the mutative ego or the I-sense undergoing modifications as 'I am the body,' 'The organs are mine,' etc.

known only the existence of Puruṣa. When even that discriminative enlightenment ceases because of supreme detachment and does not function for want of knowables, *i.e.* when the subject is relieved even of the vestige of I-sense, then the Puruṣa or Seer is said to be in isolation, *i.e.* abiding in his own nature. Buddhi then being separated becomes an object of knowledge. It is thus how everything from Buddhi downwards is regarded as an object. That which depends on another for its manifestation is an object of knowledge and that which does not depend on another for its revelation is the self-luminous principle of Consciousness. Puruṣa or the Seer is self-luminous, while Buddhi and other objects are revealed by something else. They appear as conscious under the influence of Consciousness or the Self. This is the nature of the subject and the object. The subject (Draṣṭā) is like the proprietor and the object (Dṛśya) is like his property. The process of realisation of Buddhi etc. will be described later.

(5) The beginningless association between Puruṣa and the object, which is due to want of true knowledge is the cause of the awareness by Puruṣa of all the modifications of the mind whether they are Sāttvika, Rājasika or Tāmasika.

———

भाष्यम्—ताः पुनर्निरोद्धव्या बहुत्वे सति चित्तस्य—

वृत्तयः पञ्चतय्यः क्लिष्टाऽक्लिष्टाः ॥ ५ ॥

क्लेशहेतुकाः कर्माशयप्रचयक्षेत्रीभूताः क्लिष्टाः, ख्यातिविषया गुणाधिकार-विरोधिन्योऽक्लिष्टाः। क्लिष्टप्रवाहपतिता अप्यक्लिष्टाः, क्लिष्टच्छिद्रेष्वप्यक्लिष्टा भवन्ति, अक्लिष्टच्छिद्रेषु क्लिष्टा इति। तथाजातीयकाः संस्कारा वृत्तिभिरेव क्रियन्ते, संस्कारैश्च वृत्तय इति, एवं वृत्तिसंस्कारचक्रमनिशमावर्त्तते, तदेवम्भूतं चित्तमवसिताधिकारमात्मकल्पेन व्यवतिष्ठते प्रलयं वा गच्छतीति ॥ ५ ॥

Although the controllable modifications are many,

**They Fall Into Five Varieties Of Which Some Are 'Kliṣṭa' And The Rest 'Akliṣṭa'. 5.**

The 'Kliṣṭas' are those mental processes which have their bases in Kleśas like Avidyā etc. (1) and are the sources of all latencies (2). The 'Akliṣṭas', on the other hand, are those that concern final discriminative enlightenment (Khyāti) and are opposed to the operation of the Guṇas (3). Some Vṛttis may be Akliṣṭa and may yet have their place in the stream of Kliṣṭa-vṛttis (4). There may arise Akliṣṭa-vṛttis in the intervals (5) of Kliṣṭa-vṛttis and *vice versa*. Latent impressions are left equally by mental processes which lead to misery as well as those which lead to freedom therefrom. These latent impressions again give rise to fluctuations of the mind (6). In this way until absolute concentration is attained by a mind in a suppressed state, the wheel of fluctuations and impressions goes on revolving. When mind is freed from the operation of the Guṇas, *i.e.* freed from the seeds of disturbance, it abides in itself, *i.e.* exists only in its pure being or again, becomes reabsorbed in its own matrix (7).

(1) The mental fluctuations which are based on the five afflictions like Avidyā etc. (*vide* Sūtras II.3-9) are the 'Kliṣṭa' ones. If any of the afflictions, namely, wrong knowledge or nescience, the cognition of Buddhi as the pure Self, attachment or passion, antipathy or aversion, and fear of death, causes a fluctuation or modification of the mind, then that is called 'Kliṣṭa'. It is so called because the impression that is left behind by such a modification, produces an afflicted mental state. It is because these Vṛttis cause 'Kleśa' or sorrow that they are also called 'Kleśa' or afflictions.

(2) For the foregoing reason, the afflicted states have been described as the breeding ground of the Saṁskāras or the latent impressions of actions. Vijñāna-bhikṣu has explained Vṛtti as that which provides the wherewithal for one to live. Chitta-vṛtti implies the various knowing states of the mind. As the mind ceases to function without these states, they are called its Vṛttis.

(3) Through wrong knowledge, the adjuncts of Puruṣa in the shape of body, mind, etc. are constantly undergoing changes or they exist in a dormant state or move in a flow of births and deaths. This is what is meant by Guṇavikāra or the changes in the Guṇas. When through correct knowledge nescience etc. are destroyed, the mental fluctuations connected with this correct knowledge counteract the operation of the Guṇas and are, therefore, known as Akliṣṭa-vṛttis or those which do not

lead to sorrow. For example, an illusion like the cognition that 'I' am the body, or the fluctuations of the mind arising out of actions done under the influence of such an illusion, are harmful processes founded on nescience. Deep contemplation or conduct based on correct knowledge that 'I' am not the body gives rise to processes which are free from afflictions. As the sequence of such fluctuations might terminate the assumption of the body, *i.e.* of the chain of births and deaths and thus of incorrect knowledge, these are called harmless or beneficial modifications conducive to the elimination of the operation of the Guṇas. When through the final discriminative knowledge, nescience is destroyed, the state of mind arising therefrom is the Akliṣṭa *par excellence*. The mediate cognition of the distinction between Puruṣa and Buddhi through verbal instruction, study and contemplation without any actual realisation of the same, is also an Akliṣṭa-vṛtti, but only in a secondary sense.

(4 & 5) It might be urged that it is hardly possible for creatures with a preponderance of 'harmful' Vṛttis to have at all any 'beneficial' ones, or for the latter to prove effective in the welter of the 'harmful' modifications of the mind. In reply, the commentator explains that the 'beneficial' modifications, though mixed with the harmful ones, remain distinct from them as a shaft of light coming into a dark room remains distinct from the surrounding darkness. The intervening period of practice of right conduct and detachment might be fruitful in giving rise to 'beneficial' modifications. In the same manner through the loopholes in the stream of 'beneficial' fluctuations, the 'harmful' ones might also creep in. As the overt modifications continue to exist as latent impressions, the 'beneficial' ones arising amongst the 'harmful' ones might gradually become stronger and eventually shut out the flow of 'harmful' fluctuations.

(6) Fluctuations whether harmful or 'beneficial' give rise to latent impressions of a corresponding nature. The retention in mind of any particular experience is called its Saṁskāra or latent impression or latency. In what follows it is being shown which Vṛttis are harmful and which are not. True knowledge (Pramāṇa) like Viveka-khyāti and valid cognition conducive to it is free from harm while the opposite is harmful. At the time of Viveka-khyāti or when a Nirmāṇa-chitta (see IV.4) is created, unreal knowledge (Viparyaya) like the I-sense and those modifications which lead to Viveka-khyāti are harmless, while, at other times these are harmful. Ideas or concepts which though ultimately unreal (Vikalpa), contribute to the acquisition of the final absolute knowledge, are harmless while their opposites are harmful.

The recollection (Smṛti) of discriminative knowledge and of those cognitions relating to Self which lead to such knowledge is harmless while the opposite one is harmful. The slumber (Nidrā) which is reduced by the practice of retaining discriminative knowledge in the mind and of recollection relating to Self, and which is conducive to the development of such knowledge, is harmless, whereas ordinary sleep is not so. The slumber, before and after which the thought of Self predominates or which gets reduced in intensity by such thought and which is just enough for health during spiritual practice, is harmless sleep.

(7) That which is, or exists, is never destroyed. That is why what looks like existing in a reasonable empirical view, will, as long as such outlook persists, continue to appear as existing. All phenomenal objects are mutable. They do not always exist in the same form. Their material assumes different forms, *e.g.* what is a clod of earth to-day becomes a pot tomorrow. In the pot the earth is not destroyed ; only the earth has changed form and is existing in the form of a pot. Thus everything ordinarily visible is existing in one form or another. We cannot think of the total absence of anything. In this change the form in which the thing existed before is called the continuing cause of the subsequent form, as the earth is of the pot. When a thing is reduced to its causal substance then it is said to be destroyed. Therefore, 'destruction' means dissolution of a thing in its original causal substance. Thus in the ordinary view a liberated mind will be presumed to be existing as merged in its principal matrix, the Avyakta. From the spiritual standpoint, when the threefold misery ceases effectively, then, there being no more chance of its being manifested, the mind lapses and looks like having disappeared. The mind then remains in a state which is the equilibrium of the three Guṇas, only the cause of misery, *viz.* the co-relation of the Self and the object, disappears for good.

In the Dhyāna or contemplation known as Dharmamegha the mind abides in its real nature, *viz.* as pure Sattva, is free from the incubus of Rajas and Tamas principles ; while in Kaivalya or the state of final isolation or liberation the mind merges into its constituent cause. Freedom of the mind from the incubus of Rajas and Tamas does not mean freedom from those principles, but freedom from such functioning on their part as stands in the way of discriminative knowledge.

———

भाष्यम्—ताः क्लिष्टाश्चाक्लिष्टाश्च पञ्चधा वृत्तयः—

प्रमाण-विपर्यय-विकल्प-निद्रा-स्मृतयः ॥ ६ ॥

Those harmful and harmless modifications are of five kinds, namely—

**Pramāṇa, Viparyaya, Vikalpa, Sleep And Recollection** (1). **6.**

(1) It might be urged that when dreamless sleep is being counted as a fluctuation of the mind, why are not waking state and dream state being so counted ? Why are not volition etc. also mentioned ? In reply, it is to be stated that the waking state is occupied mainly with Pramāṇa, though Vikalpa etc. are also present ; while a dream state is primarily one of Viparyaya, though Vikalpa, recollection and Pramāṇa might also form part of it. The states of waking and dream have not been mentioned separately as by the mention of the other four, *viz*. Pramāṇa, Viparyaya, Vikalpa and Smṛti (recollection) as well as by the fact that the stoppage of such fluctuations will bring about a stoppage of the waking state and dream state, they have been included automatically. Similarly, volition has not been specifically mentioned because it arises through modifications of cognition and stops with the shutting out of such modifications. By the five false cognitions, volition has also been implied, as resolutions are formed through attachment, hatred, aversion, etc. In reality the author of the Sūtra has mentioned only the fundamental modifications which should be controlled. That is why the feelings or states of fluctuation like happiness or misery have not been included. Happiness or sorrow cannot be controlled by itself ; it is to be eliminated by shutting out valid cognition etc. which give rise to them.

In the Yoga philosophy the word Vṛtti has been used technically to imply cognition or conscious mental states. Of them, Pramāṇa is correct cognition, Viparyaya is incorrect cognition, Vikalpa is the cognition of a thing which does not exist and which is other than Pramāṇa and Viparyaya ; Nidrā or dreamless sleep is indistinct awareness of the state of suppression ; and Smṛti or memory is the awareness again of previous cognitions. The dominantly active or inert states of the mind are always associated with cognition which prevails over all types of fluctuations ; hence the stoppage of cognitive modifications leads to the cessation of all mentation. Therefore the fluctuations to be controlled in Yoga are the cognitive fluctuations or Pratyayas. Yogins attain the arrested state of mind by stopping the cognitive fluctuations. The Vṛttis in Yoga mean the variations of Prakhyā or the Sattva-element of the mind. Chitta or the mind is the internal power which cognises, wills and retains by blending together the knowledge relating to sound, touch, light, taste and smell brought in by the five sense-organs, the experience relating to movement of objects brought in by the organs of action, the perception of inertness of outside elements by the five Prāṇas or the vital forces of the body and the perception of pleasure and pain as inherent in the internal organs. The following examples will make the idea clear. You see an elephant. The eyes only see a black mass ; its other properties are not known by the eyes. Knowledge about its power of carrying loads, its power of movement, its mode of life, its toughness, its trumpets had been gathered before by your appropriate sense-organs and retained in the mind. The inner faculty which combines all these fragments of knowledge after the elephant is seen and produces the concept that it is an elephant, is Chitta. The feeling of satisfaction or pleasure that you may have at the sight of the elephant is also an action of Chitta or mind-stuff and is only a reappearance of the feeling of pleasure which you have experienced before.

By its movements or fluctuations the existence of the mind is felt ; the absence of fluctuations can only mean the lapse of Chitta. The modifications of the mind can be divided into several main heads according to the three constituent principles or Guṇas. Out of them only the principal controllable ones have been mentioned by the author of the Sūtras as being five in number so far as Yogic practice is concerned. All students of this science should particularly remember the following points, regarding Chitta : Chitta or the mind is the internal organ with three functions, *viz.* cognition (*i.e.* knowing), conation (*i.e.* willing), and retention. Retention is the subliminal or latent impression. The feeling or impression of things seen, of things retained in the mind (as memory), of things willed, of pleasure or pain acutely felt, are modifications of the mind, known as Pratyayas. Conation or willing being a cognised or conscious function is also of the nature of Pratyaya. Saṁskāras or latent, *i.e.* subliminal impressions are unconscious functions. Thus mind has two properties, *viz.* Pratyaya and Saṁskāra. Of these, Pratyaya is called Chitta-vṛtti or the modification of the mind. In this science the fluctuations or modifications taken collectively are ordinarily known as Chitta or mind. Since the fluctuations are cognitive by nature of knowledge, they are the transformations of Buddhi which is the transformation of Sattva. That is why the words Chitta and Buddhi have been used in the same sense at many places. That Buddhi or intellect is not the Buddhi as a Tattva or principle. Similarly, 'Chitta-vṛtti' or 'modification of the mind' has been designated 'Buddhi-vṛtti' or modification of Buddhi. The words 'Chitta' and 'Manas' have been used in the same sense in many places, but really speaking, Manas is the sixth sense. In other words, the awareness that is necessary for the internal effort, for the setting in motion of the external senses and for the inner awareness of mental states is the work of the mind. Mental perception is due to that awareness just as visual knowledge is due to the eye. Thus mind, the instrument of conation, is the internal centre of the organs of knowledge and action, while Chitta-vṛtti or modification or fluctuation of the mind is nothing but knowledge itself. The specific knowledge of things cognised, done or retained by the mind is Chitta-vṛtti. It should be remembered that this is the ancient division of the mind.

---

भाष्यम्—तत्र—

प्रत्यक्षानुमानागमाः प्रमाणानि ॥ ७ ॥

इन्द्रियप्रणालिकया चित्तस्य बाह्यवस्तूपरागात्तद्विषया सामान्यविशेषात्मनोऽर्थस्य विशेषावधारणप्रधाना वृत्तिः प्रत्यक्षं प्रमाणम्। फलमविशिष्टः पौरुषेयश्चित्तवृत्तिबोधः। बुद्धेः प्रतिसंवेदी पुरुष इत्युपरिष्टादुपपादयिष्यामः।

अनुमेयस्य तुल्यजातीयेष्वनुवृत्तो भिन्नजातीयेभ्यो व्यावृत्तः सम्बन्धः, यस्तद्विषया सामान्यावधारणप्रधाना वृत्तिरनुमानम्। यथा, देशान्तरप्राप्तेर्गतिमच्चन्द्रतारकं चैत्रवत्, विन्ध्यश्चाप्राप्तिरगतिः।

आप्तेन दृष्टोऽनुमितो वार्थः परत्र स्वबोधसंक्रान्तये शब्देनोपदिश्यते, शब्दात्तदर्थविषया वृत्तिः श्रोतुरागमः। यस्याऽश्रद्धेयार्थो वक्ता न दृष्टानुमितार्थः स आगमः प्लवते, मूलवक्तरि तु दृष्टानुमितार्थे निर्विप्लवः स्यात्॥ ७॥

Of these,

**Perception, Inference And Testimony Constitute The Pramāṇas (1). 7.**

Perception is that modification of the mind which is caused by its contact (2) with an outward object through the sense-channel and which is concerned mainly (3) with the special features of the object that is characterised by the special as well as by certain general features. The outcome (4) of this perceptual modification is the Self's awareness of this modification as undistinguished from the Self. That the Self is the reflector of Buddhi (5) will be established later on.

Inference is that kind of mental modification which is based on the general characteristics of a knowable and is concerned with the entity (*viz.* the mark) (6) that is present in the instances where the probandum occurs and is absent from the instances where the probandum does not occur. For example, the moon and the stars have motion as Chaitra (name of a person) has, for they, like him, change their position ; the Vindhya Hills do not change its location and so it has no motion.

The mental modification arising from hearing the words of a reliable person who desires to convey his cognition to the hearer is Āgama-pramāṇa, *i.e.* authoritative testimony to the hearer (7). That testimony may be false, *i.e.* cannot at all be a Pramāṇa, if the person communicating the knowledge is not trustworthy or is deceitful or is one who has neither seen nor experienced what he seeks to communicate. That transferred cognition which has its basis in the direct experience of the first authoritative exponent or in his correct inference is genuine and perfectly valid (8).

(1) Pramā is uncontradicted knowledge about a real object. The instrument of Pramā, *i.e.* the way of getting correct knowledge is Pramāṇa. Pramāṇa is making sure of a real thing which was unknown before ; in other words, Pramāṇa is the process of Pramā in regard to an unknown thing. This definition of Pramāṇa might give rise to the doubt that when the absence of fire is established by an inference, then the definition of Pramāṇa cannot cover that inference. In reply it has to be stated that cognition of a non-existent thing is really the cognition of existent things other than that one and is just a 'Vikalpa'. The absence of a thing is in reality some other positive thing and is asserted only in relation to something present. About the knowledge of non-existence it has been said in the Śloka-vārttika by Kumārila Bhaṭṭa, that it is

formed mentally and independently of the senses by perceiving a positive entity and then remembering that which is asserted to be absent. For example, when we do not see a pot in a place, we first see a vacant and illuminated place, and then we form an idea in the mind that the pot is absent. In fact, no knowledge can be formed without reference to an object. All the knowledge that we have of things that exist is mainly of two kinds, *viz.* Pramāṇa and experience. Of these, Pramāṇa relates to things which are outside the sense-organs or accepted as outside the sense-organs. Perception, inference and testimony—all these Pramāṇas are characterised by this feature. Experience relates to what occurs inside the sense-organs, *e.g.* cognition of memories, of pleasure, etc. Realisation of something not known before is also called Pramā ; its instrument is called Pramāṇa. The definition of Pramāṇa distinguishes it from memory. In this science of Yoga, certain experiences have been taken to be mental 'perception' and thus included in the category of Pramāṇa. Recollection is not, however, mental perception because it is the feeling again of things felt before. Therefore, Pramāṇa and recollection are different.

(2) Mental fluctuations vary with differences in the external objects. That is why these objects affect or modify the mind. When the mind comes into contact with an object through the sense-channel, then the mind is affected or changed. Each modification of the mind-stuff is one piece of knowledge. Chitta comes into contact with objects through six sense-channels. The five external sense-organs and the sixth internal one, called Manas, are the channels recognised by the science of Yoga. Through the external sense-channels we get only an inchoate elementary sensation, which is just a form of reception. For example, what we get through the ear is only an inchoate sensation, *e.g.* the cawing sound. Then with the help of the other functions of the mind we ascertain that it is the voice of the crow. This complete knowledge is mental perception.

In the perception of mental objects, we get adequate knowledge of cognition, *i.e.* by collecting the experience imparted by the senses we become aware of the cognition. The sensation of pleasure etc. is inchoate mental knowledge. The full knowledge thereof which follows is the adequate knowledge of a mental object. Like the action of external sense-organs, the mind receives the impressions first ; next when the mind-stuff is affected thereby, *i.e.* other mental functions like memory etc. co-operate, then mental perception takes place. Thus in all mental perceptions, reception comes first and then comes the full perception. Therefore, the sure awareness of a thing outside the senses is Pramāṇa. This definition is applicable to all direct perceptions.

(3) The feature and form of external objects are called their Viśeṣa (special characteristics). Every object has its peculiar properties of sound, touch, etc. different from those possessed by others ; they are called their feature (Mūrti) while Vyavadhi is their special form. Take the case of a piece of brick. Its colour and shape cannot be exactly described by howsoever large a number of words we may use ; but when we see it we can at once have the exact cognition. That is why direct apprehension mainly relates to Viśeṣa, *i.e.* form and feature. The word 'mainly' has been used to imply that some awareness of the general features is present therein, though knowledge of the special properties and features predominates. That which is present in many things is called Sāmānya or generality. Words like fire, water, etc. are used in a general sense. On account of nature and shape, fire may be of many kinds though their general name is 'fire'. Existence is a common feature of all things. In direct apprehension knowledge of such general features is also present in a modified form. In the following instances of inference and verbal communication, however, the awareness is only of the general features, because they are established by words, signs, etc. It cannot be said that in the case of 'Chaitra (name of a person) exists'—a case established by inference or verbal communication—we have an instance of the knowledge of a particular object ; because if Chaitra had been seen before, the mention of the word 'Chaitra' will only bring the recollection (which is not a Pramāṇa) of Chaitra. The knowledge of 'existing at a certain place' will only fall under the category of Pramāṇa. If Chaitra was not seen before, the statement will not convey any particular information about Chaitra. Inference or verbal communication can only convey general and partial information.

(4) Outcome = Result of the perceptual process. Vijñāna-bhikṣu says it is the 'effect of Vṛtti as Karaṇa'. In illustrating the expression, 'the self's awareness of this modification', he says that it is like the cognition of 'I am knowing the pot.' But that kind of cognition might be of two kinds. In direct apprehension, the perception is—'This is a pot' or 'The pot exists.' But as it contains a reference to the knower, it can be analytically expressed in words as 'I am seeing the pot.' Again, while seeing a pot one feels 'I am seeing a pot.' The first awareness, *viz.* of 'the pot exists' is primarily unreflective perception and the second one, *viz.* of 'I am seeing the pot' is predominantly reflective perception. The first, 'This is a pot' or 'The pot exists' is direct perception. In that direct perception there function three ideas—'I', 'the pot' and 'seeing', but when the pot is being seen then it is felt only that the pot exists ; and the Seer,

the act of seeing and the object seen are not felt separately. The knowledge of 'I am the Seer' being absent, and the presence only of the pot being felt, the Seer implied in the ego and the aprehended 'pot' appear to be undifferentiated. This has been stated already in the 4th Sūtra. The mental modification due to direct perception may last for a moment and may be followed by the stream of similar states. But when the perceptual modification concerning 'a pot' arises, then it is not differentiated as 'I am seeing the pot,' there is only the feeling that the 'pot' is present. In knowing the pot, the Seer behind it is present ; that is why the Seer can be said to exist in an undifferentiated form in the awareness of the pot, though as a matter of fact they are really different.

This can be understood in another way. All knowledge is a transformation of Ahaṁkāra or the cognition of 'I' and 'mine'. Of these, perceptual knowledge is the transmutation of the I-sense due to the action of an external object. Therefore, knowledge of a pot is only a modifiction of the I-sense. But the Seer is included in the 'I', that is why in the perception of the pot, the transmutation of the I-sense in the shape of knowledge of the pot and the Seer are undifferentiated. Of course, by reflection and reasoning we can understand the difference between the Seer and the pot, but that is not possible in a mental fluctuation like the unreflective perception relating to the pot.

'The Self's awareness' means the manifestation of the knowledge of which Puruṣa or the knower is the witness. It may be urged that if the Puruṣa is the illuminator of various modifications then he must have variety or he must be subject to change. This contention would have been valid if variability could affect Puruṣa. But this is not so. It is only the senses and the mind which are subject to variations. If objects are analysed one comes upon only subtle activity which is appearing and disappearing every moment. Under its influence Buddhi or the pure I-sense is also undergoing subtle change from moment to moment. Puruṣa is the illuminer of the momentary phases of the mutation of Buddhi. Buddhi is co-existent with mutation and Puruṣa is what remains when such mutation ceases. That is why that mutation cannot reach Puruṣa. This is really how a Yogin realises the principle of Puruṣa. First, he realises Tanmātra, *e.g.* the light Tanmātra, taste Tanmātra, out of the various gross elements, *i.e.* the variety in colours or in tastes etc. Then gradually by deep meditation he realises the disappearance of those principles in the I-sense. By realising that the subtle principles of Tanmātra are nothing but variations of the I-sense, he arrives at the pure awareness of the 'I' as a principle or category and then with discriminative knowledge he realises the Puruṣa principle. Thus by gradually shutting out subtle and yet more subtle mutations he is established in that principle, *i.e.* gets a clear idea of that principle.

(5) 'The Self is the reflector of Buddhi,' this description is of a deep import. Reflection generally means change of direction of a ray of light after striking a surface like that of a mirror. Similarly, 'reflection' here implies a change or seeming change in the character of a perception or cognition caused by its contact with some other reagent. The perception or cognition, at a given moment of Buddhi is reflected at a later moment as ego. The root cause of this reflection is Puruṣa. To be able to think 'I exist' is also the result of such reflection. For all lower physical sensations or perceptions of objects, the centre of reflection is Buddhi or the organs below it. But the reflector of Buddhi, which is the highest form of the phenomenal Self, is beyond Buddhi ; that is the immutable Consciousness or Puruṣa. This idea of reflection is the way of reaching the Puruṣa principle. After realising the principle of the pure I-sense by force of concentration, its reflector the Puruṣa principle has to be realised by a process of meditation. This really is Viveka-khyāti or final discriminative knowledge.

(6) Concomitance and non-concomitance are the two kinds of relationship in an inference. Concomitance means agreement in presence or agreement in absence, while non-concomitance implies non-agreement in presence or absence. Broadly speaking, having realised the nature of these kinds of relationship and having known one of the two related things, to know the rest is inference. When non-existence of something is inferred, it implies the knowledge of the existence of some other things ; this has been explained before. Cognition of a non-existent or negative thing has no place in this science.

(7) The knowledge from sentences composed of the cases and verbs gives their purport but does not necessarily give the assurance of its absolute certitude. In every case there may not be a correct cognition. In some instances doubts arise and in some others the doubts are dispelled through inference. For example, 'So and so is reliable, when he says it, it must be true.' From study also one can make sure. This is inferential proof. From this many think that Āgama or verbal testimony is not a separate source of valid knowledge. But it is not so. Some men are found naturally to possess the power to find out what is in another mind, or can communicate his own thought to another. They are called thought-readers. They also possess the power of thought-transference. Telepathy is of this class. If you think that a book is in such and such a place, that thought will at once rise in their mind, *i.e.* they will come to have a

knowledge of the existence of the book in that place. How does the cognition come to the thought-readers ? Not by direct perception. The words uttered mentally by one person and the sure knowledge arising out of their meaning affects the other mind and produces similar knowledge in that mind. That must be admitted to be a cognition different from direct perception or inference. With ordinary men this power of thought-reading not being fully developed they cannot comprehend what is in another mind unless the words are uttered. We generally express our thoughts by words ; that is why we have to express the thoughts by words if we wish to impress others by it. There are men whose sure knowledge of things seen or experienced by them will not carry conviction with you, but there are others whose words as soon as uttered will impress you. They possess such power that their ideas conveyed to you through their words get fixed in your mind. Famous orators are like that. People, whose words are accepted without question, are called Āpta or reliable persons. When the word uttered by an Āpta conveys his sure knowledge to your mind and produces a similar sure knowledge therein, it is called Āgama or verbal testimony. All the Śāstras were originally taught by such persons who had realised the various ultimate principles. That is why these are called Āgamas. But that is not strictly so, because in cognition by verbal communication there must be a speaker and a listener. As inference and direct perception might be faulty at times, so if there is any error in the Āpta, his communication would be erroneous. Only verbal knowledge, *i.e.* the meanings of uttered words, is not an Āgama or transferred cognition. In an Āgama-pramāṇa an unknown thing is made known with the help of the words used by an Āpta. Abhinava Gupta has called it transfer of power through affection. According to Plato, "No philosophical truth could be communicated in writing at all, it is only by some sort of immediate contact that one soul could kindle the flame in another (***Burnet***)."

(8) Just as a faulty premise leads to an invalid inference, defect in the senses to defective perception, so verbal communication is also liable to be defective.

———

विपर्ययो मिथ्याज्ञानमतद्रूपप्रतिष्ठम् ॥ ८ ॥

भाष्यम्—स कस्मान्न प्रमाणम् ? यतः प्रमाणेन बाध्यते, भूतार्थविषयत्वात् प्रमाणस्य, तत्र प्रमाणेन बाधनमप्रमाणस्य दृष्टम्, तद्यथा द्विचन्द्रदर्शनं सद्-

विषयेणैकचन्द्रदर्शनेन बाध्यत इति। सेयं पञ्चपर्वा भवत्यविद्या, अविद्याऽस्मिता-रागद्वेषाभिनिवेशाः क्लेशा इति, एत एव स्वसंज्ञाभिस्तमोमोहो महामोहस्तामिस्रः अन्धतामिस्र इति, एते चित्तमलप्रसङ्गेनाभिधास्यन्ते ॥ ८ ॥

**Viparyaya Or Illusion Is False Knowledge Formed Of A Thing As Other Than What It Is. 8.**

Why is Viparyaya not Pramāṇa ? Because that is demolished by correct knowledge of a thing which exists in reality. In other words, the object of Pramāṇa is real while the object of illusory cognition is its opposite. False cognition is sublated by correct knowledge, *e.g.* the illusion of seeing the moon double is contradicted by the valid knowledge of one moon. This wrong knowledge or Viparyaya that causes affliction has five parts. They are nescience, Asmitā or egoism, attachment, hate and fear of death—the five 'Kleśas'. They are also known technically as Tamas, Moha, Mahāmoha, Tāmisra and Andhatāmisra. These will be explained in connection with the impurities of the mind.

(1) Viparyaya is knowing a thing as different from what it really is ; Vikalpa is based on words suggesting a non-existing thing ; deep (dreamless) sleep is based on obscurity or inertia ; recollection is based on only matters felt before. Fluctuations of mind thus vary according to the basis on which they are founded. Pramā is the mental power which exhibits a real thing. Knowledge derived through concentration is the highest form of Pramā. Delusion (or knowing a thing as different from what it is) which is shut out by Pramā, is commonly known as Viparyaya or false cognition. Nescience etc. are the five forms of false cognition. Their common feature is misconception and these can all be shut out by correct knowledge. Viparyaya is the general name for all forms of incorrect knowledge. Kleśas like nescience etc. though classed as Viparyaya are really technically so called in relation to spirituality when the total extinction of all miseries is dealt with. Any misapprehension can be called a Viparyaya, but those misconceptions which Yogins consider to be the roots of miseries and eliminable, are regarded as Viparyayas of the nature of affliction (Kleśa).

शब्दज्ञानानुपाती वस्तुशून्यो विकल्पः ॥ ९ ॥

भाष्यम्—स न प्रमाणोपारोही, न विपर्ययोपारोही च, वस्तुशून्यत्वेऽपि शब्दज्ञानमाहात्म्यनिबन्धनो व्यवहारो दृश्यते, तद्यथा चैतन्यं पुरुषस्य स्वरूपमिति, यदा चितिरेव पुरुषस्तदा किमत्र केन व्यपदिश्यते, भवति च व्यपदेशे वृत्तिर्यथा चैत्रस्य गौरिति। तथा प्रतिषिद्धवस्तुधर्मो निष्क्रियः पुरुषः, तिष्ठति वाणः स्थास्यति स्थित इति गतिनिवृत्तौ धात्वर्थमात्रं गम्यते। तथा अनुत्पत्तिधर्मा पुरुष इति, उत्पत्तिधर्मस्याभावमात्रमवगम्यते न पुरुषान्वयी धर्मः, तस्माद्विकल्पितः स धर्मस्तेन चास्ति व्यवहार इति ॥ ९ ॥

**The Modification Called 'Vikalpa' Is Based On Verbal Cognition In Regard To A Thing Which Does Not Exist. (It Is A Kind Of Useful Knowledge Arising Out Of The Meaning Of A Word But Having No Corresponding Reality.)** (1). **9.**

Vikalpa does not fall within the category either of Pramāṇa or of false cognition (Viparyaya) ; because though there is no reality behind Vikalpa, yet it has its use through the power of verbal cognition. For example, 'Chaitanya (Consciousness) is the nature of Puruṣa.' Now what is here predicated and of what, seeing that Consciousness is Puruṣa itself? There must always be a statement of the relationship of one to another in predication, as in the phrase 'Chaitra's cow' (2). Similarly, Puruṣa is inactive and devoid of characteristics of matter. In the phrase 'Puruṣa has the character of not being created,' no positive quality relating to Puruṣa is being indicated but the mere lack of the property of being created is implied. That is why that characteristic is regarded as 'Vikalpa' and the term is used to indicate an idea which has no existence beyond the word.

(1) There are expressions and words which have no answering reality. From hearing those words or expressions, an ideation takes place in our minds. That is Vikalpa-vṛtti or modification due to vague notion. Those creatures who express their ideas through language have to depend largely on such notions. 'Ananta' (infinite) is an expression conveying a

vague notion. We use that word often and understand its import to some extent. It is, however, not possible to comprehend the real significance of that word. We can understand the significance of 'finite' and from that an insubstantial and vague ideation takes place in our mind through the word 'infinite'. The words 'infinite', 'innumerable', etc. are also used in a different sense, *e.g.* whose limit cannot be reached by measurement, or whose measure cannot be arrived at by counting. In this sense 'infinite' and 'innumerable' are not verbal delusion or vague ideation. But if we take 'infinite' as the measure of a totality, then it will be a verbal delusion because the moment we speak of a whole, we will be thinking of a 'finite' thing. When Yogins attempt to gain correct knowledge of internal and external matter through wisdom acquired by concentration, then they have to give up Vikalpa-vṛttis, because these are all ultimately unreal. Essential cognition or knowledge filled with truth (Ṛtambharā Prajñā, Sūtra I.48) is antagonistic to Vikalpa *i.e.* cognition of things that have no existence beyond the word. In reality until imaginary cognition disappears from the thought process, real Ṛta or realised truth cannot be perceived.

Vikalpa can be divided into three parts—vague notion of things, vague notion of action and vague notion of nothingness. Example of the first is 'Chaitanya is the nature of Puruṣa.' In this, although the two are the same, for usage their separate mention is an instance of Vikalpa. When a non-agent of an action is used as an agent, then it is an instance of Vikalpa of action. Modification of the mind arising out of words or expressions indicative of nothingness is vague notion relating to nihility. For example, 'Puruṣa is devoid of the property of being created.' Void is an unreality ; by it no real object can be predicated ; that is why the modification of the mind caused by such expression does not relate to something real. So long as we go on thinking with the help of words, the Vikalpa or vague cognition will continue.

The word 'Vikalpa' has various meanings ; for example, (i) as explained above, modification caused by verbal delusion or vague cognition, (ii) in the sense of vā, *i.e.* 'or' as in 'Īśvara-praṇidhānād-vā' in Sūtra I.23, (iii) manifested world, as in Vedāntic 'Nirvikalpa-samādhi', (iv) imposition of an imaginary concept as in the case of the image of 'I' in I-sense.

(2) The phrase 'Chaitra's cow' creates a definite impression in the mind ; the expression 'Chaitanya is the nature of Puruṣa,' although it has no significance in reality, creates a similar impression in the mind through the usage of words. Because it is a little difficult to understand, the

commentator has given several examples of Vikalpa-vṛtti. In fact, it is not possible to follow the significance of Nirvitarka and Nirvichāra Samādhi unless Vikalpa-vṛtti is understood clearly. Viparyaya or false cognition has no usefulness but Vikalpa or vague notion always serves a purpose.

---

अभावप्रत्ययालम्बना वृत्तिर्निद्रा ॥ १० ॥

भाष्यम्—सा च संप्रबोधे प्रत्यवमर्शात् प्रत्ययविशेषः। कथं, सुखमहमस्वाप्सं प्रसन्नं मे मनः प्रज्ञां मे विशारदीकरोति, दुःखमहमस्वाप्सं स्त्यानं मे मनो भ्रमत्यनवस्थितं, गाढ़ं मूढ़ोऽहमस्वाप्सं गुरूणि मे गात्राणि क्लान्तं मे चित्तमलसं (अलमिति पाठान्तरम्) मुषितमिव तिष्ठतीति। स खल्वयं प्रबुद्धस्य प्रत्यवमर्शो न स्यादसति प्रत्ययानुभवे, तदाश्रिताः स्मृतयश्च तद्विषया न स्युः। तस्मात् प्रत्ययविशेषो निद्रा। सा च समाधावितरप्रत्ययवन्निरोद्धव्येति ॥ १० ॥

**Dreamless Sleep Is The Mental Modification Produced By Condition Of Inertia As The State Of Vacuity or Negation (Of Waking And Dreaming). 10.**

Since we can remember when we wake up that we had been sleeping, sleep is called a mental modification, as indicated in the feelings expressed by phrases such as 'I slept well, I am feeling cheerful, it has cleared my brain' or 'I slept poorly ; on account of disturbed sleep, my mind has become restless, and is wandering unsteadily,' or 'I was in deep sleep as if in a stupor, my limbs are heavy, my brain is tired and languid, as if it has been stolen by somebody else and lying dormant.' If during sleep there was no cognition of the inert state, then on waking, one would not have remembered that experience. There would not also have been recollection of the state in which the mind was in sleep. That is why sleep is regarded as a particular kind of mental state, and should be shut out like other cognitions when concentration is practised (1).

(1) When one is awake, the sense-organs, the organs of action and the seat of thinking (a particular part of the brain), all work actively. In the dream-state the sense-organs and the organs of action become inactive, only the seat of thinking goes on acting. But in dreamless sleep all the three become inactive. The feeling of insensibility that comes on the body immediately before sleep, is inertia or Tamas. In nightmare sometimes the sense-organs become active but the organs of action remain inactive. One can partly hear and see but cannot move one's limbs as though they are frozen. This frozen feeling is Tamas referred to above. The mental modification which is subject to that Tamas is sleep. Since activity is stopped in sleep under the influence of inertia caused by Tamas, it is a sort of calmness but it is exactly opposite to the calmness of concentration. State of sleep is neither voluntary nor transparent calmness while concentration is both. Sleep is like calm but turbid water while concentration is like calm and clear water.

With the help of examples the commentator has brought out the threefold composition of sleep due to the three Guṇas and its nature as a Vṛtti. In some instances of sleep there is an indistinct feeling which produces the memory of sleep. As a matter of fact, for inducing sleep we only recollect the feeling of sleep experienced before. Compared to waking and dreaming, sleep is a Tāmasa modification. From the Śāstras also we know that sleep is a Tāmasa attribute. It has been said before that modification of the mind is a sort of cognition. In deep sleep an inert, obscure feeling comes over the organs of the body and the mental modification caused thereby, is only a knowledge thereof. In waking and dreaming, mental modification, *i.e.* Pramāṇa etc. arises, but in deep sleep there is no such modification. Sleep is a state relating to the power of retention, or in other words, the languid sensation in the body causing an obscure feeling in the organs is sleep and the knowledge of that feeling is the mental modification or the Chitta-vṛtti called sleep.

To stop the mental modification due to sleep, the first thing to be practised is constant calmness of the body. By that, sleep, which is the reaction for making up the loss due to bodily waste, becomes unnecessary. Even when the body remains calm, one-pointedness and Smṛti-sādhana (or cultivation of constant remembrance according to prescribed method) are necessary for resting the brain. That is the chief practice for overcoming sleep and is called Sattva-saṁsevana (cultivation of self-cognition). Constant watchfulness directed towards self-knowledge, *e.g.* 'I won't forget myself,' is called Samprajanya Only such steady and unobstructed practice all day and night long can lead to conquest of sleep, and single-mindedness towards this leads to Samprajñāta-yoga. Only after attaining and then superseding the latter can one attain Asamprajñāta concentration.

As under ordinary conditions some extraordinary powers manifest themselves in some persons, so also some persons may attain sleeplessness (not insomnia). But as this is not accompanied by stoppage of other mental fluctuations, it cannot be regarded as Yoga. When practising Smṛti-sādhana, some people get deep sleep or their minds stop fluctuating. Their heads droop, some stay erect but they breathe like one in sleep. Often an indistinct sense of felicity prevails due to absence of any effort in the system and there is no recollection of anything else. These have to be got rid of through Sattva-saṁsevana mentioned before.

———

अनुभूतविषयासम्प्रमोषः स्मृतिः ॥ ११ ॥

भाष्यम्—किं प्रत्ययस्य चित्तं स्मरति, आहोस्विद् विषयस्येति। ग्राह्योपरक्तः प्रत्ययो ग्राह्यग्रहणोभयाकारनिर्भासस्तथाजातीयकं संस्कारमारभते। स संस्कारः स्वव्यञ्जकाञ्जनस्तदाकारामेव ग्राह्यग्रहणोभयात्मिकां स्मृतिं जनयति। तत्र ग्रहणाकारपूर्वा बुद्धिर्ग्राह्याकारपूर्वा स्मृतिः सा च द्वयी भावितस्मर्तव्या चाऽभावितस्मर्तव्या च स्वप्ने भावितस्मर्तव्या, जाग्रत्समये त्वभावितस्मर्तव्येति। सर्वाः स्मृतयः प्रमाण-विपर्यय-विकल्पनिद्रास्मृतीनामनुभवात् प्रभवन्ति। सर्वाश्चैता वृत्तयः सुखदुःखमोहात्मिकाः सुखदुःखमोहाश्च क्लेशेषु व्याख्येयाः। सुखानुशयी रागः, दुःखानुशयी द्वेषः, मोहः पुनरविद्येति। एताः सर्वा वृत्तयो निरोद्धव्याः। आसां निरोधे संप्रज्ञातो वा समाधिर्भवति असंप्रज्ञातो वेति ॥ ११ ॥

**Recollection Is Mental Modification Caused By Reproduction Of The Previous-Impression Of An Object Whithout Adding Anything From Other Sources** (1). **11.**

Does the mind remember the process of knowing which took place before or the object which produced the knowledge (2) ? Though knowledge is of an object, yet it reveals both the nature of the object and the process of knowing and produces latent impressions of the same kind. These latencies manifest themselves when excited (3) by external cause and assume in recollection the form of the object as well as of the process of knowing. Of these, the reappearance in the mind of a thing taken in before is called recollection, while the display of the power of original cognition is named 'Buddhi' or Pramāṇa. Of the two, in Buddhi the cognitional aspect appears to be prominent, while in memory or recollection the object-aspect attains prominence. Memory is of two kinds, *viz.* remembrance of things only imagined (*i.e.* unreal) and of things not imagined (*i.e.* real). In a dream-state memory of imagined things appear (4) while in a waking state memory of real things appear. All memories arise out of impressions whether of right cognition, misapprehension, vague ideation, deep sleep or of former memory. The foregoing fluctuations are of the nature of pleasure, pain or stupefaction (5). These will be explained in connection with Kleśas or afflictions. Attachment follows pleasure, aversion follows pain, while stupefaction is nescience. All these fluctuations must be shut out. When they are eliminated, then will be reached concentration—Samprajñāta or Asamprajñāta as the case may be.

(1) Asampramoṣa = Desisting from taking things which are not really one's own. In recollection a previous experience is only reproduced without stealing from, *i.e.* accretion from, anything else.

(2) When we remember a pot do we remember only the object or the knowledge (*i.e.* the sensation of knowing or the process of knowing the pot)? In reply, the commentator affirms that both are remembered. Though knowledge is influenced by the object, *i.e.* takes after the character of the object, yet it also includes the act of knowing. In other words, only the knowledge of the pot does not arise, but it is mixed with the experience : 'I am knowing the pot.' Remembrance of a thing experienced before, unalloyed by anything else, is Smṛti ; but in that recollection of the object a new awareness : 'I am knowing this' is also present. The word 'new' here does not refer to the thing experienced before, but the process of knowing which was taking place anew in the mind is referred to. When in recollection there is such a remembrance, it must be admitted that both are present in it, *viz.* (a) knowledge of the object experienced

before and (b) the new mental process of knowing. Of these two, the first is the knowledge of a thing experienced before and the second of something not experienced before. The first is memory or recollection and the second is knowledge in the shape of Pramāṇa or correct new apprehension.

In all experiences there is an object as well as the process of knowing. Both these produce latent impressions and therefore both give rise to cognition. Of these, the modification arising out of the latent impressions of the object is recollection while that of the process of knowing is an action—a mental action, *i.e.* faculty of knowing. Therefore, that latent impression is of the faculty of knowing. The mental action arising out of the faculty of knowing is not exactly the same as before but a new knowledge which is Pramāṇa.

(3) The term 'Swavyañjakāñjana' used by the commentator means coloured by the cause of its own manifestation.

(4) Bhāvita-smartavya = Recollection of an experience, roused or imagined, of unreal cognition. For example, the imagined conception of 'I have become a king' brings in its train thoughts of palace, throne, etc. in a dream. In a waking state there is chiefly knowledge of real thoughts and objects.

(5) In fact, the sensation or feeling in which there is no capacity for clear knowledge of pleasure or pain, is stupefaction. For example, after severe pain there is a feeling of numbness devoid of the sense of pain. Stupefaction is predominantly Tamas in quality ; that is why it is akin to nescience. All comprehensions in the mind are associated either with pleasure, pain or Moha (delusion). Therefore, these can be called fluctuations of the state of the mind relating to cognition. Attachment, hate and fear, all give rise to actions of the mind, hence they are modifications of the state of the mind relating to conation. Waking, dreaming and deep sleep are modifications relating to the state of retention.

———

भाष्यम्—अथासां निरोधे क उपाय इति—

अभ्यासवैराग्याभ्यां तन्निरोधः ॥ १२ ॥

चित्तनदी नाम उभयतोवाहिनी, वहति कल्याणाय, वहति पापाय च। या तु कैवल्यप्राग्भारा विवेकविषयनिम्ना सा कल्याणवहा। संसारप्राग्भारा अविवेक-

विषयनिम्ना पापवहा। तत्र वैराग्येण विषयस्रोतः खिलीक्रियते, विवेकदर्शनाभ्यासेन विवेकस्रोत उद्घाट्यते। इत्युभयाधीनश्चित्तवृत्तिनिरोधः ॥ १२ ॥

What are the means of stopping them ?

**By Practice And Detachment These Can Be Stopped. 12.**

The river of mind flows in both directions—towards good and towards evil. That which flows down the plane of Viveka or discriminative knowledge ending in the high ground of Kaivalya or liberation, leads unto good ; while that which flows up to the plateau of cycles of re-birth down the plane of non-discrimination leads unto evil. Among these, the flow towards sense-objects is reduced by renunciation, and development of a habit of discrimination opens the floodgate of discriminative knowledge. The stopping of mental modifications is thus dependent upon both (1).

(1) Practice and renunciation are the commonest means of attaining Mokṣa or salvation. All other methods are included in them. These two principles of Yoga have been quoted in Śrīmad Bhāgavad Gītā. The commentator has mentioned only the practice of discriminative knowledge because it is the principal means. One will get as much benefit as one practises. Concentration with strong mental, moral and physical discipline is the aim of practice. One should not be deterred on account of the difficulties in the way but proceed steadfastly. Many, finding the path of practice difficult and being unable to subdue the tumult of the inner nature, try to find solace in the idea 'I am being impelled by God to follow the path of attachment.' But it should be remembered that whether under God's direction or otherwise, the result of practising evil is bound to be misery, while the practice of good would lead to happiness. In fact, the development of the feeling : 'I am doing everything at the bidding of God' is also a matter of practice. If this feeling prevails in one's all actions, then there would be justification for such an attitude and it would be a blessing. But if it is used for justifying actions under the promptings of violent passions, then what else other than dire misery can be expected ?

तत्र स्थितौ यत्नोऽभ्यासः ॥ १३ ॥

भाष्यम्—चित्तस्य अवृत्तिकस्य प्रशान्तवाहिता स्थितिः, तदर्थः प्रयत्नः वीर्यमुत्साहः तत्सम्पिपादयिषया तत्साधनानुष्ठानमभ्यासः ॥ १३ ॥

**Exertion To Acquire Sthiti Or A Tranquil State Of Mind Devoid Of Fluctuations Is Called Practice. 13.**

Absence of fluctuations or undisturbed calmness of the mind (1) is called Sthiti or tranquillity. The effort, the energy and the enthusiasm, *i.e.* the repeated attempt for attaining that state, is called practice.

(1) The continuity of the mind devoid of all fluctuations is called Praśānta-vāhitā. That is the highest state of tranquillity of the mind ; the other forms of calmness are only secondary. As the practice improves, the tranquillity also increases. With one's aim fixed on Praśānta-vāhitā the effort to hold on to whatever placidity has been attained by one is called practice. The greater the energy and enthusiasm with which the effort is made, the sooner will the practice be established. In the Muṇḍaka Upaniṣad it is stated : "This Self is realised not by one who has no energy, nor by one who is subject to delusion, nor by knowledge devoid of real renunciation, but when the wise man exerts himself in this way (*i.e.* with energy, knowledge and renunciation), his soul reaches the abode of Brahman."

———

स तु दीर्घकालनैरन्तर्यसत्कारासेवितो दृढभूमिः ॥ १४ ॥

भाष्यम्—दीर्घकालासेवितो निरन्तरासेवितस्तपसा ब्रह्मचर्येण विद्यया श्रद्धया च सम्पादितः सत्कारवान् दृढभूमिर्भवति, व्युत्थानसंस्कारेण द्रागित्येव अनभिभूतविषय इत्यर्थः ॥ १४ ॥

**That Practice When Continued For A Long Time Without Break And With Devotion Becomes Firm In Foundation. 14.**

Continued for a long time and constantly practised in a devoted way, *i.e.* with austerity, continence, learning and reverence, it is said to have been done with earnest attention and it gets firmly established. In other words, in that state the calmness which is aimed at in practice is not easily overcome by any latent impressions of the fluctuating state (1).

(1) The word 'constantly' implies practice, daily and, if possible, every moment. Practice which is not broken by its opposite habit of restlessness, is constant practice. Tapasyā is giving up of worldly pleasure by strong mental, moral and physical discipline. Learning refers to knowledge of truth. When these are done, the practice will no doubt be a reverent one. It is said in the Chhāndogya Upaniṣad : "That which is done with proper knowledge, with devotion and in conformity with the scriptures, *i.e.* done in the proper method, becomes more forceful."

———

दृष्टानुश्रविकविषयवितृष्णस्य वशीकारसंज्ञा वैराग्यम् ॥ १५ ॥

भाष्यम्—स्त्रियः अन्नपानम् ऐश्वर्यम् इति दृष्टविषयवितृष्णस्य, स्वर्गवैदेह्यप्रकृतिलयत्वप्राप्तावानुश्रविकविषये वितृष्णस्य दिव्यादिव्यविषयसंप्रयोगेऽपि चित्तस्य विषयदोषदर्शिनः प्रसंख्यानबलाद् अनाभोगात्मिका हेयोपादेयशून्या वशीकारसंज्ञा वैराग्यम् ॥ १५ ॥

**When The Mind Loses All Desire For Objects Seen Or Described In the Scriptures It Acquires A State Of Utter Desirelessness Which Is Called Detachment. 15.**

When the mind becomes indifferent to things seen, *e.g.* women, food, drinks, power etc. and does not hanker after objects or states promised in scriptures such as going to heaven or having the 'discarnate' state (1) or of dissolution into primordial matter, or even when in the presence of such things the mind finds out their defects and by virtue of the acquisition of discriminative knowledge (2) maintains complete freedom from their influence and is indifferent to good or evil, it is said to have reached a controlled state of Buddhi without

Vikalpa (3) called Vaśīkāra-saṁjñā and this is Vairāgya (detachment).

(1) 'Discarnate' state and dissolution into primordial matter will be explained in the notes to Sūtra I.19.

(2) Prasaṁkhyāna = Attainment of Viveka-khyāti or ultimate discriminative knowledge. Anābhoga = opposed to Ābhoga which denotes the state of a mind fully engrossed in a matter as happens, for instance, to a mind in concentration. In a disturbed state of the mind it is occupied with ordinary affairs which breed trouble. In objects to which we are fully attached or in which we willingly engage ourselves, we get Ābhoga. When the attachment disappears the mind is freed from their incubus. Then we hardly think of them, nor are we inclined towards them.

(3) When through discriminative knowledge one comes to realise the power of worldly things in breeding the three-fold misery, then one realises that enjoyment of worldly objects is similar to being scorched by fire. The difference between getting to know about the demerit of things through study and reflection alone and the wisdom through discriminative knowledge is like the difference in experience between hearing that fire burns and actually getting burnt. When through this knowledge the demerit of everything is realised and a complete state of detachment prevails in the mind, that state is technically called the state of Vaśīkāra which is Vairāgya (detachment).

The Vaśīkāra stage of mind is not reached at once. There are three other antecedent states of detachment. (1) Yatamāna, (2) Vyatireka and (3) Ekendriya are the three previous stages. To go on attempting not to indulge in sensuous enjoyments is Yatamāna detachment. When that becomes successful to some extent, *i.e.* when attachment towards some things disappears altogether and in respect of others it becomes feeble, then by a process of elimination, a spirit of renunciation can be maintained partially, that is known as Vyatireka abnegation. When by practice that is mastered, when the sense-organs are completely weaned away from objects and only the tendency to attachment remains in the mind, then it is called Ekendriya. Ekendriya means that which resides in one sense-organ—here, the mind. Later when the adept Yogin has no longer to control his tendency to attachment, when naturally his mind and his senses remain aloof from worldly objects and even from supermundane matters, then that is called the state of Vaśīkāra which is Vairāgya or complete detachment. That is a state of absolute indifference to the things of the world.

———

तत् परं पुरुषख्यातेर्गुणवैतृष्ण्याम् ॥ १६ ॥

भाष्यम्—दृष्टानुश्रविकविषयदोषदर्शी विरक्तः पुरुषदर्शनाभ्यासात् तच्छुद्धि-प्रविवेकाप्यायितबुद्धिर्गुणेभ्यो व्यक्ताव्यक्तधर्मकेभ्यो विरक्त इति, तद्द्वयं वैराग्यं, तत्र यदुत्तरं तज्ज्ञानप्रसादमात्रम्। यस्योदये प्रत्युदितख्यातिरेवं मन्यते 'प्राप्तं प्रापणीयं, क्षीणाः क्षेतव्याः क्लेशाः, छिन्नः श्लिष्टपर्वा भवसंक्रमः, यस्य अविच्छेदाज्जनित्वा म्रियते मृत्वा च जायते,' इति। ज्ञानस्यैव परा काष्ठा वैराग्यम् एतस्यैव हि नान्तरीयकं कैवल्यमिति ॥ १६ ॥

**Indifference To The Guṇas Or The Constituent Principles Achieved Through A Knowledge Of The Nature Of The Puruṣa Is Called Paravairagya (Supreme Detachment). 16.**

Through the practice of the effort to realise the Puruṣa-principle, the Yogin having seen the faulty nature of all objects visible or described in the scriptures, gets a clarity of vision and steadiness in Sāttvika qualities. Such a Yogin edified with a discriminative knowledge (1) and with sharpened and chastened intellect becomes indifferent (2) to all manifest and unmanifested states of the three Guṇas or constituent principles (3). There are thus two kinds of detachment. The last one is absolute clarification of knowledge (4). When detachment appears in the shape of clarified knowledge, the Yogin, with his realisation of the nature of Self, thinks thus : 'I have got whatever is to be got ; the afflictions which have to be eliminated have been reduced ; the continuous chain of birth and death, bound by which men are born and die, and dying are born again, has been broken.' Detachment is the culmination of knowledge, and Kaivalya (or liberation) and detachment are inseparable.

(1) & (2) 'Praviveka' means the highest form of knowledge. Only the attainment of an arrested state of mind does not bring about Kaivalya or liberation. When the arrested state of mind, which is usually broken through natural causes or on account of latent impression, is no longer broken, then it is called the state of liberation. For achieving such

uninterrupted arrested state of mind, detachment is necessary. For detachment, knowledge of the constituent principles (Puruṣa is also a principle) is necessary. After withdrawing the mind from objects through Vaśīkāra, concentration in an arrested state of the mind through the knowledge about Puruṣa has to be practised. When the knowledge of the nature of Puruṣa dawns, the mind becomes free from thoughts of worldly objects, and is only occupied with matters relating to discrimination. Those who withdraw their minds from external objects by detachment (Vaśīkāra) and concentrate on the unmanifested or the void as the final principle not noticing at the same time the distinction between Puruṣa and 'Buddhi' are not on the right path. Since they have failed to discover the distinction between Puruṣa and 'Buddhi', their state of concentration is not complete and does not bring them towards the final state of 'Nirodha' or ultimate dissolution of the mind. This is due to the fact that while their abnegation might be complete in respect of worldly things, it is incomplete in regard to unmanifested things. That is why they rise again after being merged in Prakṛti or the ultimate constituent principle, because not having realised the distinction between unmanifested Prakṛti and Puruṣa, their knowledge remains incomplete. From that subtle seed of ignorance they rise or are born again. That is why Yogins first practise Vaśīkāra, then the act of contemplating on Puruṣa followed by a realisation of the difference between the conscious-like Buddhi and the alsobute knower Puruṣa and thus become averse to the unmanifested and all the mutations thereof, *i.e.* they become indifferent to the three Guṇas whether in their manifest or unmanifested (like void) state.

(3) Attachment is a function of Buddhi or the inner senses. Hence non-attachment is also its function. In Pravṛtti or attachment we get predilection, while in Nivṛtti or detachment we get aloofness or cessation. That Buddhi which brings about a realisation of the Puruṣa-principle is called Agryā Buddhi or the highest form of intellect. Kaṭha Upaniṣad says : "Subtle-minded sages realise Him through Agryā Buddhi." When knowledge of the nature of Puruṣa is acquired, then there is no more inclination in the satisfied mind to be engrossed in the unmanifested Prakṛti or the void ; on the other hand, it develops a desire to engage itself in the contemplation of the Puruṣa-principle and thus get perpetual peace or be submerged in its constituent cause. A complete separation from the Guṇas and their mutations then arises. Para-vairāgya or the highest detachment and un-adulterated knowledge of the Puruṣa-principle are inseparable. Only by that means Kaivalya or liberation, in the shape of complete cessation of the mind, is attainable.

(4) Jñānaprasāda or clarification of knowledge indicates the highest purification of knowledge. Man's knowledge is directly or indirectly conducive to elimination of misery. That knowledge which brings about final and entire cessation of all sorrows is the highest form of knowledge. Then there cannot be anything higher to know. By Para-vairāgya or supreme renunciation sorrows can be prevented fully and finally ; that is why it is the last stage of knowledge or its extreme purification. Moreover, it is absolute knowledge. There is no sense of attachment in it, and without attachment consequent tendency to action being absent, the mind will be placid and nothing but knowledge of the Puruṣa-principle will be there. Consequently, there will be nothing but purified knowledge without any tinge of attachment. When the state of mind is free from the tendency to activity and of inertia, that is illumination of knowledge. By the words 'I have got whatever is to be got' etc., the commentator has indicated detachment and refinement of knowledge only. Regarding Para-vairāgya, Kaṭha Upaniṣad says : "The wise, knowing of the eternal bliss, do not look for the immutable in ephemeral things."

———

भाष्यम्—अथ उपायद्वयेन निरुद्धचित्तवृत्तेः कथमुच्यते सम्प्रज्ञातः समाधिरिति ?—

वितर्कविचारानन्दास्मितारूपानुगमात् सम्प्रज्ञातः ॥ १७ ॥

वितर्कः चित्तस्य आलम्बने स्थूल आभोगः, सूक्ष्मो विचारः, आनन्दः ह्लादः, एकात्मिका संविद् अस्मिता। तत्र प्रथमश्चतुष्टयानुगतः समाधिः सवितर्कः। द्वितीयो वितर्कविकलः सविचारः। तृतीयो विचारविकलः सानन्दः। चतुर्थस्तद्विकलः अस्मितामात्र इति। सर्वे एते सालम्बनाः समाधयः ॥ १७ ॥

What is Samprajñāta-samādhi of the mind whose fluctuations have been arrested by the two methods (practice and detachment) mentioned before ? (1)

**When Concentration Is Reached With The Help Of Vitarka, Vichāra, Ānanda And Asmitā, It Is Called Samprajñāta-Samādhi. 17.**

When the concentrated mind (2) is filled with the grosser form of perceptibles, *i.e.* realises them, then it is called Vitarka.

Similarly, Vichāra concentration relates to subtle objects (3). The third, Ānanda, is the feeling of felicity—a blissful feeling filling the mind (4). Asmitā is I-sense or awareness of individual personality (5). Of these, in the first, *viz.* Savitarka-samādhi there is the presence of all the four objects. The second, *i.e.* Savichāra-samādhi is free from Vitarka (6). The third, *i.e.* Sānanda-samādhi is free from Vichāra (7). The fourth is Asmitā-mātra or pure I-sense, and it is free even from the sense of bliss (8). All these states of concentration have, however, an object concentrated upon (9).

(1) The description of Samprajñāta concentration given in the commentaries on the first Sūtra should be recalled in this connection. The successful concentration attained in the habitually one-pointed state of the mind which brings knowledge cutting at the root of all afflictions is called Samprajñāta-yoga. Those Samādhis or concentrations which bring forth such realisable knowledge have four distinct divisions. The object of contemplation marks their differences, while the classification of the knowledge derived therefrom, *viz.* Savitarka and Nirvitarka or Savichāra and Nirvichāra, is based both on the object contemplated upon and on the nature of the contemplation (see Sūtra I.41-44).

(2) If the modification of the mind caused by the verbal delusion (Vikalpa), consisting in the mingling of the name of an object, the object itself and its knowledge relates to any gross matter, then it is called Vitarkānvayī or depending on Vitarka. The things which we see around us like cow, pot, blue, yellow etc. which are taken in by our sense-organs, are gross objects. As a matter of fact, when sound, colour etc. taken in by the senses are mingled and presented to our mind as a single entity, what we perceive is a gross object. A cow, for example, is a conglomeration of several features perceptible by our senses which are comprehended as a single entity. When such gross matter along with the words indicating it becomes the object of concentration then that is called Savitarka-samādhi, while when there is no such Vitarka, it is called Nirvitarka-samādhi. Both are Samprajñāta-samādhi relating to Vitarka.

(3) When concentration relating to gross objects is mastered, full insight is obtained of subtle principles by a special process of mental analysis with the help of the knowledge gained during the state of concentration. This is Savichāra-samprajñāta. Analytic thinking cannot be conducted without the help of words ; that is why this Savichāra-samādhi

is also characterised by the vagueness due to mingling of words *viz.* name of the object, the object itself and its knowledge, even though it be in respect of subtle objects. Meditative analysis is its special feature. It is, therefore, free from gross objects. Subtle matter and subtle faculties of reception are the objects of this concentration. As in such concentration subtle objects of contemplation are realised by Vichāra or analysis, it is called Savichāra. This and Nirvichāra are cases of concentration related to Vichāra (analysis). It is the kind of meditative analysis through which we have to pass in arriving at Prakṛti from Vikṛti or its modifications. Similarly, knowledge of Heya (things to be avoided), Heyahetu (causes of avoidables), Hāna (avoidance), Hānopāya (means of avoidance) which dawns through concentration, is also attained by analysis. As the fundamental principles and subtle Yogic ideals are realised through such thinking, the concentration on subtle objects is called Vichārānugata-samādhi.

(4) Concentration on bliss is free from Vitarka and Vichāra. It is not in respect of gross or subtle things. The object or basis of this concentration is a particular feeling of Sāttvika happiness felt all over the mind and the senses due to a particular state of calmness. The body is the receptacle of the mind, the sense-organs, organs of action and the Prāṇas or vital forces. Consequently, that sense of happiness is like a natural feeling of tranquillity or Sāttvika calmness of the whole body. Thus Sānanda-samādhi (or concentration on the felicity of mind) really relates to the sense-organs or instruments of cognition. That peace, *i.e.* inactivity of the bodily organs, gives more happiness than their being engaged in action is known from this kind of Samādhi. A Yogin who has realised this bliss, quietens his sense-organs in this manner and thus conserves his energy.

Through a special kind of Prāṇāyāma (breath control) or by concentration on vital parts of the body, the body becomes calm when a feeling of bliss pervades the body. If concentration is practised on that feeling alone, a feeling of bliss gradually comes over all the sense-organs. That is the practice of Sānanda-samādhi. There is not so much dependence on spoken words as in the case of Vitarka, because it is a matter of feeling, of bliss felt. Nor is there any need in it for thinking as in the case of approach to Tanmātras from the Bhūtas, not even of subtle Bhūtas which is the basis of concentration where Vichāra prevails. That is why this concentration on bliss is free from Vitarka and Vichāra. Spoken in terms of Samāpatti, it is the subject of Nirvichārā Samāpatti or engrossment free from reasoning. It is said in the scriptures that the happiness that is derivable from making the senses free from the influence of their corresponding worldly objects by constant practice and lumping them up in the mind is not comparable to anything obtainable from heavenly or worldly things attainable through personal exertion.

(5-8) Concentration with Vitarka and Vichāra is dependent on and relates to knowable objects. Concentration based on a feeling of felicity relates to the organs of cognition, while that based on pure I-sense relates to the knower. As the latter relates only to the cogniser, *i.e.* to conceptions like 'I am the cogniser of the bliss,' and thus concerns only the 'I', it is free from the touch of bliss. This implies a state beyond the feeling of bliss and not the lack of it. Being of the nature of peace (quiescence) it is a more coveted state than bliss. In Sānanda-dhyāna or meditation with the blissful feeling as its basis, the feeling of happiness or bliss pervades the organs. In concentration based on the I-sense, the object of concentration is not the feeling of bliss but its recipient. This is the difference between Sānanda-samādhi and Sāsmita-samādhi. Puruṣa or pure Consciousness is not the object of any concentration. Asmitā-mātra or pure I-sense is the object of this concentration. This I-sense is called Grahītā or the cogniser. It is manifested with the help of Puruṣa. The object concentrated upon in Sāsmita-samādhi is not the real Puruṣa but its imitation—the mutative ego or the Mahat. In the Sāṁkhya philosophy it is called the Mahat-tattva. It is Buddhi shaped after Puruṣa, a feeling of 'I know myself,' a sort of feeling of identity between the pure Consciousness and Buddhi.

Buddhi-tattva or the principle of Buddhi is the first phenomenon to be manifested. However subtle the knowledge might be, existence of knowledge implies a knower. When knowledge disappears, *i.e.* the mind gets into an arrested state, then the knower-knowable relationship or the ego terminates, and the Puruṣa abides in himself.

The author of the Sūtra has said that Asmitā-kleśa is the identification of Puruṣa with Buddhi. There is a subtle connection between Puruṣa and Buddhi and when that is eliminated through Viveka-khyāti, Buddhi disappears. Therefore, Sāsmita-samādhi or concentration on the pure I-sense is the ultimate realisation of the principle of I-sense, that is, of the 'I' of common usage, the receiver.

(9) In Samprajñāta-samādhi the mind is not entirely arrested but is in a partially arrested state. Therefore, it is inevitable that it will require a basis (object) of concentration.

———

भाष्यम्—अथासंप्रज्ञातसमाधिः किमुपायः किंस्वभावो वेति ?—

विरामप्रत्ययाभ्यासपूर्वः संस्कारशेषोऽन्यः ॥ १८ ॥

सर्ववृत्तिप्रत्यस्तमये संस्कारशेषो निरोधश्चित्तस्य समाधिः असंप्रज्ञातः, तस्य परं वैराग्यमुपायः। सालम्बनो हि अभ्यासस्तत्साधनाय न कल्पते इति, विरामप्रत्ययो निर्वस्तुक आलम्बनीक्रियते, स च अर्थशून्यः, तदभ्यासपूर्वं चित्तं निरालम्बनमभावप्राप्तमिव भवतीति एष निर्वीजः समाधिरसंप्रज्ञातः ॥ १८ ॥

What is the means of attaining Asamprajñāta-samādhi and what is its nature ?

**Asamprajñāta-Samādhi Is The Other Kind Of Samādhi Which Arises Through Constant Practice Of Para-Vairāgya Which Brings About The Disappearance Of All Fluctuations Of The Mind Wherein Only The Latent Impressions Remain. 18.**

When all fluctuations cease, the arrested state of mind with only the latencies (1) in them is known as Asamprajñāta-samādhi. Supreme detachment is the means of attaining it, because it cannot be attained when an object is the basis of concentration. Complete cessation of fluctuations (2) emanates from Para-vairāgya or supreme detachment which is free from any material cogitation. It is totally devoid of all objects and its practice makes the mind independent of any object, and non-existent as it were. This kind of Nirvīja or objectless Samādhi (3) is Asamprajñāta-samādhi.

(1) Saṁskāra-śeṣa = Where only the latencies persist. There is no cognised modification in the arrested state, but only the latent impression of a break in cognition. Mind has two functions, cognition and retention. In an arrested state there is no cognition, but since cognition might re-appear, it must be admitted that the latent impression of fluctuation exists in the mind. Therefore, the expression 'Saṁskāra-śeṣa' implies the state of the latent impressions both of fluctuations and of the arrested state. The latency of the arrested state means the cessation of the latencies of fluctuations. Saṁskāra-śeṣa, therefore, is that state wherein the latency of arrested state renders the latencies of fluctuations inoperative.

(2) The means of attaining such cessation is the practice, *i.e.* constant awareness in mind, of the idea of supreme detachment. How cessation of fluctuation can be brought about by supreme detachment is explained below. In Samprajñāta-yoga, one reaches the pure I-sense gradually, after having mastered the antecedent principles beginning from gross matter. Then focusing on the idea that 'I' do not want even the pure I-sense, if the mind acquires a momentum for the arrested state, fluctuations will no longer arise in the mind. Then the mind would appear to be a void. That is called the 'moment' of arrested state, in other words, the interval between two states of fluctuation. That is the state in which the Seer abides in himself. Then the pure Consciousness is not arrested but the knowledge of non-self disappears ; consequently, the knower of non-self, *viz.* the I-sense, also disappears.

(3) Nirvīja-samādhi (*i.e.* without an object to meditate upon) is not necessarily Asamprajñāta-samādhi. Concentration with an object is not always Samprajñāta-samādhi. Samprajñāta means the constant awareness of the knowledge acquired through concentration in a one-pointed state of the mind. Similarly, Asamprajñāta-samādhi is that wherein concentration is attained in a habitually arrested state of the mind after having realised abiding knowledge by Samprajñāta. Then non-receptivity becomes the habit of the mind. This difference should be noted carefully. Asamprajñāta-samādhi leads to Kaivalya or the state of liberation, but Nirvīja-samādhi does not always lead to liberation. This point has been amplified in the next Sūtra.

The exact nature of a habitually arrested state of the mind has to be understood clearly. Shutting out states of knowledge is an arrested state. This is of two kinds : (i) an arrested state in which the latencies remain and which assert themselves when the opportunity arises, and (ii) in which there is not even those latencies and the arrested state is perpetual. In the former case again two states are possible : (a) When there is a break in the process of knowing an object and that knowledge passes on to the state of latent impression. This is happening every moment and is part and parcel of the fluctuating state of the mind. This is not noticeable. (b) Arresting, through concentration, the process of knowing. This is known as Nirodha concentration.

In Sabhaṅga-nirodha as the above class (i) is called, only the intake of knowledge is stopped but the latencies remain and they appear and disappear. In the state of complete stoppage of fluctuating knowledge and the latencies for all time to come, the mind dissolves itself into its constituent principles and this is known as the state of Kaivalya or liberation ;

with the elimination of the latencies all knowledge is shut out, and the mind resolves itself into its constituent principles. In a state of fluctuation, latent impressions are rousing cognitive modifications and cognition is receding to latencies in quick succession. In this process, the disappearance of cognition is hardly noticeable, and it seems that the flow of cognised modification is continuous. When through the practice of concentration, the rise of the latent impression is completely stopped, and the flow of the disappearance of modifications continues, then that is called Nirodha-samādhi, or concentration in an arrested state of the mind.

----

भाष्यम्—स खल्वयं द्विविधः, उपायप्रत्ययो भवप्रत्ययश्च, तत्र उपायप्रत्ययो योगिनाम्भवति—

भवप्रत्ययो विदेहप्रकृतिलयानाम् ॥ १६ ॥

विदेहानां देवानां भवप्रत्ययः, ते हि स्वसंस्कारमात्रोपयोगेन ( -मात्रोपभोगेन इति पाठान्तरम् ) चित्तेन कैवल्यपदमिवानुभवन्तः स्वसंस्कारविपाकं तथाजातीयकमतिवाहयन्ति, तथा प्रकृतिलयाः साधिकारे चेतसि प्रकृतिलीने कैवल्यपदमिवानुभवन्ति यावन्न पुनरावर्तते अधिकारवशाच्चित्तमिति ॥ १६ ॥

That (Nirvīja) Samādhi is of two kinds, *viz.* that attained by (prescribed) effort (1) and that through Bhava or nescient latencies which bring about the cycle of births. Of these, the Yogins adopt the prescribed means of effort.

**While In The Case Of The Videhas Or The Discarnates And Of The Prakṛtilayas Or Those Subsisting In Their Elemental Constituents, It Is Caused By Nescience Which Results In Objective Existence. 19.**

In the Videhas or discarnate Devas (2) it is caused by objective existence, because they live in a state which is like Kaivalya (the state of liberation) with a mind functioning only so far as its own residual latencies are capable of, and who live through the state of life brought about by their latent impressions. Similarly, the Prakṛtilayas (3), or those whose minds retaining latent impressions (4) remain resolved in Prakṛti (primary constituent principle), remain in a state like that of Kaivalya, until by force of those latent impressions their minds assert themselves in fluctuation.

(1) Effort = The means like devotion etc. prescribed in the next Sūtra (I.20) for attainment of, or as the means of bringing about, discriminative knowledge. The word 'Bhava' has been variously explained by different commentators. It refers, however, to those subtle subliminal impressions of nescience which are responsible for discarnate existence as a Deva etc. Birth is only resurgence of self under the influence of previous latent impressions, its existence for a limited period and its destruction afterwards. The life of Devas, or of those who are in their elemental principles, can therefore be called birth. In the Sāṁkhya-sūtras it has been stated that those who are in their elemental state emerge again as submerged men do from water. Therefore, Bhava is that latent impression of nescience which is responsible for birth. What is the reason for a discarnate's birth? It is the non-realisation of the Self or Puruṣa as distinct and separate from Prakṛti and its mutations. The discarnates attain that state by force of the impressions of their concentration. Thus the subtle latent impression of nescience involving rebirth is the Bhava of the discarnates etc. Subtle nescience means that which is neither gross like the nescience of those who have not experienced concentration nor completely destroyed by realisation of discriminative enlightenment. The Bhava of ordinary sentient beings is the unattenuated latent impressions of nescience in the shape of afflictive Karmāśaya or latencies inspiring continued activity.

(2) Discarnate Devas = When a Yogin, having realised through concentration the true nature of the gross elements, delights in abandoning their pursuit and considers merely such abnegation to be the highest attainment and having grown indifferent to sights, sounds, etc. completely shuts them out, his organs dry up for want of contact with knowables, because the organs cannot remain manifest for a moment without contact with their corresponding objects. Thus having shut out all contacts with sensory objects, *i.e.* having acquired non-afflictive latencies, such Yogins, when they give up their bodies, resolve their organs into the constituent elements and get into a state of objectless concentration and thus enjoy a state analogous to the state of Kaivalya or liberation for a limited period according to the strength of their latencies. These are the discarnate Devas. On the other hand, Yogins who without trying to shut out all

contacts with objects, remain satisfied with the contemplation of the constituent principles relating to the organs of reception and the felicity experienced thereby, go into different Lokas or heavenly abodes when they give up their mortal existence and enjoy the pleasure of contemplation during the period of their divine existence. Not having realised the supreme Puruṣa, the discarnate Devas carry within them the germ of A-darśana or non-awareness of the ultimate truth and thus they are born again and fail to secure perpetual peace.

(3) Prakṛtilaya = Merging into Prakṛti the primary constituent principle. According to Āchārya Gauḍapāda the expression 'Vairāgyāt Prakṛtilayaḥ' (merging into elemental principles through detachment) means that those who practise detachment but have not acquired the knowledge of the constituent principles, on account of their ignorance, merge after their death into one or other of the main principles, *viz.* Pradhāna, Buddhi, Ahaṁkāra and the five Tanmātras. Of these, Prakṛtilaya mentioned in this Sūtra should be taken to mean submergence into Pradhāna or the primary constituent principle because the mind can only be lost in this, *i.e.* the concentration can only then be 'seedless' or objectless.

(4) When the mind acquires Viveka or discriminative enlightenment its tendency to fluctuation ceases, *i.e.* by such knowledge the inclination to experiences which keeps the mind alive or in a state of fluctuation, is burnt out altogether. Its other name is Charitārthatā or complete attainment of the desired object. Experience and liberation are the two objectives of Puruṣa. With the acquisition of discriminative enlightenment, the objectives are fulfilled. Until such knowledge is acquired inclination to modifications does not cease and the mind goes on fluctuating in accordance with the natural law.

———

श्रद्धावीर्यस्मृतिसमाधिप्रज्ञापूर्वक इतरेषाम् ॥ २० ॥

भाष्यम्—उपायप्रत्ययो योगिनां भवति। श्रद्धा चेतसः संप्रसादः, सा हि जननीव कल्याणी योगिनं पाति, तस्य हि श्रद्दधानस्य विवेकार्थिनः वीर्यमुपजायते, समुपजातवीर्यस्य स्मृतिरुपतिष्ठते, स्मृत्युपस्थाने च चित्तमनाकुलं समाधीयते, समाहितचित्तस्य प्रज्ञाविवेक उपावर्तते, येन यथावद् वस्तु जानाति, तदभ्यासात् तद्विषयाच्च वैराग्याद् असंप्रज्ञातः समाधिर्भवति ॥ २० ॥

**Others (Who Follow The Path Of The Prescribed Effort) Adopt The Means Of Reverential Faith, Energy, Repeated Recollection, Concentration And Real Knowledge (And Thus Attain Asamprajñāta-Samādhi). 20.**

Yogins adopt this means. Tranquillity that is experienced by the mind through reverential faith (1) sustains a Yogin like a loving mother. This kind of faith gives a seeker after discriminative knowledge, energy (2) which brings him the (sustained) memory (3) which makes the mind undisturbed and collected and conducive to concentration (4). In such a mind dawns the light of discriminative knowledge, by which the Yogin understands the real nature of things. By retaining such knowledge and by cultivating detachment towards all knowables he thus attains Asamprajñāta-samādhi (5).

(1) Śraddhā = Tranquillity (with a feeling of reverence) of the mind or certitude in the desire for the object of pursuit. In many cases the knowledge obtained from the Śāstras or from preceptors merely satisfies one's curiosity. Such knowledge for satisfying one's curiosity, is not Śraddhā. Knowledge accompanied by tranquillity is Śraddhā. From such an attitude, a tendency arises to find out more and more the good points about the object of reverence and thus love for the object is generated.

(2) Enthusiasm leading to sustained effort is Vīrya* or energy. When the mind is tired and wants to drift to a different subject, the power which can bring it back to devotional practice is called Vīrya. Where there is Śraddhā there is Vīrya. As in physical culture when a man wants to lift a heavy weight, he practises it by gradually lifting progressively heavier weights, so when one gives up laziness and practises discipline of the organs his energy is increased. By referring to seekers after discriminative knowledge, it is implied that the Śraddhā and Vīrya mentioned here relate to the means for attainment of Kaivalya. There may be Śraddhā and Vīrya for other objects but they do not bring about Yoga or the state of liberation.

(3) Smṛti = Memory or repeated recollection is the principal item in devotional practice. This practice may be termed Smṛti-sādhana. It

* It is difficult to find an exact equivalent of Vīrya in English. It denotes a combination of energy, fortitude and stamina.

consists in recalling the feeling experienced at the time of contemplating an object and in feeling that it is being remembered and will be remembered. When this is achieved memory is retained firmly in the mind which is the only means of getting into the habitual state of one-pointedness of mind. One-pointedness is attained when the memory becomes permanently established.

God and the various constituent principles are the objects of contemplation. Smṛti is to be practised on them. The method of Smṛti-sādhana relating to God is as follows :

First, try to remember the co-relation between the name indicative of God and God Himself. When the repetition, either mental or oral, of the indicative name (which is OM and called Praṇava) brings before the mind the conception of an eternally emancipated God, then will the memory of co-relation be properly fixed. Then imagine that such a God is residing within your inner self and go on repeating the indicative name, remembering at the same time that you are repeating the name with the recollection of God and that you will continue to remember it. In the preliminary stage remembrance of God by the indicative name might be replaced by a more descriptive, wordy Mantra.

Similarly, when practising contemplation on the various Tattvas or principles, *i.e.* Bhūta-tattva, Tanmātra-tattva, Indriya-tattva, Ahaṁkāra-tattva and Buddhi-tattva (respectively the principles of gross elements, subtle monads, the organs, the I-sense and the pure I-sense), their peculiar features should be envisaged and recollected for purposes of Smṛti-sādhana. The highest practice relates to constant remembrance of the discrimination between Puruṣa and Prakṛti, the pure Consciousness and the knowable. While practising this, the thoughts arising in the mind should be kept before the mind as it were, *i.e.* your thought-process should always be the subject of your scrutiny and no extraneous idea, *i.e.* nothing other than that which is being thought of, should be allowed to crop up therein, and you should go on watching what your mind is receiving. This is the chief means of cleansing your mind, *i.e.* for attaining self-purification. This is the best form of Smṛti-sādhana.

Without Smṛti-sādhana pure Consciousness cannot be realised. Cultivation of memory can be practised in the midst of all actions, even while walking, sitting or lying down. If when we are engaged in worldly pursuits, we can keep in mind the object of spiritual contemplation and carefully notice that it is never absent from the mind, we may be said to be working, established in a Yogic state.

In Smṛti-sādhana we must always watch what is rising in the mind, and abandoning the disturbed state must keep the mind undisturbed and in a volitionless state. That is the correct way of purifying the mind and attaining tranquil knowledge. When the memory becomes firmly established, *i.e.* when one never ceases to be aware of one's self, the Samādhi that ensues from being engrossed in self only, is real Samprajñāta-yoga.

For purposes of developing and preserving memory, careful practice is necessary. When through practice, watchfulness becomes a habit then is memory established. In the Buddhist texts too prominence has been given to memory (Smṛti). These also point out that without memory and its careful development, mind cannot be arrested at will. In Bodhicharyāvatāra it has been said that constant watchful observation of the body and the mind, in whatever state they may be at different times, is Samprajanya. This kills self-forgetfulness, reveals the slightest fluctuation of the mind and gives the power to stop such fluctuation. It thus enables one to concentrate on constituent principles, especially those pertaining to one's own self. It might be questioned that this habit of watching the different fluctuations of the mind is not one-pointedness but multi-pointedness. In reply it can be said that though in respesct of the knowables it is multi-pointed, in respect of the instrument of reception it is one-pointed, because the intellect is then occupied with one thought only, *viz.* 'I shall be watchful and shall remain watchful.' This is the basic one-pointedness, and on its attainment the achievement of one-pointedness in respect of the knowables also becomes easy. By attaining one-pointedness only in respect of knowables, one-pointedness in respect of the reflector of the mind (the superior Self) may not be achieved.

While practising this, the Yogin does not cease to have knowledge of outside objects, but he goes on observing things with a disinterested mind. Things which are coming to the mind are not escaping his notice and he is noticing the impressions that are being left on the ego through the senses. In this way when the mind-stuff is purified and the organs become quiet or inactive, *i.e.* lose their distinctive features, then the outside objects fail to make any impression on the ego. In that state the fact of not noticing any object is not forgetfulness but full remembrance of self or I-sense free from the impact of unwanted objects and this is real Samprajñāta-yoga or true concentration. As the self-remembrance becomes purer and subtler, the realisation of the subtle principles is achieved more and more. Devotees should carefully understand the difference between not noticing outside objects under the stress of agitated thoughts, and shutting out their knowledge at will by sterilising the senses as described above. Again, voluntary stoppage of the action of the organs and shutting out contact with their objects is not stopping fluctuations of the mind. The mind can then still remain steeped in the thought of objects. In such a condition, by recollection of self and careful introspection the mind has to be purified and freed from volitions. Then the mind has to be moulded into homogeneity and stopped from functioning.

It should, however, be remembered that this sort of stoppage of fluctuations of mind or Nirodha-samādhi or arrested state of mind does not necessarily mean the attainment of the goal. The Bhava-pratyaya-nirodha referred to in the previous Sūtra, is an arrested state of mind of this category. The completely arrested state of mind, which is effected after acquiring discriminative enlightenment, *i e.* Smṛti about the Seer, the reflector of the ego, is the state leading to attainment of Kaivalya or liberation.

(4) Śraddhā leads to Vīrya. People who have no reverential faith in their objectives cannot apply any energy to attain them. By fixing the mind repeatedly on a subject, notwithstanding the attending discomfort, memory or recollection thereof is obtained. When it gets fixed, it leads to concentration. Concentration brings forth supreme knowledge, through which true knowledge of things to be avoided arises and thus Kaivalya is attained. This is the way to Mokṣa or liberation. Whatever be the devotional path followed, no one can side-track these general methods. Lord Buddha said in the Dhammapada that all sorrows can be cured through good conduct, reverential faith, enthusiasm, remembrance, concentration and correct knowledge.

(5) What we conceive of as a performer, knower and supporter of things other than the self, is what is known as Mahān Ātmā. It is the pure I-sense, when one speaks of being the doer, the knower and retainer of a thing or an object. The fact that the I-sense which is a phase of Buddhi is not Puruṣa (or metempiric Self or pure Consciousness) has to be realised first in a mind, made calm and clear through concentration ; then by shutting out therefrom all other knowledge the ability to remain absorbed in the knowledge about Puruṣa, is Viveka-khyāti or discriminative enlightenment. Through Viveka, Buddhi ceases to act, *i.e.* Nirodha-concentration ensues. It also brings about the knowledge of discernment such as omniscience. When by renouncing even that power and practising Nirodha-concentration, the arrested state of mind becomes habitual through force of latent impression thereof, it is called Asamprajñāta-samādhi. It is so called because in that state all Samprajñāna or knowledge, even discriminative enlightenment, is shut out.

———

भाष्यम्—ते खलु नव योगिनः मृदुमध्याधिमात्रोपाया भवन्ति, तद्यथा मृदूपायः, मध्योपायः, अधिमात्रोपाय इति। तत्र मृदूपायोऽपि त्रिविधः मृदुसंवेगः, मध्यसंवेगः, तीव्रसंवेग इति। तथा मध्योपायस्तथाधिमात्रोपाय इति। तत्राधिमात्रोपायानाम्—

तीव्रसंवेगानामासन्नः ॥ २१ ॥

समाधिलाभः समाधिफलं च भवतीति ॥ २१ ॥

Yogins (of previous Sūtra) are of nine kinds according as their methods of practice are slow, moderate and speedy. These methods have again three degrees each, *viz.* of gentle ardour, of medium ardour and of intense ardour (1). Of those speedy methods,

**Yogins With Intense Ardour Achieve Concentration And The Result Thereof Quickly. 21.**

(1) The word 'Saṁvega' is a technical term in the science of Yoga. We find it in Buddhist literature also. It means not only detachment, but also aptitude combined with a feeling of reverence in devotional practice and the resultant ardour to hasten forward. It is like gathering momentum as you proceed. Endowed with latent impression of detachment and full of enthusiasm and energy, when the devotee constantly engages himself with intensity in attaining the path of liberation, he acquires momentum as he advances.

———

मृदुमध्याधिमात्रत्वात्ततोऽपि विशेषः ॥ २२ ॥

भाष्यम्—मृदुतीव्रः, मध्यतीव्रः, अधिमात्रतीव्र इति, ततोऽपि विशेषः, तद्विशेषान्मृदुतीव्रसंवेगस्यासन्नः, ततो मध्यतीव्रसंवेगस्यासन्नतरस्तस्मादधिमात्रतीव्रसंवेगस्याधिमात्रोपायस्यासन्नतमः समाधिलाभः समाधिफलं चेति ॥ २२ ॥

**On Account Of The Methods Being Slow, Medium And Speedy, Even Among Those Yogins Who Have Intense Ardour, There Are Differences. 22.**

The difference is of varying degrees, *viz.* mild, medium, and deepest ardour. On account of this difference, the attainment of concentration and its results by Yogins with mild ardour is imminent, with medium ardour more imminent and with deepest ardour the most imminent (1).

(1) Sāttvika Śraddhā or Śraddhā (reverential faith) which is established as the chief means for practising concentration is the quickest method. So for energy. The most intense form of energy is to give up all other pursuits and to be occupied in bringing about concentration of mind. Constant remembrance (knowledge) of the constituent principles, *i.e.* of realities, and of God is the best form of knowledge. Of concentrations, Samprajñāta is the highest form amongst the Savīja types while amongst the Nirvīja ones, Asamprajñāta is the best. These are the best means of attaining Kaivalya or liberation which is the principal object of concentration.

———

भाष्यम्—किमेतस्मादेवासन्नतमः समाधिर्भवति, अथास्य लाभे भवति अन्योऽपि कश्चिदुपायो न वेति—

ईश्वर-प्रणिधानाद्वा ॥ २३ ॥

प्रणिधानाद् भक्तिविशेषाद् आवर्जित ईश्वरस्तमनुगृह्णाति अभिध्यानमात्रेण, तदभिध्यानादपि योगिन आसन्नतमः समाधिलाभः फलं च भवति इति ॥ २३ ॥

Does concentration become imminent from this (earnest desire to concentrate on principles) alone, or is there any other means ?

**From Special Devotion To Īśvara Also (Concentration Becomes Imminent). 23.**

Through a special kind of devotion (1) called Īśvara-praṇidhāna, on the part of the devotee, Īśvara inclines towards him and favours him with grace for fulfilment of his wish. From such grace also a Yogin obtains concentration and its result, the attainment of the state of liberation, becomes imminent.

(1) Previously it has been stated that the mind can be made one-pointed through contemplation on Grāhya (knowables), Grahaṇa (instruments of reception) and Grahitā (receiver), and it has been indicated that therewith Samprajñāta-yoga can be practised. There is yet another way, for making the mind one-pointed or stable. Praṇidhāna is a special form of devotion. It consists in feeling the existence, in the innermost core of the heart, of God as described later and to rest content by surrendering oneself to Him. To feel always that I am doing everything as if (though not in reality) being prompted by Him is, what is known as surrendering everything to God. The saying, "Whatever I do, willingly or unwillingly, I am offering its fruits, whether happiness or misery, to you" means that 'I do not want either happiness or sorrow nor shall be perturbed by either. Everything is being done by you.' To make oneself disinterested in everything one should follow this devotional practice. This frame of mind banishes all egotistic feelings and brings about a perpetual faith in God.

(2) Being touched by his devotion, God desires that the wishes of a whole-hearted and dependent devotee may be fulfilled. Naturally God's grace would be directed towards conferment of the highest benefit on the devotee, *viz.* attainment of Mokṣa or the state of liberation and not worldly pleasures, which it is best not to seek from God. Worldly pleasures or misery arise out of one's action. From Īśvara-praṇidhāna spiritual knowledge is obtained through God's grace. Through contemplation on God, as on a liberated being, the mind in the normal course also becomes calm and thereby concentrated. From knowledge derived through such concentration, the spiritual needs of a Yogin are met. He does not have to wait for special favour from God ; while Yogins who surrender all the fruits of their labour to God and seek knowledge from Him, get it through His grace.

भाष्यम्—अथ प्रधानपुरुषव्यतिरिक्तः कोऽयमीश्वरो नामेति ?—

क्लेशकर्मविपाकाशयैरपरामृष्टः पुरुषविशेष ईश्वरः ।। २४ ।।

अविद्यादयः क्लेशाः, कुशलाकुशलानि कर्माणि, तत्फलं विपाकस्तदनुगुणा वासना आशयाः । ते च मनसि वर्तमानाः पुरुषे व्यपदिश्यन्ते स हि तत्फलस्य भोक्तेति, यथा जयः पराजयो वा योद्धृषु वर्तमानः स्वामिनि व्यपदिश्यते । यो ह्यनेन भोगेन अपरामृष्टः स पुरुषविशेष ईश्वरः । कैवल्यं प्राप्तास्तर्हि सन्ति च बहवः केवलिनः, ते हि त्रीणि बन्धनानि छित्त्वा कैवल्यं प्राप्ताः, ईश्वरस्य च तत्सम्बन्धो न भूतो न भावी यथा मुक्तस्य पूर्वा बन्धकोटिः प्रज्ञायते नैवमीश्वरस्य, यथा वा प्रकृति-लीनस्य उत्तरा बन्धकोटिः संभाव्यते नैवमीश्वरस्य । स तु सदैव मुक्तः सदैवेश्वर इति । योऽसौ प्रकृष्टसत्त्वोपादानादीश्वरस्य शाश्वतिक उत्कर्षः स किं सनिमित्तः ? आहोस्विन्निर्निमित्त इति । तस्य शास्त्रं निमित्तम् । शास्त्रं पुनः किन्निमित्तम् ? प्रकृष्टसत्त्वनिमित्तम् । एतयोः शास्त्रोत्कर्षयोरीश्वरसत्त्वे वर्तमानयोरनादिः सम्बन्धः । एतस्मात् एतद्भवति सदैवेश्वरः सदैव मुक्त इति ।

तच्च तस्यैश्वर्यं साम्यातिशयविनिर्मुक्तं, न तावद् ऐश्वर्यान्तरेण तदतिशय्यते, यदेवातिशयि स्यात्तदेव तत्स्यात्, तस्माद् यत्र काष्ठाप्राप्तिरैश्वर्यस्य स ईश्वरः । न च तत्समानमैश्वर्यमस्ति, कस्माद् द्वयोस्तुल्ययोरेकस्मिन् युगपत् कामितेऽर्थे नवमिदमस्तु पुराणमिदमस्तु इत्येकस्य सिद्धौ इतरस्य प्राकाम्यविघातादूनत्वं प्रसक्तं, द्वयोश्च तुल्ययोर्युगपत् कामितार्थप्राप्तिर्नास्त्यर्थस्य विरुद्धत्वात् । तस्मात यस्य साम्यातिशयविनिर्मुक्तमैश्वर्यं स ईश्वरः, स च पुरुषविशेष इति ।। २४ ।।

Now, who is this Īśvara, other than Puruṣa and Prakṛti ? (1)

**Īśvara Is A Particular Puruṣa Unaffected By Affliction, Deed, Result Of Action Or The Latent Impressions Thereof. 24.**

Kleśa or affliction (=nescience etc.), good or bad deeds and the result thereof as well as the subliminal impressions of the result of action, though subsisting in the mind, are imputed to Puruṣa. That is why Puruṣa (Self or Ātmā) is imagined to be experiencing them just as victory or defeat gained or suffered by the soldiers in the field is attributed to their commander. The special Puruṣa, who, on account of His eternal liberation, is unaffected even by the touch of enjoyment or suffering, is called Īśvara. There are many Puruṣas who have attained the state of liberation, cutting asunder the threefold bondage (2). Īśvara had no such bondage in the past nor will He have any in future. Liberated persons are known to have had a previous state of bondage (3), but Īśvara's case is not like that. The Prakṛtilīnas have the possibility of bondage in future, but in the case of Īśvara there is no such possibility. Īśvara is always free and always supreme. The question, therefore, arises whether this perpetual supremacy of Īśvara, on account of the excellence of His Self (4), is something of which there is proof, or is it something without any proof? The reply is: 'The scriptures are its proof.' What is the proof of the genuineness of the scriptures? Their genuineness is based on supreme wisdom. The Śāstras and their sublime wisdom which are present in the mind of Īśvara and His pre-emience are eternally related to each other (5). For these reasons Īśvara is always Īśvara, *i.e.* omniscient and always liberated.

His pre-eminence is never equalled nor excelled. The commentator explains it by saying that the excellence of Īśvara is the highest excellence unsurpassable by anybody else's and without any equal. That is why the person whose eminence has reached the limit is Īśvara. There is no pre-eminence equal to His, because if there were two persons with equal eminence but contradictory desires—one wishing a thing to be new and the other wishing the same thing at the same time to be old—then the fulfilment of the directives of one will impair the equality of power of the other or if both are equally powerful, their directives will be inoperative. For that reason (6) the Puruṣa whose excellence has no equal or is never excelled is Īśvara and He is that special Puruṣa.

(1) It should be clearly understood that Īśvara is neither the Puruṣa principle nor the Pradhāna principle but is made up of both. He is a

particular Being and His godly attributes are based on the ultimate constituent principles. In fact, such attributes witnessed by Puruṣa, as have from time without beginning attained perfection in the forms of omniscience and omnipotence, are godly attributes. Yogins desirous of spiritual attainment concentrate only on such pure and perfect aspects of God and practise special devotion to Īśvara.

(2) The three forms of bondage are Prākṛtika, Vaikārika and Dākṣiṇa. In the case of those who remain merged in elemental principles the bondage is Prākṛtika. In the case of the discarnates, the bondage is Vaikārika because they cannot reach the basic constituent principles. Their minds, when they reappear, are concerned only with the modifications of the elemental principles. The third is the bondage of those who receive sacrificial gifts because they are attached to objects of enjoyment here and hereafter.

(3) It is known that Ṛṣis like Kapila and others were not free to start with but were liberated afterwards ; some Prakṛtilīna beings who are now apparently liberated will have to reappear with superior attributes. It is quite different in the case of Īśvara, as He has no such bondage and will never have any. In the past or future, as far as we can see or think of, the Being in respect of whom we can trace no bondage, is Īśvara.

(4) God is most sublime and has unsurpassable excellence. On account of His eternal discriminative enlightenment He has the eternal attributes of omniscience and omnipresence. We can only conjecture the existence of God but we know from the Śāstras that in the beginning some one propounded the spiritual knowledge. Ṛṣis like Kapila were the original teachers of the religion of salvation. These Ṛṣis, as we know from the Upaniṣad, got their knowledge from Īśvara. Ṛṣis propounded the Śāstras ; these have thus been derived from God. From Īśvara came the Śāstras and from Śāstras the knowledge of Īśvara ; this cycle of cause and effect goes on eternally.

(5) Supreme spirituality signified by the qualities like eternal freedom, omniscience attributed to Īśvara and the excellent religion of liberation are eternally related to each other like cause and effect.

(6) There are many persons who have special powers. Īśvara is One such, but His special feature is that no one has as much power as He has, nor can anybody else's power exceed His ; that is why He is called Īśvara.

———

भाष्यम्—किंच—

तत्र निरतिशयं सर्वज्ञवीजम् ॥ २५ ॥

यदिदमतीतानागतप्रत्युत्पन्नप्रत्येकसमुच्चयातीन्द्रियग्रहणमल्पं बहु इति सर्वज्ञवीजम्, एतद्धि वर्द्धमानं यत्र निरतिशयं स सर्वज्ञः। अस्ति काष्ठाप्राप्तिः सर्वज्ञवीजस्य सातिशयत्वात् परिमाणवदिति, यत्र काष्ठाप्राप्तिः ज्ञानस्य स सर्वज्ञः स च पुरुषविशेष इति। सामान्यमात्रोपसंहारे कृतोपक्षयमनुमानं न विशेषप्रतिपत्तौ समर्थमिति तस्य संज्ञादिविशेषप्रतिपत्तिरागमतः पर्यन्वेष्या। तस्यात्मानुग्रहाभावेऽपि भूतानुग्रहः प्रयोजनं ज्ञानधर्मोपदेशेन कल्पप्रलयमहाप्रलयेषु संसारिणः पुरुषानुद्धरिष्यामीति। तथा चोक्तम् 'आदिविद्वान् निर्माणचित्तमधिष्ठाय कारुण्याद्भगवान् परमर्षिरासुरये जिज्ञासमानाय तन्त्रम् प्रोवाच' इति ॥ २५ ॥

Besides,

**In Him The Seed Of Omniscience Has Reached Its Utmost Development Which Cannot Be Exceeded. 25.**

The supersensuous knowledge, vast or little, that is found in any being, in respect of the past, present and future (affairs), singly or collectively, is the seed of omniscience (1). When this sort of supersensuous knowledge in a person goes on increasing and reaches a stage which cannot be exceeded that person is called omniscient. (The argument is as follows :)

The seed of omniscience has grades of development and thus is capaple of increasing from more to still more. The person in whom it has reached its highest point is a particular being who knows everything.

Inference which is concerned with proving certain general features proves that an omniscient Being exists and there it ends ; and it cannot give any specific information about Him. Therefore, His description etc. are to be ascertained from Āgama or the Śāstras. Although He has no need of His own, the motive of His action is to be found in His compassion for living beings, in His desire to save, at the time of the dissolutions of the universe, through His instructions in knowledge and piety, men who are caught up in the vortex of worldly existence (*i.e.* cycle of birth and death). For this sort of compassion, His inclination (2) is necessary. Pañcha-śikha has said in this connection : "The first enlightened one, the great Ṛṣi (Kapila), through compassion, assumed a created mind and instructed the enquiring Āsuri the Tantra (Sāṁkhya philosophy)."

(1) Here the method of inferring the existence of Īśvara is being shown.

(*a*) If an immeasurable thing is divided into parts, then the parts would be innumerable. For example, if immeasurable time is divided into measured hours, the result will be innumerable hours.

(*b*) If the parts of an immeasurable thing are taken as progressively increasing then in the end it would be a thing bigger than which nothing exists, *i.e.* nothing bigger than that can be conceived. That is the greatness more than which does not exist.

(*c*) The basic ingredient of our cognitive faculty is Prakṛti which is immeasurable. In every created being the power of knowledge that is seen, whether less, more or still more, is but a modified form of that immeasurable omniparous cause. According to (*a*) above, the parts of an immeasurable thing must be innumerable. Therefore, the faculties of knowledge, or the individual selves must be innumerable.

(*d*) From a worm to man, the faculty of knowledge goes on increasing ; so it is progressive (*i.e.* not fixed). From (*b*) above, it would appear that the parts of an immeasurable thing going on increasing becomes so big that nothing can exceed it. The constituent cause of the variable faculty of knowledge is limitless (Prakṛti). Therefore, the extent of knowledge will ultimately reach a stage more than which there would be none.

(*e*) The particular Being whose power of knowledge is so excessive, so non-pareil, is Īśvara.

From the Sūtra and the commentary only a general idea of Īśvara is derived, *i.e.* only this much comes to be known that there is a Being of that description. From the Śāstras, *i.e.* from the sayings of those who have realised Him through special devotion (Praṇidhāna) the particulars of Īśvara are to be gathered.

(2) Ordinary human mind goes on fluctuating continually and in-

voluntarily under the influence of previous latent impressions. It cannot be stopped even if someone wants to stop it. When a Yogin after having acquired discriminative enlightenment can bring the mind to an arrested state by extinguishing the latent impressions, he can, if necessity arises, shut out the working of the mind for a specified period, after which the arrested state will cease and the mind will reappear. Being freed from latent impressions of nescience, the mind will emerge, not uncontrolled as in the case of an ordinary being, but with correct knowledge for the benefit of the Yogin. Such a mind will also arise or disappear at the bidding of the Yogin, except in the case of a Yogin who shuts out his mind for ever, there will be no chance of a created mind to appear.

That liberated persons can work with such created minds is the finding of the Sāṁkhya philosophy. The commentator has quoted Pañchaśikha in support of this view. Īśvara also favours creatures in this way. Yogins assume a created mind only when the need for it arises. 'I shall liberate the creatures from the snares of birth and death by giving them proper knowledge' is the incentive for the emergence of Īśvara's created mind. In the opinion of the commentator, Īśvara assumes such a mind at the time of dissolution of this creation.

———

भाष्यम्—स एषः

पूर्वेषामपि गुरुः कालेनानवच्छेदात् ॥ २६ ॥

पूर्वे हि गुरवः कालेन अवच्छेद्यन्ते, यत्रावच्छेदार्थेन कालो नोपावर्त्तते स एष पूर्वेषामपि गुरुः। यथा अस्य सर्गस्यादौ प्रकर्षगत्या सिद्धस्तथा अतिक्रान्तसर्गादिष्वपि प्रत्येतव्यः ॥ २६ ॥

He is

**The Teacher Of Former Teachers, Because With Him There Is No Limitation By Time (To His Omnipotence). 26.**

The former teachers of knowledge and of piety are limited by time, but He to whom time as a limiting factor is not applicable, was the teacher of the former teachers. As He was present with His full powers in the beginning of the present cycle of creation, so was He at the beginning of the past creations.

———

तस्य वाचकः प्रणवः ॥ २७ ॥

भाष्यम्—वाच्य ईश्वरः प्रणवस्य। किमस्य संकेतकृतं वाच्यवाचकत्वम्, अथ प्रदीपप्रकाशवदवस्थितमिति। स्थितोऽस्य वाच्यस्य वाचकेन सह सम्बन्धः। संकेतस्तु ईश्वरस्य स्थितमेवार्थमभिनयति, यथा अवस्थितः पितापुत्रयोः सम्बन्धः संकेतेनावद्योत्यते—अयमस्य पिता अयमस्य पुत्र इति। सर्गान्तरेष्वपि वाच्य-वाचकशक्त्यपेक्षस्तथैव संकेतः क्रियते सम्प्रतिपत्तिनित्यतया नित्यः शब्दार्थसम्बन्ध इत्यागमिनः प्रतिजानते ॥ २७ ॥

**The Sacred Word Designating Him Is Praṇava Or The Mystic Syllable OM. 27.**

Īśvara is indicated by the mystic syllable. Is this relationship a matter of convention or is it always necessarily existing as between the lamp and the light ? The relationship between a word and its object is always there, and the convention in reference to Īśvara expresses what is inherent in Him. For example, the relationship between the father and the son exists and is indicated by the words 'this is that person's father, that is this person's son.' In other creations too convention dependent on the relationship between the denoting words and the object denoted has been in use (1). Sages, who know the Śāstras, say that on account of similarity of usage, the relationship between a word and the object indicated by it is eternal (2).

(1) There are many things (*viz.* perceivables) which are denoted by names, *i.e.* uttered sounds, but absence of such a name does not interfere with knowing the things. There are other things again which are only understood by the thought raised by the expressed word. Those names are also conventional but the significance of those words is the setting-up

of a current of thought. The example of the first kind is Chaitra, Maitra (names of persons), etc. Even if those names are not there, there would be no difficulty in knowing them. The example of the second kind of words is 'father', 'son', etc. The word 'father' indicates a person of whom a son is born. 'Maitra is Chaitra's father,' in this phrase the name 'Chaitra' will indicate only the existence of a person known as Chaitra. Looking at Chaitra without knowing his name will also bring similar knowledge. If Chaitra has been seen before, mention of the name will bring up the recollection of Chaitra. Even if the name is forgotten, he can be remembered and kept in mind. But the relationship between Chaitra and Maitra, *i.e.* what is meant by the word 'father', cannot be thought of without the use of the symbolic word, *i.e.* language. The meaning of the word 'father' is the result of a thinking process. As the presence of a lamp indicates illumination, so the utterance of the word 'father' indicates the relationship. Unless there is a thought-process or a symbol thereof, the full significance is not understood.

Īśvara is also the product of a similar thought-process. Unless certain faculties implied by words are thought of, no conception can be had of Īśvara. The thought-process associated with Īśvara has been symbolised by the word OM. Although words and their meanings are invariably related, the same words cannot always have the same meanings, because men might change the convention from time to time. According to commentators, the word OM has been used to imply Īśvara not only in this creation but also in previous creations. The symbol has been re-introduced in this creation by omniscient persons or by persons who have recollection of their previous births. The particular reason why in the Śāstras framed by Ṛṣis the word OM is so much liked is that there is no other word which can bring about calmness of mind as this word can.

Consonants cannot be pronounced in prolonged continuity, vowels however can be so pronounced. The syllable OM is comparatively easy to pronounce. When this word is uttered mentally, a sort of effort moves from the throat to the brain which Yogins utilize towards contemplation. Continuity of thought in the mind cannot be mastered without continuity in the utterance of words. Thus the symbol OM is useful in all respects.

(2) Sampratipatti = similarity of usage. It has been stated before that a particular meaning can be conveyed by different words as men wish, but it is imperative that ideas which are to be understood through verbal thought-process, should be indicated by symbols or words. [See in this connection comments on Sūtra III.17 (2) (H).]

———

भाष्यम्—विज्ञातवाच्यवाचकत्वस्य योगिनः—

तज्जपस्तदर्थभावनम् ॥ २८ ॥

प्रणवस्य जपः प्रणवाभिधेयस्य च ईश्वरस्य भावना। तदस्य योगिनः प्रणवं जपतः प्रणवार्थश्च भावयतश्चित्तमेकाग्रं सम्पद्यते। तथा चोक्तम् 'स्वाध्यायाद्योगमासीत योगात्स्वाध्यायमामनेत् (स्वाध्यायमासते)। स्वाध्याययोगसम्पत्त्या परमात्मा प्रकाशते' इति ॥ २८ ॥

Yogins having understood the relationship between the verbal symbol and the thing expressed will

**Repeat It And Contemplate Upon Its Meaning. 28.**

Repetition of the symbol (OM) and contemplation on its object—Īśvara—bring one-pointedness (1) to the mind of the Yogin who is engaged in repeating the symbol and contemplating on its meaning. It has been said : "Through contemplative repeating of Mantras, Yoga should be consolidated and through Yoga chanting of Mantras improved. Through the glory of such chanting and of such Yoga, the supreme soul is revealed (2)."

(1) The verbal concept which has to be formed in order to comprehend the meaning of God has been symbolised by the syllable OM. Consequently, if the import of OM is correctly remembered, thought of God will dawn on the mind. When with the utterance of the word OM the significance of Īśvara is fully brought to the mind, it will be clear that the relationship between the symbol and the object has been clearly comprehended. A devotee has to practise carefully at first this method of raising the thought of the relationship. This is done by repeating the word OM and recollecting simultaneously its significance. Then when the symbol and its import come naturally to the mind, Īśvara-praṇidhāna mentioned before can be taken to be well established.

The principles of Grahītā (receiver) and Grahaṇa (instruments of reception) are parts of oneself ; so they can be felt or realised. Therefore, although at first a verbal concept is necessary for their realisation, they can be thought of without reference to words. Nirvitarka and

Nirvichāra contemplations (detailed later in I.43 and 44 Sūtras) are of that nature. But to form a concept of God, who is outside the I-sense, help of words is necessary. That concept is again the recollection of certain words implying qualities—One who is free from affliction, activity, etc. But for the purpose of concentrating on Him, thinking of such diverse qualities will not be helpful.

What we can think of or feel as an entity, is one or other of the three principles of receiver, instrument of reception, and object received, *i.e.* knowable. In other words, it must be thought of either as gross knowables such as light, sound, etc. or as subtle instruments of reception, *e.g.* Buddhi, I-sense, etc. Therefore, to conceive a thing outside of us, we have to think of it as endowed with colour, sound, etc. or if we conceive it as part of ourselves, *i.e.* if we think of it as residing within us, we cannot help thinking of it as part of our Buddhi, I-sense, etc. Therefore, to think of God as an outside object, we have to think of Him as endowed with form, etc. The beginners in Yoga system adopt this method.

Buddhi, I-sense, etc. are realised as parts of oneself, because we cannot ascertain or realise someone else's Buddhi, I-sense, etc. If, therefore, God has to be thought of as part of oneself He has to be thought of as 'I am He.' This method is supported by the Śāstras.

In effect, the process of Īśvara-praṇidhāna has to be practised inside the heart. The inner part of the chest wherein one feels pleasure if there is love or happiness, and sadness, if there is unhappiness or fear, is called the heart. As a matter of fact, the location of the heart has to be determined by following the feeling. It cannot be located by analysing the body anatomically. The feeling of attachment, etc. produces a reflex action which is cognised in the heart, but we cannot locate where the mental modification takes place. That is why it is easier to get to the cogniser by meditation on the region of the heart. That region is the centre of the I-sense related to one's body. The brain is no doubt the centre of mental actions but if mental fluctuations are stopped for a time, it can be felt that the sense of ego is going down to the heart. When by meditation on the region of the heart, the subtle I-sense is realised and it is pursued upward into the brain, then can the subtlest centre of 'I' be located. Then the heart and the brain become one and the same.

Beginners who find it easier to practise Īśvara-praṇidhāna with a God having a figure should imagine a luminous figure of God inside their hearts. As a liberated person is calm in mind and is blissful in face on account of his highest attainment, so should the contemplated holy figure in one's heart be imagined to be and it should be contemplated that one is fully associated with that figure. In repeating the mystic syllable OM, one should think oneself to be within the emblem—calm, restful and felicitous.

When after some practice the mind of the devotee becomes somewhat calm and carefree and he is able to rest in a feeling of godliness, then a transparent white limitless luminous sky should be imagined by him within his heart. Then knowing that the omnipresent God is pervading that space, the devotee should contemplate that his I-sense, *i.e.* his whole self is in the God who is present in his heart. The next step would be to merge his mind in the mind of the Īśvara residing in the void-like space within his heart and rest in a state of contentment, without any care or thought. In the Muṇḍaka Upaniṣad the method has been beautifully described as follows : "Brahman or the God within the heart, is the target ; the mystic syllable OM is the bow ; and the self or ego is the arrow. With an undistracted mind one should hit the mark and be completely absorbed by getting the self into Brahman." In other words, one should contemplate that one is completely within the God in one's heart.

When the above process of meditation is mastered the devotee has a sort of blissful feeling in his heart. Then he should recollect that the blissful feeling, arising out of a sense of staying in God, is 'I' and he should bring his mind to a state of calmness and blissfulness after the mind of God. If this is practised with ardent devotion, carefully and continuously, the ultimate result of Īśvara-praṇidhāna, *viz.* realisation of one's own Self is achieved (see next Sūtra).

In repeating the mystic syllable OM, the 'O' is pronounced comparatively short and 'M' long—prolonged without break. It is better to repeat it mentally, instead of articulately.

In practising Īśvara-praṇidhāna it has, of course, to be done with reverence. When the remembrance of God brings happiness, the feeling of attachment arising out of that sense of happiness and of God's greatness is reverence.

There is another way of repeating the mystic syllable. It is this. When 'O' is pronounced, bring to mind the reverential feeling and when the elongated 'M' is uttered continuously, persist in the reverential feeling. After getting into this way, if it is practised with breathing, it gives better result. In inhaling the normal breath, mentally utter 'O' and bring to mind a recollection of the object of reverence, then exhale slowly, mentally uttering 'M' continuously and continue in the feeling of the revered object.

By this sort of practice, *i.e.* repeating the mystic syllable with remembrance, the mind soon becomes one-pointed. From one-pointedness comes Samprajñāta concentration and from that Asamprajñāta-yoga is achieved.

(2) The meaning of the verse quoted, is as follows : Through Svādhyāya, *i.e.* through recollection of the meaning of the mystic syllable during the process of repetition, get fixed in Yoga, *i.e.* make the mind one-pointed. When the mind gets one-pointed, the inner meaning of the Mantra (abbreviated token name) that is being repeated is realised. Then again go on repeating the Mantra, remembering its inner meaning. By that, when its still finer and purer significance becomes clear, then the repetition should be continued in the same way. In this way, with a gradual increase of Yoga through repetition and of repetition through Yoga, the process results in firmly establishing the best form of concentration.

———

भाष्यम्—किं चास्य भवति—

ततः प्रत्यक्चेतनाधिगमोऽप्यन्तरायाभावश्च ॥ २९ ॥

ये तावदन्तराया व्याधिप्रभृतयस्ते तावदीश्वरप्रणिधानान्न भवन्ति, स्वरूपदर्शनमप्यस्य भवति, यथैवेश्वरः पुरुषः शुद्धः प्रसन्नः केवलोऽनुपसर्गस्तथायमपि बुद्धेः प्रतिसंवेदी यः पुरुष इत्येवमधिगच्छति ॥ २९ ॥

What else happens ?

**From That Comes Realisation Of The Individual Self** (1) **And the Obstacles Are Resolved. 29.**

Obstacles like illness etc. are removed through Īśvara-praṇidhāna and the Yogin realises his own Self. As God is pure (free from piety or sin), blissful (free from afflictions like nescience), isolated (free from attributes like Buddhi etc.), and thus an unencumbered (free from possibility of birth, span of life and experience) Being, so is Puruṣa (2) who is the reflector of Buddhi of the devotee. This is how the individual Self is realised.

(1) The word 'Pratyak' is used in different senses. What is underlying everything, that is Īśvara, is Pratyak. The word also means ancient ; therefore, ancient Being Īśvara is Pratyak. In the present case the meaning is different. Here Pratyak means knower of the opposite object. Vāchaspati Miśra explains the word as 'Knower of non-self as opposed to self'. That sort of consciousness is Pratyak-chetana, or Puruṣa. The word 'Puruṣa' when used by itself might refer to a free being, an unliberated person, Īśvara etc. But Pratyak-chetana means the true Self of a person who has nescience (and thus of one who is free from nescience also). This should be carefully noted. The consciousness which is opposed to objects, *i.e.* knowables, and is directed towards one's Self is Pratyak-chetana. Every Puruṣa with the adjunct of Buddhi or the enjoyer, observer, knower, is Pratyak-chetana. One's own Self is Pratyak-chetana.

(2) This has been explained fully in note (1) of Sūtra I.28. Īśvara by Himself is Consciousness only. So mind cannot remain in Him as He is not comprehensible as a perceivable object. Awareness is self-cognizant and does not admit of objective apprehension, as something external to us What is external to self is knowable. If absolute Awareness is taken as a knowable then it would no longer be awareness in itself, it would be a thing occupying space and made up of light, sound, etc. In reality when thinking of God in the manner described above we come ultimately to our own Consciousness, that is conceiving God in the self. 'Realising the soul in the self' is practically the same. The significance of these expressions becomes clear by contemplating that Īśvara is free from all nescience, established in Himself and in His own Self. To understand a thing which is self-cognizant is to be like that thing. This is how Īśvara-praṇidhāna brings knowledge of one's own self.

The composer of the Sūtra has shown how Praṇidhāna of a Nirguṇa eternally liberated Īśvara can bring about salvation, as that is the principal item in the practice of Karma-yoga. It includes also the Praṇidhāna of the Saguṇa Īśvara. The Praṇidhāna of Saguṇa Īśvara or Hiraṇyagarbha was also in vogue amongst the Sāṁkhya-yoga sect. To get to the Nirguṇa Īśvara through the Saguṇa Īśvara and to go to the Nirguṇa ideal straight are in effect the same thing. The Saguṇa Īśvara of Sāṁkhya-yogins is a calm, absorbed Being engaged in the contemplation of Self. So His Praṇidhāna is conducive to attainment of concentration and discriminative knowledge or Viveka and this method may be helpful to some. Although the two methods divided the devotees into two sects, there was no difference of opinion regarding the aim. The result of thinking of a reposed, self-cognizant, absorbed being inside the heart will be a similar feeling of those attributes in the devotee's heart and this will lead him eventually from knowables to the instruments of knowing by having a current of self-cognizance flowing through him. On realisation of the pure 'I', the Yogin gets a feeling as if he is in everything and everything is in him or that he is a manifestation of the Saguṇa Brahman.

———

भाष्यम्—अथ केऽन्तराया ये चित्तस्य विक्षेपकाः, के पुनस्ते कियन्तो वेति ?—

व्याधि-स्त्यान-संशय-प्रमादालस्याविरति-भ्रान्तिदर्शनालब्धभूमिकत्वानवस्थितत्वानि चित्तविक्षेपास्तेऽन्तरायाः ॥ ३० ॥

नव अन्तरायाश्चित्तस्य विक्षेपाः सह एते चित्तवृत्तिभिर्भवन्ति, एतेषामभावे न भवन्ति पूर्वोक्ताश्चित्तवृत्तयः। व्याधिर्धातुरसकरणवैषम्यं, स्त्यानमकर्मण्यता चित्तस्य, संशय उभयकोटिस्पृग्विज्ञानं स्यादिदमेवं नैवं स्यादिति, प्रमादः समाधिसाधनानामभावनम्, आलस्यं कायस्य चित्तस्य च गुरुत्वादप्रवृत्तिः, अविरतिश्चित्तस्य विषयसंप्रयोगात्मा गर्द्धः, भ्रान्तिदर्शनं विपर्ययज्ञानम्, अलब्धभूमिकत्वं समाधिभूमेरलाभः, अनवस्थितत्वं यल्लब्धायां भूमौ चित्तस्याप्रतिष्ठा, समाधिप्रतिलंभे हि तदवस्थितं स्यात्। इत्येते चित्तविक्षेपा नव योगमला योगप्रतिपक्षा योगान्तराया इत्यभिधीयन्ते ॥ ३० ॥

What are those impediments which disturb the mind? What are these called and how many are these?

**Sickness, Incompetence, Doubt, Delusion, Sloth, Non-Abstention, Erroneous Conception, Non-Attainment Of Any Yogic Stage, And Instability To Stay In A Yogic State, These Distractions Of The Mind Are The Impediments. 30.**

These nine obstacles cause distraction of the mind. They arise with the fluctuations of the mind. In their absence, the fluctuations do not arise. Sickness is disorder of the humours, secretions and the organs of the body. Incompetence or listlessness is incapacity of the mind. Doubt is a kind of thinking touching on both sides, such as : 'It can be this or it cannot be this.' Delusion is not thinking of the processes for concentration. Sloth is disinclination arising out of heaviness of the body and the mind. Non-abstention arises out of thirst for or addiction to worldly objects. Erroneous conception is false knowledge. Non-attainment of any (Yogic) stage means not being firmly established in any of the Yogic states of concentration. Inability to remain in a state relates to failure to maintain the attained state (of concentration). When concentration is established, the mind-stuff remains firm in the attained state. These nine kinds of disturbance are called foes of Yoga or obstacles to Yoga (1).

(1) Destruction of the impediments and the mind being fully concentrated are the same thing. When the body ails, effort at Yoga or concentration cannot be made fully. Bodily disturbance and illness should be removed by wholesome and measured diet taken only after the food previously taken is digested. This is the sure way of killing illness. By special devotion to God, refinement and good sense will come which will prompt the Yogin to take good and limited quantity of food at proper intervals and he will take proper care of his health, so that he will never lose that good sense. In spite of a proper sense of duty, when on account of restlessness the mind cannot be kept engaged in devotional work like contemplation etc. that is incompetence. Unpleasant though it might appear, constant Vīrya will remove listlessness. If there is doubt, appropriate Vīrya is not possible. Without firmness and Vīrya it is not possible to get success in Yoga ; for attaining that, one must get rid of doubts. By listening to instructions, by contemplation and by being in the company of a calm and sure-minded preceptor, doubts can be removed. Instead of thinking of the practice of concentration, to be engaged in worldly affairs through self-forgetfulness is delusion. Disinclination to engage oneself in devotional practice on account of dullness of body and mind is sloth. While in incompetence the mind roams about uncontrolled and cannot be applied to devotional practice, in sloth, the mind on account of a preponderance of Tamas (obtuseness) remains torpid—this is the difference between the two impediments. Moderation in diet, wakefulness and enthusiasm can conquer sloth. Remaining aloof from worldly affairs and giving up interest therein, remove non-abstention. Not knowing what is

to be really forsaken or removed and not knowing the means of doing it, to consider the lower stage to be higher and *vice versa* is called false or erroneous conception. There are various kinds of erroneous conception. Through profound devotion to God as well as to the preceptor and study of sacred scriptures, false conception is removed.

Non-attainment of stages of concentration such as Madhumatī etc. is referred to here. To get established in a stage, realisation of the 'principles' is necessary ; otherwise there will be retrocession.

Through Īśvara-praṇidhāna the impediments mentioned above disappear, because whatever are antidotes to such obstacles are obtained through special devotion to God, whereby pure Sāttvika intellect is developed and the Yogin gradually gains powers with which he is able to resist such obstacles.

———

दुःखदौर्म्मनस्याङ्गमेजयत्व-श्वास-प्रश्वासा विक्षेपसहभुवः ॥ ३१ ॥

भाष्यम्—दुःखमाध्यात्मिकम् आधिभौतिकम् आधिदैविकं च। येनाभिहताः प्राणिनस्तदुपघाताय प्रयतन्ते तद्दुःखम्। दौर्म्मनस्यमिच्छाभिघाताच्चेतसः क्षोभः। यदङ्गान्येजयति कम्पयति तदङ्गमेजयत्वम्। प्राणो यद्बाह्यं वायुमाचामति स श्वासः, यत् कौष्ठ्यं वायुं निःसारयति स प्रश्वासः, एते विक्षेपसहभुवो विक्षिप्तचित्तस्यैते भवन्ति, समाहितचित्तस्यैते न भवन्ति ॥ ३१ ॥

**Sorrow, Dejection, Restlessness Of Body, Inhalation And Exhalation Arise From (Previous) Distractions. 31.**

Sorrow is of three kinds—Ādhyātmika (arising within oneself), Ādhibhautika (inflicted by some other creature) and Ādhidaivika (through natural calamity). Sorrow is that which upsets creatures who try for its removal. Dejection is caused through non-fulfilment of desire or when wished-for things do not happen. The upsetting of bodily equilibrium or steadiness results in shakiness of the body. The ordinary process of taking in the breath and exhaling the same (1) is also associated with mental distraction. These disturbances generally take place in a distracted state of mind. They do not appear in a reposeful mind.

(1) The natural process of inhalation and exhalation is referred to here. When this is done unconsciously or unwillingly it is detrimental to concentration. But the regulated breathing, *i.e.* controlled inhalation and exhalation which is practised for bringing about concentration through Prāṇāyāma is not likely to produce disturbance or obstacles. In complete concentration, breathing generally stops but the flow of inner consciousness resulting from Prāṇāyāmic breathing continues and if recollection thereof is consciously maintained, it brings about concentration on that object.

———

भाष्यम्—अथ एते विक्षेपाः समाधिप्रतिपक्षास्ताभ्यामेवाभ्यासवैराग्याभ्यान्निरोद्धव्याः। तत्राभ्यासस्य विषयमुपसंहरन्निदमाह—

तत्प्रतिषेधार्थमेकतत्त्वाभ्यासः ॥ ३२ ॥

विक्षेपप्रतिषेधार्थमेकतत्त्वावलम्बनं चित्तमभ्यसेत्। यस्य तु प्रत्यर्थनियतं प्रत्ययमात्रं क्षणिकं च चित्तं तस्य सर्वमेव चित्तमेकाग्रं नास्त्येव विक्षिप्तम्। यदि पुनरिदं सर्वतः प्रत्याहृत्य एकस्मिन्नर्थे समाधीयते तदा भवत्येकाग्रमिति, अतो न प्रत्यर्थनियतम्। योऽपि सदृशप्रत्ययप्रवाहेण चित्तमेकाग्रं मन्यते तस्य यदेत्रकाग्रता प्रवाहचित्तस्य धर्मस्तदैकं नास्ति प्रवाहचित्तं क्षणिकत्वाद्, अथ प्रवाहांशस्यैव प्रत्ययस्य धर्मः स सर्वः सदृशप्रत्ययप्रवाही वा विसदृशप्रत्ययप्रवाही वा प्रत्यर्थनियतत्वादेकाग्र एवेति विक्षिप्तचित्तानुपपत्तिः। तस्मादेकमनेकार्थमवस्थितं चित्तमिति। यदि च चित्तेनैकेनानन्विताः स्वभावभिन्नाः प्रत्यया जायेरन् अथ कथमन्यप्रत्ययदृष्टस्यान्यः स्मर्त्ता भवेत्, अन्यप्रत्ययोपचितस्य च कर्माशयस्यान्यः प्रत्यय उपभोक्ता भवेत्? कथंचित् समाधीयमानमप्येतद् गोमयपायसीयं न्यायमाक्षिपति।

किं च स्वात्मानुभवापह्नवश्चित्तस्यान्यत्वे प्राप्नोति, कथं यदहमद्राक्षं तत्स्पृशामि यश्च अस्प्राक्षं तत्पश्यामीति अहमिति प्रत्ययः सर्वस्य प्रत्ययस्य भेदे सति प्रत्ययिन्यभेदेनोपस्थितः, एकप्रत्ययविषयोऽयमभेदात्मा अहमिति प्रत्ययः कथमत्यन्तभिन्नेषु चित्तेषु वर्तमानः सामान्यमेकं प्रत्ययिनमाश्रयेत्? स्वानुभवग्राह्यश्चायमभेदात्माऽहमिति प्रत्ययः, न च प्रत्यक्षस्य माहात्म्यम्प्रमाणान्तरेणाभिभूयते, प्रमाणान्तरं च प्रत्यक्षबलेनैव व्यवहारं लभते। तस्मादेकमनेकार्थमवस्थितञ्च चित्तम् ॥ ३२ ॥

These distractions which are antagonistic to concentration can be checked by practice and renunciation mentioned before. Of these, the object of practice is summed up by this Sūtra which says that—

**For Their Stoppage (i.e. Of Distractions) Practice Of (Concentration on) A Single Principle Should Be Made. 32.**

For the elimination of distractions, the mind should be fixed on one principle (1) for purposes of practice. For those who hold that the mind (2) is nothing but one state limited to one object (A) and is without a substrate—only a momentary impression and thus transitory—, the mind will always be one-pointed, for then there cannot be a distracted or disturbed mind. But the mind becomes one-pointed only when it is withdrawn from various objects and set on only one object. For this reason it is to be held that it is not occupied with one object only (B). Again, those who hold that the mind becomes one-pointed through the continuous flow of discrete but similar ideas, would have to say that one-pointedness is a character of the flow of such ideas. But that also cannot be true, because in their own view the mind itself is momentary and how in that case can there be a flow (of one mind) ? If, on the other hand, it is held that one-pointedness is the characteristic of each component of a continuous flow of ideas,—flow whether of similar ideas or dissimilar ideas—then each component idea will be individually one-pointed. If that happens there will be no such thing as a distracted mind. Hence, the mind has to be regarded as one, as being occupied with many objects and as being a substrate of all modifications. Further, if ideas which are unrelated, distinct and totally different are born (C) without a common substrate, then how can one idea remember something cognised by another ? Also, how can the state which holds within it the impressions of past actions be different from the state which enjoys the fruits of action ? Howsoever the matter might be explained, it would be no better than an exemplification of the logic of Gomaya-pāyasa (3).

Moreover, if each idea of the mind is considered to be uniquely different from every other idea, then that would mean the repudiation of the feeling of one's own self (D). How that would happen is being explained. In cognitions like the following, 'The 'I' that saw is the 'I' which is touching it and the 'I' that touched is the 'I' that is seeing it',—although the sensations of touch and sight are different, the feeling of the 'I' persists in an identical form. How can this sense of personal identity have any identity with the differing sensations of touch and sight ? This self-same sense of ego is experienced by one through one's own feelings. The superiority of direct perception cannot be impugned by any other proof ; the other proofs gain acceptance only when supported by perception. Therefore mind is one, takes in many objects and is stable, *i.e.* is not a void (baseless) but a continuous entity.

(1) The phrase 'a single principle or reality' has been differently interpreted by different commentators. Vāchaspati Miśra says it refers to Īśvara, Vijñāna-bhikṣu says it refers to some gross principle, whereas Bhojarāja says it refers to a specially selected principle. In fact, there is no indication here in respect of the object of contemplation but only in respect of the quality of contemplation. Whatever might be the object contemplated upon—Īśvara or anything else—that should be taken up as the sole principle. God can be contemplated upon in various ways and gradually, *e.g.* when we sing hymns in praise of God, keeping in mind the meanings thereof, the mind wanders to different objects depicting the glory of God. Practising on one principle is not like that. When God is thought of as present within oneself, or as an idea contemplated upon, then that kind of concentrated attention is called the meditation on one principle. Such practice is opposed to fluctuations, and by it, the fluctuations of the mind are removed. The same rule applies to the contemplation of other principles.

For practice of one principle, Īśvara and I-sense are the best. 'I am the observer of all the modifications that are taking place every moment in the mind'—a recollection of such an 'I' as a support of contemplation is very soothing to the mind. This is what the Upaniṣads call the contemplation on I-sense.

If contemplation on God only had been intended, the author of the Sūtra would not have used the phrase 'one principle'. Further it has been said that through special devotion to God all obstacles are removed. Therefore, practice of contemplation on one principle is only a particular method. That which in the aggregate of all physical actions like breathing etc. gives rise to the recollection of one thought is called one principle. Such thought is best when it relates to God or to I-sense. It might relate to something else. As a matter of fact, when the object concentrated upon collectively becomes a sort of one idea in the mind, then that is adoption of one principle. By its practice the mind easily gets tranquil. When it is co-ordinated with inhalation and exhalation of breath, ordinary breathing turns into Yogic breathing and when that is mastered, one is not easily perturbed by afflictions. As it becomes a natural and pleasant support, it can remove sullenness. Further, as there is an underlying attempt to keep still, it decreases shakiness or restlessness of the body. In this way disturbance and its concomitants disappear and the mind becomes gradually tranquil.

(2) It is laid down that a disturbed mind should be made one-pointed. The commentator here controverts the opinion of those who hold that the mind is a momentary thing.

(A) Such people think that the mind comes into existence with a thought and disappears with it, and that it is only a state or a modification without any substratum and is wholly transitory.

(B) If the mind is transitory, there cannot be any justification for calling a mind disturbed, one-pointed, etc., because each mind is, on this view, separate and short-lived, and each must therefore be one-pointed as each mind has only one object to think upon.

(C) If the thoughts are separate and unconnected, the remembrancer or cogniser of one knowledge or action cannot be the same as of another. If it is urged that the latent impression of knowledge or action is retained and reappears in a subsequent thought then its existence in some form would be postulated which would be contrary to the basic proposition that mind comes into existence with a thought and disappears with it. Consequently, the Sāṁkhya view that knowledge is but the different states of the same basic entity, *viz.* the mind, appears to be correct.

(D) There is yet another argument in support of this view. 'The 'I' that saw is the 'I' that is touching' or 'The 'I' that touched is the 'I' that is seeing'—this sort of identifying perception reveals the identity of the knower 'I' in all the experiences.

(3) It is fallacious to hold that cow-dung and milk-pudding are the same, because both of them come from the same source, *viz.* a cow.

---

भाष्यम्—यस्येदं शास्त्रेण परिकर्म निर्दिश्यते तत्कथम् ?

मैत्रीकरुणामुदितोपेक्षाणां सुखदुःखपुण्यापुण्यविषयाणाम्भावनातश्चित्तप्रसादनम् ॥ ३३ ॥

तत्र सर्वप्राणिषु सुखसंभोगापन्नेषु मैत्रीं भावयेत्, दुःखितेषु करुणां, पुण्यात्मकेषु मुदिताम्, अपुण्यात्मकेषु उपेक्षाम्। एवमस्य भावयतः शुक्लो धर्म उपजायते, ततश्च चित्तं प्रसीदति प्रसन्नमेकाग्रं स्थितिपदं लभते ॥ ३३ ॥

The method of cleansing the mind prescribed in the Śāstras—what is it like ?

**The Mind Becomes Purified By The Cultivation Of Feelings Of Amity, Compassion, Goodwill And Indifference Respectively Towards Happy, Miserable, Virtuous And Sinful Creatures. 33.**

Of these, a spirit of friendliness should be entertained towards those who have experienced happiness, a spirit of compassion towards those who are in distress, a spirit of goodwill towards those who are treading the path of virtue and a spirit of (benevolent) indifference towards those who are steeped in vice (by overlooking their faults). This sort of thought gives rise to cleaner virtue and thus the mind becomes pure. A purified mind becoming one-pointed eventually attains serenity (1).

(1) We generally feel envious when we find people, in whom we are not interested or by whom our self-interest is jeopardised, to be happy; similarly a cruel delight is felt when we find an enemy to be unhappy or in distress. Reputation of a pious person of a different persuasion often

excites jealousy and displeasure. When a person in whom we are not interested is found to be leading a sinful life we feel sorry or angry or become cruel towards him. Such feelings of envy, cruel delight, malevolence or anger disturb the mind and prevent its attaining concentration. That is why if by cultivating feelings of amity etc., the mind can be kept pleasant and happy, free from any disturbing element, then it can become one-pointed and tranquil. When necessary the devotee should think of it in this way. First recall to mind the pleasure that you would feel when you find your friend to be happy. Then imagine that you would feel equally happy when you find your enemies and others happy, whose happiness you now envy. Similarly, when you delight at the distress of your enemies, remember how you would take compassion when your dear ones suffer and get into the habit of feeling equally compassionate towards your enemies. As you feel pleased with a person of your persuasion when he acts piously, you should feel equally happy when a person of a different persuasion behaves in a virtuous way. To overlook the lapses of others is indifference. It is not a positive thinking but restraining the mind from dwelling on the frailties of others. These four practices are called Brahmavihāra by the Buddhists and these, they say, lead to the Brahmaloka.

---

प्रच्छर्दनविधारणाभ्यां वा प्राणस्य ॥ ३४ ॥

भाष्यम्—कौष्ठ्यस्य वायोर्नासिकापुटाभ्यां प्रयत्नविशेषाद् वमनं प्रच्छर्दनम्, विधारणं प्राणायामः। ताभ्यां वा मनसः स्थितिं सम्पादयेत् ॥ ३४ ॥

**By Exhaling And Restraining The Breath Also (The Mind Is Calmed). 34.**

Exhaling or expulsion (1) is the ejection of the internal air through the apertures of the nose by a special kind of effort. Restraining or Prāṇāyāma is retention of the breath. The mind can also be calmed or stabilised by these methods.

(1) For calming the mind, it should be made to hold on to something. Therefore, practising breathing only without attempting to settle the mind, would never result in calmness. In fact, if Prāṇāyāma is

practised without Dhyāna (deep meditation) the mind instead of becoming calm would get more disturbed. That is why for every effort for control of breath, the mind should be made one-pointed with a particular thought with every inhalation. The Śāstras say that the breath should be attuned to a conception of the void. In other words, when exhaling, it should be supposed that the mind is vacant, has no thought in it. Exhalation with such thought calms the mind ; otherwise not. The effort with which breath is exhaled has three steps. First, the effort to exhale it slowly ; secondly, the effort to keep the body still and relaxed ; and thirdly, the effort to keep the mind vacant or without any thought. This is how the breath is to be exhaled. Then, to remain as far as possible in that vacant state of the mind is Prāṇāyāma. In this method there is no effort to take in the breath, which will take place naturally, but it should be watched that the mind continues to remain vacant at that time also.

That the ego is disentangling itself from the body and the 'feeling of self' in the core of the heart is moving on to the wordless, thoughtless state of concentrated 'OM'—this thought is possible only at the time of exhalation and not at the time of inhalation. That is why no reference to inhalation has been made in the Sūtra. In exhalation and retention of breath, the nerves of the body get relaxed and the mind gets into a sort of vacant, inactive state which is not possible at the time of inhalation. To practise this method, the breath should be exhaled with prolonged and appropriate effort. The whole body and the chest should be kept still and inhalation and exhalation should be done by the movement of abdominal muscles. When this is practised assiduously for some time, a happy feeling or feeling of lightness spreads all over the body. Further practice is to be continued with this feeling, and when that is mastered, retention need not be practised after each exhalation, but at intervals, which will not tire the devotee excessively. When the practice is advanced, gradually it might be easier to have retention after each exhalation.

The special feature of this practice is to arrive at a unification of exhalation and retention so that the two can be achieved in the same process, and no separate effort has to be made for each. At the time of exhalation the entire volume of internal air need not be ejected. When some air remains, the exhalation should be reduced and passed on to retention. Carefully mastering this, it should be watched that both the body and the mind remain still and in a vacant state, specially at the time of natural inhalation in none too fast a manner. When with practice, it can be continued for a long time without interruption, and can be done whenever wanted, then the mind gets settled without any fluctuation and this may lead to the state of concentration (Samādhi). With breathing, in one effort, a disturbed mind can be easily anchored to a particular place internally ; that is why it is one of the approved ways of achieving stability of the mind. This sort of Prāṇāyāma can be practised constantly, it is very suitable for attaining tranquillity.

———

विषयवती वा प्रवृत्तिरुत्पन्ना मनसः स्थितिनिबन्धनी ॥ ३५ ॥

भाष्यम्—नासिकाग्रे धारयतोऽस्य या दिव्यगन्धसंवित् सा गन्धप्रवृत्तिः, जिह्वाग्रे दिव्यरससंवित्, तालुनि रूपसंवित्, जिह्वामध्ये स्पर्शसंवित्, जिह्वामूले शब्दसंविदित्येताः प्रवृत्तय उत्पन्नाश्चित्तं स्थितौ निबध्नन्ति संशयं विधमन्ति समाधिप्रज्ञायां च द्वारीभवन्तीति। एतेन चन्द्रादित्यग्रहमणिप्रदीपरत्नादिषु प्रवृत्तिरुत्पन्ना विषयवत्येव वेदितव्या। यद्यपि हि तत्तच्छास्त्रानुमानाचार्योपदेशैरवगतमर्थतत्त्वं सद्भूतमेव भवति एतेषां यथाभूतार्थप्रतिपादनसामर्थ्यात्तथापि यावदेकदेशोऽपि कश्चिन्न स्वकरणसंवेद्यो भवति तावत्सर्वं परोक्षमिवापवर्गादिषु सूक्ष्मेष्वर्थेषु न दृढां बुद्धिमुत्पादयति। तस्माच्छास्त्रानुमानाचार्योपदेशोपोद्बलनार्थमेवावश्यं कश्चिद्विशेषः प्रत्यक्षीकर्त्तव्यः। तत्र तदुपदिष्टार्थैकदेशस्य प्रत्यक्षत्वे सति सर्वं सुसूक्ष्मविषयमपि आ अपवर्गात् सुश्रद्धीयते एतदर्थमेवेदं चित्तपरिकर्म निर्दिश्यते। अनियतासु वृत्तिषु तद्विषयायां वशीकारसंज्ञायामुपजातायां चित्तं समर्थं स्यात्तस्य तस्यार्थस्य प्रत्यक्षीकरणायेति तथा च सति श्रद्धावीर्यस्मृतिसमाधयोऽस्याप्रतिबन्धेन भविष्यन्तीति ॥ ३५ ॥

**The Development Of Higher Objective Perceptions Called Viṣayavatī (1) Also Brings About Tranquillity Of Mind. 35.**

The subtle perception of smell which one gets when concentrating on the tip of the nose is the higher smell-perception. Similarly, concentration on the tip of the tongue gives supersensuous taste, that on the palate supersensuous colour, that on the tongue supersensuous touch and that at the root of the tongue supersensuous sound. The awakening of these higher perceptions stabilises the mind firmly, removes doubts and forms the gateway to knowledge acquirable through concentration. Such perceptions of the sun, the moon, the planets, jewels, or lamps etc. are also regarded as objective perceptions. The Śāstras, inference and verbal instructions of preceptors can no doubt produce veridical knowledge of things, yet until by the foregoing method an object is brought within the purview of one's own perception such knowledge would remain an indirect knowledge, and not helpful in producing firm conviction in respect of subtle things like the state of salvation, etc. That is why, for the removal of doubts in respect of instructions and knowledge acquired from teachers or the Śāstras, or by inference, some specific feature of the object must be definitely perceived. If a part of the knowledge acquired from the Śāstras is proved to be true by direct perception, then faith is developed in subtle matters like salvation, and that is why such training for purifying the mind has been prescribed. In the midst of unsettled modifications of the mind such special knowledge of smell, sound, etc. arising in the above-mentioned manner and Vaśīkāra-saṁjñā, *i.e.* complete renunciation arising therefrom, the mind becomes capable of having a complete realisation of such matters. When that happens, faith, energy, remembrance and concentration come to the mind without any interruption.

(1) The term Viṣayavatī or 'relating to objects' refers to objects of the senses. 'Higher sense-perception' indicates such modification of the mind as would produce perception of the supersensuous aspects of the objects of the senses. If the mind is fixed on the tip of the nose, a strange novel perfume pervades the air breathed, and this can be experienced easily.

The optic nerve is situated above the palate. On the tongue the sense of touch is most developed. The root of the tongue is closely related to the ear for purposes of articulation. Therefore, concentration on these points develops a finer power of perception of the sense-organs. When the eyes are shut after looking intently at the moon or the stars for some time, their image continues in the mind. Contemplating on that, higher perception thereof is produced, because these are included in the category of colour, etc. This kind of supersensuous power is called Kasin by the Buddhists

Unless such contemplation is practised continuously for a day or two, its effects are not realised. Practising this by slow degrees for some time before practising it more intensely in a state of fasting or on meagre diet at a place where there are no interruptions and with no other thought, by holding the mind concentrated on the tip of the nose, etc. the higher sense-perception is developed. That this sort of realisation induces deep faith in Yoga and a renunciation of earthly sounds, etc. has been clearly explained by the commentator.

———

विशोका वा ज्योतिष्मती ॥ ३६ ॥

भाष्यम्—प्रवृत्तिरुत्पन्ना मनसः स्थितिनिबन्धनीत्यनुवर्त्तते। हृदयपुण्डरीके धारयतो या बुद्धिसंविद् बुद्धिसत्त्वं हि भास्वरमाकाशकल्पं तत्र स्थितिवैशारद्यात् प्रवृत्तिः सूर्येन्दुग्रहमणिप्रभारूपाकारेण विकल्पते, तथाऽस्मितायां समापन्नं चित्तं निस्तरङ्ग-महोदधिकल्पं शान्तमनन्तमस्मितामात्रं भवति, यत्रेदमुक्तम् 'तमणुमात्रमात्मानमनुविद्याऽस्मीत्येवन्तावत्सम्प्रजानीते' इति। एषा द्वयी विशोका, विषयवती अस्मितामात्रा च प्रवृत्तिर्ज्योतिष्मतीत्युच्यते, यया योगिनश्चित्तं स्थितिपदं लभत इति ॥ ३६ ॥

**Or By Perception Which Is Free From Sorrow And Is Radiant** (1) **(Stability Of Mind Can Also Be Produced). 36.**

The words within brackets above are implied in this Sūtra. Contemplation practised on the innermost core of the heart brings about knowledge of Buddhi. That Buddhi is resplendent and is like the Ākāśa (or boundless void). Proficiency in being able to stay long in that contemplation develops perception in that direction whereby Buddhi is perceived as resembling effulgent sun, moon, planet or as a luminous jewel. Similarly, the mind engrossed in the thought of pure I-sense (2) appears like a waveless ocean, placid and limitless, which is pure I-sense all over. It has been said in this connection : "By the reflective meditation on the self or self in its pure atomic form, there arises the pure knowledge of 'I am'." This higher perception named Viśokā is twofold, one relating to objects, the other relating to pure I-sense. These are called Jyotiṣmatī (effulgent) and through them the mind of the Yogin attains stability.

(1) This experience is described as free from sorrow because when a very pleasant Sāttvika feeling is acquired, the mind always remains immersed in it. And it is described as radiant or effulgent because on account of Sāttvika enlightenment there is abundance of the light of knowledge. The light referred to here is not the optical light but the fine illumination of knowledge which manifests things that are subtle, covered from view or situated at a distance.

(2) The method of gradually reaching the contemplation of Buddhisattva or pure I-sense is first to imagine in the 'lotus', *i.e.* core of the heart, called the abode of Brahman, the presence of a limitless uninterrupted expanse of clear effulgence like the sky. Pure I-sense is not an object to be cognised (Grāhya) but is an instrument of cognition (Grahaṇa) ; that is why only thinking of the luminous sky does not bring about the contemplation of Buddhisattva. Conception of the instrument of reception (Grahaṇa) is mingled in the initial stage with a hazy idea of the cognisable object (Grāhya) and commonly, the effulgence in the heart remains objectively present in the contemplation of pure I-sense. Until the mind gets fully fixed on Grahaṇa, it goes on oscillating between the light and pure I-sense. This effulgence is therefore called the conceptual representation of pure I-sense. The Upaniṣad says that its size is that of a thumb (*i.e.* minute) and its appearance is like that of the sun. In the Śvetāśvatara Upaniṣad we have : "Brahma reveals himself in Yoga to one who first contemplates on an effulgence like that of the mist, smoke, sun, air, fire, fire-fly, lightning, crystal or moon."

Like contemplation on a visual form, contemplation on ideas of touch, taste, etc. might also be suggestive of the meditation on I-sense. In such a case the pleasant feeling of touch, etc. in the core of the heart might be adopted for leading on to the 'I' who is the knower of that pleasant feeling. That contemplation can be conducted in the following manner :

First imagine in your heart a limitless, sky-like or transparent effulgence ; then think that the self is within that, *i.e.* 'I am spread all over it.'

Such thought brings ineffable bliss. The transparent, radiant sense of ego radiating from the heart to infinity is called Viśokā Jyotiṣmatī or effulgent light free from sorrow. It is not pure I-sense but only a modification thereof. Pure I-sense is only Grahaṇa, but this sort of 'cognition of I' is not wholly so. Subtle things are revealed by it. Yogins focus this inner light emanating from the heart on the object which they want to know. Therefore in this kind of meditation, pure reception is not the principal thing but the particular object received. In the highest perception free from sorrow relating to pure I-sense, the principal thing is Grahaṇa ; it is the engrossment in pure I-sense. When the method of objective contemplation relating to self is mastered, contemplation on I-sense alone excluding the objects in which 'I' had been supposed to be present has to be practised which will bring about a realisation of pure I-sense. In this way the idea of space is eliminated and only the idea of the cogniser of space—pure I-sense—remains, *i.e.* the Sāttvika faculty of sentience in a current of time becomes manifest, because then there is very little sense-activity but only the state of sentience.

There is another way of arriving at pure I-sense. The centre of the I-sense pertaining to the body and all the organs is the heart. Concentrating on the heart, suspending all movements of the body, the feeling of serenity felt all over the body should be contemplated upon. When such contemplation is mastered, the sensation referred to is found to be very pleasant. The cessation of the activities of all the organs results in an unspecified pleasant state. This unspecified sensation is the undiversified sixth sense, *viz.* I-sense, Asmitā. One can realise pure I-sense by concentrating on this ego or Asmitā. It should be remembered that the awareness of one's own self is called Asmitā.

Both the methods really lead to the stabilisation of the mind on the same object. What that Asmitā-mātra or pure I-sense is, has been explained by the commentator by quoting the words of the sage Pañchaśikha. Pure I-sense can be called infinite from another point of view. Pure I-sense being the final stage of cognition in respect of reception is the illuminer of all objects. That is why it is infinite or all-pervading. As a matter of fact after contemplating this concept of infinity one has to go to the cogniser of that infinite conception, *viz.* pure I-sense.

Unless the exact nature of the contemplation on Asmitā is understood it is not possible to comprehend what the state of salvation is. That is why here it has been gone into in some detail. Practising this method of contemplation, each according to his capacity, the mind becomes tranquil. And having thus attained one-pointedness, Samprajñāta and Asamprajñāta Yogas are mastered.

In Sūtra I.17 the contemplation on the principle of I-sense has been described. In this Sūtra the stabilisation of the mind with the help of the awareness of Asmitā in the form of radiance or the infinite sky or space has been spoken of.

———

वीतरागविषयं वा चित्तम् ॥ ३७ ॥

भाष्यम्—वीतरागचित्तालम्बनोपरक्तं वा योगिनश्चित्तं स्थितिपदं लभत इति ॥ ३७ ॥

**Or (Contemplating) On A Mind Which Is Free From Desires (The Devotee's Mind Gets Stabilised). 37.**

If a Yogin meditates on a passionless mind he also attains stability of mind (1).

(1) A mind full of passion or desires finds it easy to think of objects but finds it difficult to get into a carefree self-centred state, whereas a mind free from passion finds it easy to be unattached and free. Fully realising what that state is, if the mind is set thinking on it and the habit is assiduously cultivated then the mind gradually becomes tranquil.

If contact is established with a saint, free from desires, his carefree, non-desiring mien will give an idea of what the attitude of desirelessness is. Further, imagining the mind of Hiraṇyagarbha and others free from desires, if one's mind is set on its contemplation then the result will be the same.

If one's own mind can be freed from desires, and thus free from thought, and if that state of the mind can be mastered by practice, then also the mind becomes free from attachment to objects. This is really practising detachment.

———

स्वप्ननिद्राज्ञानालम्बनं वा ॥ ३८ ॥

भाष्यम्—स्वप्नज्ञानालम्बनन्निद्राज्ञानालम्बनं वा तदाकारं योगिनश्चित्तं स्थितिपदं लभत इति ॥ ३८ ॥

**Or By Taking As The Object Of Meditation The Images Of Dreams Or The State Of Dreamless Sleep (The Mind Of The Yogin Gets Stabilised). 38.**

The Yogin who adopts for purposes of contemplation the images of dreams or the state of dreamless sleep can also get stability of mind (1).

(1) In dream, external knowledge is shut out and the ideas in the mind appear as vivid. To adopt these vivified ideas and contemplating on them, is contemplating on the images of dream. This may be very suitable for people with a certain disposition. This can be done in three ways : (*i*) To form a mental image of the object contemplated upon and to think of it as real ; (*ii*) when recolletion is practised, then even in a dream one will be aware that he is dreaming. Then the desired object should be properly contemplated upon and on awakening and at other times effort should be made to maintain that state ; (*iii*) when any good feeling or idea is felt in a dream, then immediately on awakening and thereafter that feeling should be contemplated upon. In every case a dreamlike state of shutting out the external objects should be adopted.

In dream, external cognition is shut out but mental images continue to be cognised. In deep dreamless sleep, however, both external and mental objects are obscured by Tāmasa feeling and a hazy idea of inactivity remains. Taking that inactive feeling as the object of contemplation this method is practised.

———

यथाभिमतध्यानाद्वा ॥ ३९ ॥

भाष्यम्—यदेवाभिमतं तदेव ध्यायेत्तत्र लब्धस्थितिकमन्यत्रापि स्थितिपदं लभत इति ॥ ३९ ॥

**Or By Contemplating On Whatsoever Thing One May Like (The Mind Becomes Stable). 39.**

Whatever is considered suitable (no doubt for purposes of Yoga) can be contemplated upon. If one can get the mind stabilised there, one can get stability elsewhere also (1).

(1) Such is the habit of the mind that if it can be stabilised for some length of time on any particular thing, it can be stabilised on other things also. If one can at will concentrate for an hour on a pot he can concentrate on a hillock for an hour also. Therefore on attaining stability of mind by practising meditation on any selected object, one can get engrossed in the Tattvas and gradually through their knowledge attain Kaivalya.

———

परमाणुपरममहत्त्वान्तोऽस्य वशीकारः ।। ४० ।।

भाष्यम्—सूक्ष्मे निविशमानस्य परमाण्वन्तं स्थितिपदं लभत इति स्थूले निविशमानस्य परममहत्त्वान्तं स्थितिपदं चित्तस्य। एवं तामुभयों कोटिमनुधावतो योऽस्याऽप्रतिघातः स परो वशीकारस्तद्वशीकारात्परिपूर्णं योगिनश्चित्तं न पुनरभ्यासकृतं परिकर्मापेक्षत इति ।। ४० ।।

**When The Mind Develops The Power Of Stabilising On The Smallest Size As Well As On The Greatest One, Then The Mind Comes Under Control. 40.**

Contemplating on subtle things the mind can attain stability on the minutest. Similarly, contemplating on the quality of greatness it can stabilise on the infinitely great which is limitless. Meditating between the two extremes, the mind acquires unimpeded power of holding on to whatsoever object it desires. This would be complete mastery over the mind. With that, the mind attains perfection and there is no further need for acquiring stability, nor is there any other call for purification by practice (1).

(1) Tanmātra is the minute atom or monad of gross elements like sound etc. It is the subtlest state of such gross matters. The sense-faculty and the power of cognising the Tanmātra are also subtle states.

Practising retention on any partcular object, if the stabilised mind can be held on to any minute or great object, that state is called Vaśīkāra or complete mastery. When the mind is brought under control, the process of contemplation on any particular object is completed. There remains then only the attainment of Asamprajñāta concentration by practising the shutting out of all mental fluctuations. How mastery of the mind can be acquired has been described in the following Sūtra. This is done by the realisation of the minutest state and the highest state of the receiver, the instrument of reception and the object apprehended and being engrossed therein. With this in view the characteristics of Samāpatti or engrossment (true and balanced insight of a one-pointed mind) are now being mentioned.

———

भाष्यम्—अथ लब्धस्थितिकस्य चेतसः किंस्वरूपा किंविषया वा समापत्तिरिति? तदुच्यते—

क्षीणवृत्तेरभिजातस्येव मणेर्ग्रहीतृग्रहणग्राह्येषु तत्स्थतदञ्जनता समापत्तिः ॥ ४१ ॥

क्षीणवृत्तेरिति प्रत्यस्तमितप्रत्ययस्येत्यर्थः। अभिजातस्येव मणेरिति दृष्टान्तोपादानम्। यथा स्फटिक उपाश्रयभेदात्तत्तद्रूपोपरक्त उपाश्रयरूपाकारेण निर्भासते, तथा ग्राह्यालम्बनोपरक्तं चित्तं ग्राह्यसमापन्नं ग्राह्यस्वरूपाकारेण निर्भासते, भूतसूक्ष्मोपरक्तं भूतसूक्ष्मसमापन्नं भूतसूक्ष्मस्वरूपाभासं भवति, तथा स्थूलालम्बनोपरक्तं स्थूलरूपसमापन्नं स्थूलरूपाभासं भवति, तथा विश्वभेदोपरक्तं विश्वभेदसमापन्नं विश्वरूपाभासं भवति। तथा ग्रहणेष्वपि इन्द्रियेष्वपि द्रष्टव्यम्। ग्रहणालम्बनोपरक्तं ग्रहणसमापन्नं ग्रहणस्वरूपाकारेण निर्भासते। तथा ग्रहीतृपुरुषालम्बनोपरक्तं ग्रहीतृपुरुषसमापन्नं ग्रहीतृपुरुषस्वरूपाकारेण निर्भासते। तथा मुक्तपुरुषालम्बनोपरक्तं मुक्तपुरुषसमापन्नं मुक्तपुरुषस्वरूपाकारेण निर्भासते। तदेवमभिजातमणिकल्पस्य चेतसो ग्रहीतृग्रहणग्राह्येषु पुरुषेन्द्रियभूतेषु या तत्स्थतदञ्जनता तेषु स्थितस्य तदाकारापत्तिः सा समापत्तिरित्युच्यते ॥ ४१ ॥

What the nature of engrossment of a stabilised (1) mind is and in what objects it is engrossed are being described.

**When The Fluctuations Of The Mind Are Weakened The Mind Appears To Take On The Features Of The Object Of Meditation—Whether It Be The Cogniser (Grahītā), The Instrument Of Cognition (Grahaṇa) Or The Object Cognised (Grāhya)—As Does A Transparent Jewel, And This Identification Is Called Samāpatti Or Engrossment (2). 41.**

'Weakened fluctuation' refers to the state of the mind when all modifications but one have disappeared therefrom. The case of a precious (flawless) gem has been taken as an example. As a transparent crystal influenced by the colour of an adjacent article appears to be tinged by it, so the mind resting on an object, and engrossed in it, appears to take on its nature (3). A mind set on subtle elements and being engrossed in them is coloured by the nature of such subtle elements, while a mind absorbed in gross elements is coloured by their gross nature. Similarly, the mind occupied with the infinite variety in external objects gets engrossed in such variety and becomes the reflector thereof. The same holds good in respect of the instruments of reception, *viz.* the organs of one's body. When the mind concentrates on the instruments of reception, it becomes occupied and tinged by them. When the mind is set thinking exclusively of the cogniser, it becomes engrossed in it and gets tinged with the nature of the cogniser—Grahītā. Likewise when the mind is occupied with the thought of a liberated soul, the mind displays the nature of such a soul. This sort of resting of the mind in and its shaping after the receiver, the instrument of reception and the object received, *viz.* the Grahītā (empiric self), the senses, and the elements, like a reflecting crystal, is called Samāpatti or engrossment.

(1) Set mind = one-pointed mind. When by practising Īśvara-praṇidhāna etc. the mind gets habituated in resting tranquilly on the desired object, it is said to be settled. The concentration attained in a habitually one-pointed mind is called engrossment or Samāpatti. That is how Samāpatti differs from simple concentration. The knowledge

acquired in such a state of engrossment is Samprajñāna or complete knowledge or Samprājñāta-yoga or concentration which gives complete and sustained knowledge. Buddhists also use the word 'Samāpatti' but in a different sense.

(2) The author has described in these Sūtras all possible types of engrossed mind.

Engrossment may be of three kinds according to the nature of objects contemplated upon—relating to the cogniser, relating to the instruments of cognition and relating to objects cognised. There is also difference due to the nature of the engrossment. Yogins, however, take the two together to avoid multiplicity and divide them into Savitarka, Nirvitarka, Savichāra and Nirvichāra. Their difference is shown in the table given below :—

| Nature of engrossment | Nature of the object | Name of engrossment or Samāpatti |
|---|---|---|
| (1) Mixed up with word, its meaning *i.e.* the object and its cognition. | Gross (Grāhya *i.e.* knowables and Grahaṇa *i.e.* instruments of cognition) | Savitarkā (concentration on gross objects with the help of words) |
| (2) DITTO. | Subtle (Grāhya, Grahaṇa and Grahītā *i.e.* the cogniser) | Savichārā (concentration on subtle objects with the help of words) |
| (3) In a purified mind free of words and forgetful of its own self, as it were, only the object by itself is present. | Gross (Grāhya and Grahaṇa) | Nirvitarkā (concentration on gross objects without the help of words) |
| (4) DITTO. | Subtle (Grāhya, Grahaṇa and Grahītā) | Nirvichārā (concentration on subtle objects without the help of words, on bliss, and on pure I-sense) |

Vitarka and Vichāra and matters relating thereto have been dealt with before. Now Nirvitarka will be dealt with. All sorts of Dhyāna, *i.e.* meditation which can be done by a mind which has not been arrested entirely will fall within one or the other of the engrossments mentioned in the table above, because there is nothing other than an object, instrument of cognition and the cogniser that can be contemplated.

(3) Samāpatti, *i.e.* the habituated state of engrossment of mind on the object contemplated upon through force of practice, has been fully explained by the author of the Sūtra as well as by the commentator. The latter has given examples of Samāpatti. Engrossment in respect of objects are of three kinds :—

(*i*) Those relating to worldly things—countless material objects like animals, pots, etc., (*ii*) those relating to the five gross elements and (*iii*) those relating to the five subtle elements, *viz.* sound-tanmātra, colour-tanmātra, etc. Engrossment or Samāpatti relating to instruments of cognition appertains both to the external and to the internal organs. Of these, the external organs are threefold—organs of perception, organs of action and the Prāṇas or vital forces. The internal organ, *viz.* the part of the mind which is the instrument of conation is the master of the external organs. All these are the mutations of the three principal internal organs, *viz.* Buddhi (pure I-sense), Ahaṁkāra (mutative ego) and the part of the mind which is the repository of latencies.

Engrossment relating to the cogniser = aforesaid contemplation on pure I-sense. It has been said before, that in Savīja-samādhi or concentration on an object when it relates to the cogniser, that cogniser is not the Puruṣa principle but is the empiric self (*i.e.* Buddhi) which is identified with the Self. That is why it is the assumed or empirical seer. Until the mind and all the organs completely cease to function, the state of resting in Puruṣa cannot be attained. So long as the mind continues to be affected by its modifications there would, therefore, be the impure, empirical seer. 'I am the cogniser of knowledge'—this feeling is its true character. When cognition ceases completely, the Knower of that quiescent state who remains in his own self is Puruṣa, or the real Seer.

Apart from these, Īśvara-samāpatti or engrossment in God, engrossment in a liberated soul, etc. which might be possible, come under the three kinds of engrossment, relating to the cogniser, organs of cognition and the object cognised. The image of God, mind or I-sense, etc. which is adopted as the object for contemplation for purposes of engrossment will fall within the appropriate category enumerated above.

———

भाष्यम्—तत्र—

शब्दार्थज्ञानविकल्पैः सङ्कीर्णा सवितर्का समापत्तिः ॥ ४२ ॥

तद्यथा गौरिति शब्दो गौरित्यर्थो गौरिति ज्ञानमित्यविभागेन विभक्तानामपि ग्रहणं दृष्टम्। विभज्यमानाश्चान्ये शब्दधर्मा अन्ये अर्थधर्मा अन्ये विज्ञानधर्मा इत्येतेषां विभक्तः पन्थाः। तत्र समापन्नस्य योगिनो यो गवाद्यर्थः समाधिप्रज्ञायां समारूढः स चेच्छब्दार्थज्ञानविकल्पानुविद्ध उपावर्त्तते सा सङ्कीर्णा समापत्तिः सवितर्केत्युच्यते ॥ ४२ ॥

Of them,

**The Engrossment, In Which There Is The Mixture Of Word, Its Meaning (i.e. The Object) And Its Knowledge, Is Known As Savitarkā Samāpatti (1). 42.**

To explain, the word 'cow', the object indicated by the word 'cow', the mental impression created by the word 'cow' implying its form, various uses, etc., although these are different, are generally taken together. When differentiated, the features of word, the object meant and ideation become distinct. When in the mind of a Yogin engrossed in the thought of a cow, there is the mingling of the word (cow), the object meant (the animal itself) and the idea of the cow, it is called Savitarkā Samāpatti.

(1) Engrossment and knowledge are inseparable. That is why the knowledge acquired in a particular state of concentration is called Savitarkā Samāpatti. The word 'Tarka' was used in ancient times in the sense of thought with the help of words. Vitarka is, therefore, a particular kind of Tarka. When in the knowledge acquired in Samādhi there is Vitarka it is called Savitarka-samādhi.

Tarka or thought with the help of words, when analysed, will show a mingling of words, the objects and the ideas produced thereby. Take the word or name 'cow'. The object is a quadruped animal. The idea about the animal takes place within us. It is not the same as the animal; neither has the name any identity with the knowledge about the cow nor with the animal itself, because any name might indicate an animal with such properties. Therefore, the three factors—the name, the object indicated and the knowlege thereof—are entirely distinct. But generally the name, the object indicated and the mental picture of the object are identified with the knowledge of the object also. Therefore, in spite of the fact that there is no identity of the three factors, the confused idea of their sameness that follows the utterance of the name is called Vikalpa. Thus our ordinary thought is about the word, the object and the idea—all mixed up. Since in this process an unavoidable error in the shape of Vikalpa is present, it is imperfect cognition and is, therefore, not the higher and true Yogic perception.

It is, however, through this process that the Yogin's knowledge is gained initially. As a matter of fact the Yogic knowledge derived through meditation with the help of words is Savitarkā Samāpatti.

The author of the Sūtra has analysed this Samāpatti to indicate its difference from Nirvitarkā Samāpatti described later. When Savitarkā Samāpatti is practised in respect of 'cow', all knowledge regarding the cow will be obtained and it will come with the help of words, *e.g.* whose cow, what sort of a cow, etc. etc.

Of course, Yogins do not direct their contemplation to the acquisition of knowledge in respect of ordinary objects such as a cow. The main purpose of engrossment is to gain knowledge of Tattvas, through which detachment is developed, leading gradually to the attainment of liberation.

———

भाष्यम्—यदा पुनः शब्दसंकेतस्मृतिपरिशुद्धौ श्रुतानुमानज्ञानविकल्पशून्यायां समाधिप्रज्ञायां स्वरूपमात्रेणावस्थितोऽर्थस्तत्स्वरूपाकारमात्रतयैव अवच्छिद्यते सा च निर्वितर्का समापत्तिः। तत् परं प्रत्यक्षं तच्च श्रुतानुमानयोर्वीजं, ततः श्रुतानुमाने प्रभवतः। न च श्रुतानुमानज्ञानसहभूतं तद्दर्शनं तस्मादसङ्कीर्णं प्रमाणान्तरेण योगिनो निर्वितर्कसमाधिजं दर्शनमिति। निर्वितर्कायाः समापत्तेरस्याः सूत्रेण लक्षणं द्योत्यते।

स्मृतिपरिशुद्धौ स्वरूपशून्येवार्थमात्रनिर्भासा निर्वितर्का ॥ ४३ ॥

या शब्दसंकेतश्रुतानुमानज्ञानविकल्पस्मृतिपरिशुद्धौ ग्राह्यस्वरूपोपरक्ता प्रज्ञा स्वमिव प्रज्ञारूपं ग्रहणात्मकं त्यक्त्वा पदार्थमात्रस्वरूपा ग्राह्यस्वरूपापन्नेव भवति सा निर्वितर्का समापत्तिः। तथा च व्याख्याता। तस्या एकबुद्ध्युपक्रमो ह्यर्थात्मा अणुप्रचयविशेषात्मा गवादिर्घटादिर्वा लोकः। स च संस्थानविशेषो भूतसूक्ष्माणां साधारणो धर्म आत्मभूतः, फलेन व्यक्तेनानुमितः, स्वव्यञ्जकाञ्जनः प्रादुर्भवति,

धर्मान्तरोदये च तिरोभवति, स एष धर्मोऽवयवीत्युच्यते, योऽसावेकश्च महांश्चाणीयांश्च स्पर्शवांश्च क्रियाधर्मकश्चानित्यश्च, तेनावयविना व्यवहाराः क्रियन्ते ।

यस्य पुनरवस्तुकः स प्रचयविशेषः, सूक्ष्मं च कारणमनुपलभ्यमविकल्पस्य, तस्यावयव्यभावादतद्रूपप्रतिष्ठं मिथ्याज्ञानमिति प्रायेण सर्वमेव प्राप्तं मिथ्याज्ञानमिति, तदा च सम्यग्ज्ञानमपि किं स्याद् विषयाभावाद्; यद् यदुपलभ्यते तत्तदवयवित्वेनाघ्रातं (आम्नातं) तस्मादस्त्यवयवी यो महत्त्वादिव्यवहारापन्नः समापत्तेर्निर्वितर्काया विषयो भवति ॥ ४३ ॥

When, however, the memory (1) of the conventional meaning of words disappears, the knowledge gained through Samādhi becomes free of Vikalpa contained in the ideas formed through verbal instruction or inference. The true nature of the object contemplated upon is then revealed and this state is called Nirvitarkā Samāpatti or engrossment free from verbal thinking. It is the truest perception* and is the root of inference and testimony which are derived from it (2). That perception does not arise from testimony or from inference. Consequently, the knowledge acquired by a Yogin in a state of Nirvitarka-samādhi is uninfluenced by any other mode of cognition than direct perception. The feature of this kind of engrossment is being given in the Sūtra.

**When The Memory Is Purified, The Mind Appears To Be Devoid Of Its Own Nature (i.e. Of Reflective Consciousness) And Only The Object (3) (On Which It Is Contemplating) Remains Illuminated. This Kind Of Engrossment Is Called Nirvitarkā Samāpatti. 43.**

When the memory of the conventional meaning of words and the knowledge derived from inference and testimony cease, the ensuing cognition seems to lose its nature as cognition and becomes, as it were, of the nature of the object. This is called Nirvitarkā Samāpatti. This has been explained (in the introduction to the Sūtra). The object contemplated

---

* Perception, inference and testimony constitute the Pramāṇas (vide Sūtra I.7).

upon in Nirvitarkā Samāpatti is cognised as a single unit, as an object which is real, and as an assemblage of particular atoms (4). Such assemblage (5) of all the constituent atoms represents their common characteristics and is inferred from the feel and the use of the manifested gross state. It appears in dependence on its causes. When a change in the characteristics takes place, the particular assemblage also disappears. Such assemblage of characteristics is called the 'whole', which is one, large or small, tangible, mutative and transitory, which render it usable in practical life.

Those who hold that the assemblage is not real and that its subtle components are also not perceivable in Nirvichāra-samādhi will have to conclude that in the absence of a 'whole', the cognition of an object is erroneous because it does not correspond to reality. In this way almost all cognitions will become erroneous. What then will be the fate of valid knowledge when there cannot be anything for its object ? For whatever is knowable by the senses is pronounced to be a 'whole'. For these reasons it has to be concluded that there is a 'whole' which is usable as large, small, etc. and which forms the object of Nirvitarkā Samāpatti.

(1) If the distinction between Savitarka knowledge and Nirvitarka knowledge is understood first, then it will be easy to follow the commentary. Generally, with the mention of a name the object denoted by it is remembered, and with the remembrance of the object the name (either generic or individual) is also remembered. In other words, a name and the object indicated by it are thought of together, inseparably. But the name and the object are two different entities. It is only through conventional usage and the latent impression thereof that the blending takes place in memory. By practice one may think of an object without its denotative name and thus the mixing of an object with its name may be avoided. This is what is called 'purifying' the mind of the memory of words and their objects, mixed together. It is not very difficult to realise this.

Such knowledge without the use of words is the real knowledge of a thing, because with the help of words we regard many non-existing things as existing. Take, for example, the expression 'Time is beginningless and endless.' This is taken as true. But 'beginningless' and 'endless' are negative conceptions. There is no possibility of directly perceiving them. Time, again, is merely of the nature of a container. 'Beginningless', 'endless', 'time' and other similar words give rise to merely verbal delusions but there is really no existing thing behind them which can be perceived. Thus knowledge based on words is in many instances delusive. Such knowledge is not Ṛta (a perceptual fact) but only a shadow of Satya (a conceptual fact). Knowledge from testimony and inference are cognitions with the help of words ; therefore, truths established by them are not always realisable facts. For example, from the sayings of the sages and inference it is established that 'Brahman is real, is of the nature of Consciousness and is infinite.' 'Real' means existing in fact. No mental or sense-conception can be formed from such words as 'real', 'infinite', etc. So except the words themselves there is nothing in 'reality' or 'infinity', which can be established by sense-perception or be realised by meditation. As a matter of fact, those predicating words have no connection with Brahman, nor do they help one in realising Him.

Therefore, the knowledge that is derived from inference, testimony and ordinary direct perception and which is mixed with words, is not pure, unalloyed Ṛta free of Vikalpa. But Nirvitarka knowledge, ***i.e.*** knowledge gained without the help of words and taking on the form of the object itself is Ṛta, truly perceptual fact.

(2) Both Nirvitarka and Nirvichāra are knowledge of the same kind. Ṛṣis who realised the highest truths, having acquired them through such knowledge, communicated them to others with the help of words and that is how spiritual truths and principles have been enunciated in the Śāstras dealing with salvation which have come down to us.

(3) Mind devoid of reflective consciousness = Forgetting even that 'I am knowing'. Svarūpa = Sva and Rūpa. Sva = The instrument that is knowing (which is the sentient principle), and its Rūpa or nature. In other words, when on account of intense concentration on the object to be known, the notion 'I am the knower' or 'I am knowing' seems to be effaced, the knowledge revealing the object only, almost free from any reflection, is obtained.

When knowledge is acquired with the help of words etc., the impressions of the actions of other senses and instruments of cognition remain and prevent the complete effacement of reflective consciousness of self.

It might be urged that as Samādhi has been defined as 'the state that shines with the light of the object alone and is devoid, as it were, of consciousness of self,' is not Savitarkā Samāpatti then Samādhi? No, Savitarkā Samāpatti is not merely Samādhi, it is also the state of retention of the knowledge acquired in Samādhi. Although in Samādhi there is no apparent knowledge of self, the knowledge of the object that is acquired may be with the help of words. In fact, when the mind is full of such knowledge assisted by words, that state is called Savitarkā Samāpatti. When the state of knowledge appears to be free from reflective consciousness, like the state in Samādhi devoid of the use of words, a collection of its latent impressions fills the mind and this is called Nirvitarkā Samāpatti. Thus the state of retention of impressions collected during concentration is Nirvitarkā Samāpatti and the recollection of such impressions with the help of words is Savitarkā Samāpatti.

Even when words are uttered, it might be Nirvitarka or Nirvichāra Dhyāna (meditation) free of Vikalpa, as for example, when the meaning of the words is not noticed but the words are uttered mechanically and conceived as sound only. Or, when the attention is given only to the effort made in uttering the word, it can be Dhyāna (meditation) of a knowable object without any Vikalpa. And if it is directed only to the cogniser or the instruments of cognition, then also it will be meditation without any Vikalpa even when uttering words.

(4) The knowledge of the gross object on which Nirvitarkā Samāpatti is attained is the highest truth in respect of that object. No gross object can be cognised better, because in that state all the senses are at rest and there is no Vikalpa.

'Cognition of an object as a single unit' means that the object is cognised as one. Although an object is the sum total of many components yet it is conceived as one. 'Separate entity' indicates that it is recognised as having a separate existence of its own. 'Assemblage or collection of particular atoms' implies that one object has a distinctive conglomeration of atoms, which can only be discovered by Nirvitarka concentration.

(5) 'Assemblage' is a particular combination of the constituent atoms peculiar to the object. For example, a pot is nothing more than the assemblage of particular atoms or monads of sound, colour, etc. comprising it and it follows that those atoms, *i.e.* the properties that are present in the atoms are present in the pot itself.

Therefore the substance 'pot' can be characterised as one, big or small, of tactile property, an object of the senses, liable to mutation and therefore not perpetual, *i.e.* liable to appearance or disappearance. All gross objects with characteristics as stated above are constantly being used by us, and they can form the object of Nirvitarkā Samāpatti. The highest knowledge about them is obtained through Nirvitarka engrossment.

---

एतयैव सविचारा निर्विचारा च सूक्ष्मविषया व्याख्याता ॥ ४४ ॥

भाष्यम्—तत्र भूतसूक्ष्मेष्वभिव्यक्तधर्मकेषु देशकालनिमित्तानुभवावच्छिन्नेषु या समापत्तिः सा सविचारेत्युच्यते। तत्राप्येकबुद्धिनिर्ग्राह्यमेवोदितधर्मविशिष्टं भूतसूक्ष्ममालम्बनीभूतं समाधिप्रज्ञायामुपतिष्ठते। या पुनः सर्वथा सर्वतश्शान्तोदिताव्यपदेश्यधर्मानवच्छिन्नेषु सर्वधर्मानुपातिषु सर्वधर्मात्मकेषु समापत्तिः सा निर्विचारेत्युच्यते। एवं स्वरूपं हि तद्भूतसूक्ष्मम्, एतेनैव स्वरूपेणालम्बनीभूतमेव समाधिप्रज्ञास्वरूपमुपरञ्जयति, प्रज्ञा च स्वरूपशून्येवार्थमात्रा यदा भवति तदा निर्विचारेत्युच्यते। तत्र महद्वस्तुविषया सवितर्का निर्वितर्का च, सूक्ष्मविषया सविचारा निर्विचारा च। एवमुभयोरेतयैव निर्वितर्कया विकल्पहानिर्व्याख्याता इति ॥ ४४ ॥

**By This (Foregoing) The Savichāra And Nirvichāra Engrossments Whose Objects Are Subtle Are Also Explained. 44.**

Of these (1) the engrossment that takes place in the gross forms of the subtle elements conditioned by space, time and causation is called Savichāra or reflective. In it also the object of contemplation is cognised as a single unit of a subtle element with manifested characteristics and its knowledge is acquired in the state of concentration. When, however, the Samāpatti or engrossment on subtle elements is unaffected by any mutation that might take place in them in time, *i.e.* past, present and future, (2) and refers to the object only as present when it embraces all (possible) properties of the object, and all its spatial positions (*i.e.* not conditioned by space),—this sort of all-embracing engrossment is called Nirvichāra or supra-reflective. 'The subtle element is like this,' 'this is how it has been taken for concentration'—this sort of verbal reflection colours the knowledge acquired in Savichāra or reflective concentration. And when the knowledge derived from it is free from reflective consciousness and is only of the object of engrossment it is Nirvichāra. Of the Samāpattis, those relating to gross (3) objects are either Savitarka or Nirvitarka and those relating to subtle objects are Savichāra or Nirvichāra. This is how by establishing that Nirvitarka is free of Vikalpa, such freedom of both itself and Nirvichāra is explained.

(1) What is Savichāra has been explained before (I.41). What the commentator has said is being explained here. 'Of manifested properties' means the properties which are evident in the shape of pot, picture, *i.e.* not unmanifested, being quiescent. Therefore, to practise engrossment in the subtle elements, a manifest object has to be adopted.

Space, time and causation :—If the manifest form of an object is adopted for the purpose of realising its constituent subtle elements, the space occupied by the object will come within the range of the knowables and the realisation of the Tanmātras in it will be limited by the idea of space. This knowledge will, however, relate only to its characteristics manifest at a particular point of time and not to its past or future properties.

Causation is that characteristic of an object by adopting which a particular Tanmātra is realised. In other words, the process of perceiving a particular Tanmātra by reflecting on a particular property of an object, is arriving at it through the principle of causation.

In Savichāra Samādhi or reflective concentration, the object is cognised as a single unit, *i.e.* it is considered without any admixture. The knowledge acquired in Savichārā Samāpatti is influenced by Vikalpa with the help of which reflection is made. And the knowledge thus gained relates only to the different subtle elements present at the time of reflection.

(2) After having mentioned the subject of Nirvichārā Samāpatti, the commentator speaks of its true nature. That state of mind which has only the illumination of a subtle element as the object of cognition, dissociated from any ideas derived from words or reflective thought but associated with the latent impression of this kind of concentration, is known as Nirvichārā Samāpatti.

In this state the knowledge acquired is not confined to a particular space as in the case of Savichārā Samāpatti. Moreover, the knowledge is not limited to the present time only but extends to the past, present and future simultaneously, and it is not determined by any single property of the object but reveals all its possible properties under all conditions. As Nirvitarkā Samāpatti is free from ideas created by Vikalpa, so is also Nirvichārā Samāpatti.

(3) Examples of all kinds of Samāpattis are given below :—

(First) Savitarka. Take the sun as the gross object of contemplation. If concentration on the sun is established, the mind will be full only of that, and all sorts of knowledge regarding it—its shape, distance, composition, etc. will be acquired. This knowledge will, however, be accompanied by verbal concepts, *e.g.* the sun is round, it is so far, etc. When the mind is full of such knowledge, it is said to be in the state of Savitarkā Samāpatti.

(Second) Nirvitarka. In concentrating on the sun, its luminosity will only be realised, and its other particulars would be shut out. When one meditates upon that luminosity to the exclusion of all other properties of the sun, being forgetful even of one's own self, as it were, one attains Nirvitarka knowledge. When the Yogin sees all gross objects in that light he finds that all external objects are nothing but a combination of the elements—light, sound, touch, smell and taste—and realises that the qualities which are imagined with the help of words as belonging to particular objects are nothing but illusory. The state of mind full only of such knowledge is called the state of Nirvitarka engrossment. This is the supreme knowledge pertaining to gross objects. When that state is attained, material possessions like wealth, family, etc. cease to have any charm and they always appear as mere combinations of light, sound, touch, smell, etc.

(Third) Savichāra. After realising the luminosity of the sun through Nirvitarka engrossment the Yogin apprehends the subtler state of that luminosity by a special process of calming the mind and the senses and that is the realisation of the light-Tanmātra or monad. Having first known from testimony and through inference that gross elements are made of Tanmātras, one has to proceed towards the realisation of the Tanmātras by reflecting on that knowledge and further quietening the mind. Savichāra engrossment is conditioned by words, objects and their knowledge all mixed together and is consequently affected by space, time and causation. In other words, the then location of the sun, the present or manifest condition of the sun and the present luminosity (not past and future) as observed by the eye—all these affect the knowledge derived by Savichārā Samāpatti.

When, however, the light-Tanmātra is realised, the Yogin perceives undifferentiated light monad shorn of its varieties, *i.e.* different colours. Such is also the case with sound, touch, etc. The pleasure, pain or stupefaction derived from material objects are but due to their gross properties, because there is variety in such grossness, and it is the variety which causes feelings of pleasure, pain, etc. So, when the unvarying monadic state is realised, the pleasure, pain or stupefaction brought about by variety will disappear.

Tanmātra is not the only object of Savichārā Samāpatti. Other subtle objects like Ahaṁkāra or mutative ego, Buddhi or pure I-sense, and unmanifested Prakṛti (the three Guṇas or constituent principles in equilibrium) also serve as objects of Savichārā Samāpatti.

(Fourth) Nirvichāra. When proficiency is acquired in Savichāra engrossment and the memory is freed from verbal concepts, the concentration only reveals the subtle nature of the object concentrated upon. The mind is then full only of the object free from any verbal notion or Vikalpa, and this is called Nirvichārā Samāpatti or supra-reflective engrossment.

Unmanifested Prakṛti being the merged or potential state of all phenomena, cannot be an object of meditation because it cannot be directly apprehended. Hence there cannot be any Nirvichāra engrossment on Prakṛti. Prakṛtilaya means dissolution of Chitta into its causal substance but it is not Samāpatti. However, a Yogin whose mind has once merged into Prakṛti and who holds on after its re-emergence to the idea 'I have known Prakṛti' can have Savichāra knowledge of Prakṛti. This is Savichārā Samāpatti on Prakṛti.

———

सूक्ष्मविषयत्वं चालिङ्गपर्यवसानम् ॥ ४५ ॥

भाष्यम्—पार्थिवस्याणोर्गन्धतन्मात्रं सूक्ष्मो विषयः, आप्यस्य रसतन्मात्रं, तैजसस्य रूपतन्मात्रं, वायवीयस्य स्पर्शतन्मात्रम्, आकाशस्य शब्दतन्मात्रमिति। तेषामहंकारः, अस्यापि लिङ्गमात्रं सूक्ष्मो विषयः, लिङ्गमात्रस्याप्यलिङ्गं सूक्ष्मो विषयः, न चालिङ्गात्परं सूक्ष्ममस्ति। नन्वस्ति पुरुषः सूक्ष्म इति? सत्यं, यथा लिङ्गात् परमलिङ्गस्य सौक्ष्म्यं न चैवं पुरुषस्य, किन्तु लिङ्गस्यान्वयिकारणं पुरुषो न भवति हेतुस्तु भवतीति अतः प्रधाने सौक्ष्म्यं निरतिशयं व्याख्यातम् ॥ ४५ ॥

**Subtlety Pertaining To Objects Culminates In A-Liṅga** (1) **Or The Unmanifested. 45.**

The subtle form (2) of Kṣiti-element is the smell-Tanmātra, of Ap-element is the taste-Tanmātra, of Tejas-element is the light-Tanmātra, of Vāyu-element is the touch-Tanmātra, of Ākāśa-element is the sound-Tanmātra. The subtler form or constituent of Tanmātra is Ahaṁkāra and the still subtler form of the ego is the first manifested Mahān or Mahat-tattva. The subtler form of the first manifested or Mahān is the unmanifested or Prakṛti. There is nothing subtler than the unmanifested. If it is said that Puruṣa is subtler than that, the reply is 'That is true, but the subtlety of Puruṣa is not of the same kind as that of the unmanifested Prakṛti.' Puruṣa is not the material cause of the first manifest object, *viz.* Mahat, but its efficient cause (3). That is why it has been said that subtlety has reached its limit in Pradhāna or Prakṛti (which is the state of equilibrium of the three Guṇas or constituent principles).

(1) Liṅga is that which terminates or merges into its cause. That by which anything is indicated is an indicator or Liṅga. That of which there is no cause or which has not merged in any other substance and which is not indicative of anything else is A-liṅga. Pradhāna or Prakṛti is A-liṅga.

(2) The elements of Kṣiti, Ap, etc. have two states—(i) the aggregated gross state which is felt as various kinds of smell, sound, light, etc. and (ii) the subtle state without any such variety, *e.g.* smell monad, sound monad, light monad, etc. The Tanmātras are the minutest sensations of subtle objects received by the senses. The external cause of such perception is the ego of the Great or Divine Mind known as Bhūtādi. Sensations of sound, etc. are really modifications of the mind. Tanmātra is perceived along the flow of time only because there is no perceptible space in it. When perception is along a flow of time, there must be a perceptible activity of the mind. Therefore, knowledge of Tanmātra stems from the working of the mutative component of internal senses (Antaḥkaraṇa), *viz.* I-sense. Thus mutative ego or Ahaṁkāra is the subtler form of Tanmātra which is really the minute part or unit of sensation. The flow of mutations

or change of knowledge has to be adopted for contemplation to realise Ahaṁkāra. The subtler form of mutative ego is Mahat-tattva, or pure Asmitā, or pure I-sense. The subtler form of Mahat is Pradhāna or Prakṛti.

(3) Puruṣa does not suffer any such change as Prakṛti does. The latter is changed into Mahat, etc. But as Prakṛti does not suffer mutation unless overseen by Puruṣa, so Puruṣa is regarded as the instrumental or efficient cause of Mahat, etc.

———

ता एव सवीजः समाधिः ॥ ४६ ॥

भाष्यम्—ताश्चतस्रः समापत्तयो वहिर्वस्तुवीजा इति समाधिरपि सवीजस्तत्र स्थूलेऽर्थे सवितर्को निर्वितर्कः सूक्ष्मेऽर्थे सविचारो निर्विचार इति चतुर्धोपसंख्यातः समाधिरिति ॥ ४६ ॥

**These Are The Only Kinds Of Objective Concentrations. 46.**

The four varieties of engrossment described before have external matter as their objects (1) ; that is why in spite of their being concentrations they have to depend on something to develop. Two of them, Savitarka and Nirvitarka, relate to gross objects, while the other two, Savichāra and Nirvichāra, relate to subtle things.

(1) External matter—All knowable objects, *e.g.* the cogniser, the instruments of cognition and the knowables. As all the engrossments develop round external objects concentrated upon, they are called Samādhis with external objects.

———

निर्विचारवैशारद्येऽध्यात्मप्रसादः ॥ ४७ ॥

भाष्यम्—अशुद्ध्यावरणमलापेतस्य प्रकाशात्मनो बुद्धिसत्त्वस्य रजस्तमोभ्यामनभिभूतः स्वच्छः स्थितिप्रवाहो वैशारद्यम्। यदा निर्विचारस्य समाधेर्वैशारद्यमिदं

जायते, तदा योगिनो भवत्यध्यात्मप्रसादो भूतार्थविषयः क्रमाननुरोधी स्फुट-प्रज्ञालोकस्तथा चोक्तम् 'प्रज्ञाप्रासादमारुह्याऽशोच्यश्शोचतो जनान्। भूमिष्ठानिव शैलस्थस्सर्वान्प्राज्ञोऽनुपश्यति' ॥ ४७ ॥

**On Gaining Proficiency In Nirvichāra, Purity In The Inner Instruments Of Cognition Is Developed (1). 47.**

When impurities which shade the illuminating nature of Buddhi are removed there is a transparent flow of quiescence free from the taints of Rajas and Tamas and this is called attainment of proficiency. When the Yogin gets such proficiency in Nirvichāra concentration, he achieves purity in his inner instruments of reception from which he gets the power of knowing things as they are, simultaneously, *i.e.* without any sequence of time, and in all their aspects ; or in other words, he acquires the clear light of knowledge through power of realisation (2). It has been said in this connection (in the Mahābhārata) : "As a man on the hill-top sees the man on the plains, so one having ascended the palace of knowledge and becoming free from sorrow sees others who are suffering."

(1-2) Adhyātma-prasāda is being explained. Adhyātma = inner instruments of cognition. Their Prasāda = purity. When the touch of Rajas (activity) and Tamas (dullness) is removed, Sattva or the enlightening (sentient) faculty predominates in Buddhi, and that is Adhyātma-prasāda. Buddhi is the highest instrument of cognition ; so with its purity all other senses become illumined. The sense of perception being then in the highest state of development, whatever is known at the time is the complete truth. That knowledge is not produced in quanta as ordinary knowledge is, but in that state all the properties and variations of the object to be known appear simultaneously. It has been stated earlier that knowledge derived from inference or from verbal communication, is knowledge of generalities. Direct cognition relates to particular aspects, and it attains the highest development in Samādhi. That is why the ultimate particulars are known by this process. The sages derived their knowledge in this way and communicated it to others in the form of Śrutis (scriptures). These form the philosophy of salvation.

---

ऋतम्भरा तत्र प्रज्ञा ॥ ४८ ॥

भाष्यम्—तस्मिन्समाहितचित्तस्य या प्रज्ञा जायते तस्या ऋतम्भरा संज्ञा भवति, अन्वर्था च सा, सत्यमेव बिभर्त्ति न तत्र विपर्यासगन्धोऽप्यस्तीति, तथा चोक्तम् 'आगमेनानुमानेन ध्यानाभ्यासरसेन च। त्रिधा प्रकल्पयन्प्रज्ञां लभते योगमुत्तमम्' इति ॥ ४८ ॥

**The Knowledge That Is Gained In That State Is Called Ṛtambharā (Filled With Truth). 48.**

When the instruments of cognition are purified, the knowledge that appears in the engrossed mind is called Ṛtambharā (lit. full of unalloyed truth) justifying the name given to it. It retains and sustains truth alone with no trace of misconception. It has been said in this connection : "By study of religious books, by inference and by attachment to the practice of meditation, developing intense insight in these three ways, perfect Yoga (or seedless, *i.e.* objectless concentration) is acquired (1)."

(1) The Śruti, *i.e.* the Upaniṣads also say that realisation comes through listening, contemplating and concentrating. If one learns by listening only that Ātman (the Self) is different from Buddhi (pure I-sense), or that the principles are such and such or that this sort of state is Mokṣa (cessation of sorrow), he really does not get to know much. Similarly, if by inference only one comes to know about Puruṣa and other principles, there is thereby no chance of bringing about cessation of sorrow. But when one constantly thinks of, or meditates on such matters as 'I am not the body,' 'External things are sorrowful and therefore should be forsaken,' 'I shall not resolve on worldly affairs,' etc., and fully realises their essence, then one is on the right road to liberation. If, however, one comes to learn by reasoning only that he is not the body and yet is

affected by its distress or pleasure, there is hardly any difference between him and an ignorant man.

There cannot be any better knowledge of an object than what can be acquired by Nirvichāra Samādhi. That is why it is complete truth. Ṛta means realised, *i.e.* perfect truth.

———

भाष्यम्—सा पुनः—

श्रुतानुमानप्रज्ञाभ्यामन्यविषया विशेषार्थत्वाद् ॥ ४६ ॥

श्रुतमागमविज्ञानन्तत्सामान्यविषयं न ह्यागमेन शक्यो विशेषोऽभिधातुं कस्मात्? न हि विशेषेण कृतसंकेतः शब्द इति। तथानुमानं सामान्यविषयमेव, यत्र प्राप्तिस्तत्र गतिर्यत्राप्राप्तिस्तत्र न भवति गतिरित्युक्तम्, अनुमानेन च सामान्येनोपसंहारस्तस्माच्छ्रुतानुमानविषयो न विशेषः कश्चिदस्तीति न चास्य सूक्ष्मव्यवहितविप्रकृष्टस्य वस्तुनो लोकप्रत्यक्षेण ग्रहणान्न चास्य विशेषस्याप्रामाणिकस्याभावोऽस्तीति समाधिप्रज्ञानिर्ग्राह्य एव स विशेषो भवति भूतसूक्ष्मगतो वा पुरुषगतो वा, तस्माच्छ्रुतानुमानप्रज्ञाभ्यामन्यविषया सा प्रज्ञा विशेषार्थत्वादिति ॥ ४६ ॥

And that knowledge

**Is Different From That Derived From Testimony Or Through Inference, Because It Relates To Particulars (Of Objects). 49.**

What comes from other sources, like that derived from instructions received, relates to generalities. Such instructions cannot describe particular properties fully because words cannot describe particular features as they are not meant to signify such features. So also in the case of inference as has been said before (Sūtra I.7) that wherever there is change of position it is inferred that there is motion, where there is no such change there can be no inference of motion (1). Thus through inference, only general conclusions can be arrived at. That is why no object of verbal communication or inference can be a paticular one. Besides, a thing which is subtle, hidden from view or situated at a distance, cannot be known by ordinary observation. At the same time it cannot be said that a thing particular knowledge of which cannot be obtained by verbal communication, inference or ordinary observations does not exist. The knowledge of particulars relating to the subtler elements or the Puruṣa-like receiver (Mahān) is, however, obtainable by the enlightenment acquired through Samādhi. Therefore, this particular knowledge is different from the (general) knowledge derivable from verbal communication or inference.

(1) Knowledge is obtainable of only that much for which reason can be adduced, but not in respect of other parts. For example when we see smoke we know that there is fire, but the paticulars regarding the nature or the form of the fire are not understood therefrom. Knowledge derived from verbal communication and inferential knowledge are acquired with the help of words. Words, specially those denoting qualities, are expressions of generality. So verbal knowledge is knowledge of a generality.

———

भाष्यम्—समाधिप्रज्ञाप्रतिलम्भे योगिनः प्रज्ञाकृतः संस्कारो नवो नवो जायते—

तज्जः संस्कारोऽन्यसंस्कारप्रतिबन्धी ॥ ५० ॥

समाधिप्रज्ञाप्रभवः संस्कारो व्युत्थानसंस्काराशयं बाधते, व्युत्थानसंस्काराभिभवात्तत्प्रभवाः प्रत्यया न भवन्ति, प्रत्ययनिरोधे समाधिरुपतिष्ठते, ततस्समाधिप्रज्ञा ततः प्रज्ञाकृताः संस्कारा इति नवो नवस्संस्काराशयो जायते, ततः प्रज्ञा ततश्च संस्कारा इति। कथमसौ संस्कारातिशयश्चित्तं साधिकारं न करिष्यतीति, न ते प्रज्ञाकृताः संस्काराः क्लेश-क्षयहेतुत्वाच्चित्तमधिकारविशिष्टं कुर्वन्ति, चित्तं हि ते स्वकार्यादवसादयन्ति, ख्यातिपर्यवसानं हि चित्तचेष्टितमिति ॥ ५० ॥

When knowledge is acquired through Samādhi, the Yogin gets new latent impressions of such knowledge.

**The Latent Impression Born Of Such Knowledge (1) Is Opposed To The Formation Of Other Latent Impressions. 50.**

The latent impressions of insight gained by concentration inhibit latent impressions of empirical life. When latent impressions of empirical life are subdued, no more cognised modifications can emerge therefrom. When modifications are shut out, Samādhi or concentration is achievd. From that comes Samādhic knowledge which entails latent impressions of such knowledge. This is how new latent impressions grow. It might be questioned why such profusion of latencies does not dispose the mind to mutativeness (2). The answer is that these latencies being destructive of affliction, do not create a disposition for mutativeness. On the other hand, they disincline the mind from its tendencies (of producing modifications). Mental effort exists until the acquisition of discriminative knowledge (3).

(1) The impression formed and retained of any cognitive or conative activity of the mind is called Saṁskāra or latent impression. Recollection of the impression of (previous) knowledge is called memory and resurgence of the impression of an action is called automatic action. All knowledge and action take place with the assistance of latent impressions. For an ordinary mortal it is impossible to know or to do a thing, completely abandoning previous latent impressions.

Latent impressions are divisible into two classes : harmful and beneficial, *i.e.* those arising out of nescience and those pregnant with correct knowledge. As knowledge is antagonistic to nescience, the latent impressions of true knowledge destroy such impressions of nescience. Knowledge derived through Samprajñāta-samādhi is the acme of knowledge while discriminative enlightenment is its final stage. Therefore, the latent impression of knowledge derived through Samādhi is able to destroy the latent impression of nescience. When the latent impressions of nescience get feeble, the fluctuations of the mind also are enfeebled, because the fluxes of the mind are really caused by attachment, hatred and such other nescience.

It has already been said (Sūtra I.16) by the commentator that knowledge culminates in detachment. That is how from the knowledge of the fundamental principles derived through Samprajñāta-samādhi and Viveka-khyāti or discriminative enlightenment, detachment becomes complete.

(2) Inclination towards mutation arises from the latent impressions in the mind. It might appear, therefore, that the latent impressions derived through Samprajñāta-yoga will also dispose the mind towards such mutation. That, however, is not the case. The latent impressions of Samprajñāta are really such impressions as prevent the reception of objects by mind, which results in misery. As Samprajñāta impressions get stronger, the working of the mind slows down to a stop.

(3) When Samprajñāta-yoga reaches its highest stage in Viveka-khyāti or discriminative enlightenment the activity of the mind ceases. Through that, on the realisation of the distinction between Buddhi, the receptacle of all sorrows, and Puruṣa, the immutable cogniser, the highest form of detachment is achieved and the mind ceasing to act, the Seer is said to be in a state of Kaivalya or liberation.

---

भाष्यम्—किञ्चास्य भवति—

तस्यापि निरोधे सर्वनिरोधान्निर्बीजस्समाधिः ॥ ५१ ॥

स न केवलं समाधिप्रज्ञाविरोधी प्रज्ञाकृतानां संस्काराणामपि प्रतिबन्धी भवति। कस्मात्; निरोधजः संस्कारः समाधिजान्संस्कारान्बाधत इति। निरोधस्थिति-काल-क्रमानुभवेन निरोधचित्त-कृतसंस्कारास्तित्वमनुमेयम्। व्युत्थान-निरोधसमाधिप्रभवैः सह कैवल्यभागीयैः संस्कारैश्चित्तं स्वस्यांप्रकृताववस्थितायांप्र-विलीयते, तस्मात्ते संस्काराश्चित्तस्याधिकारविरोधिनो न स्थितिहेतवो यस्मादवसि-ताधिकारं सह कैवल्यभागीयैः संस्कारैश्चित्तं विनिवर्त्तते। तस्मिन्निवृत्ते पुरुषः स्वरूपप्रतिष्ठः अतः शुद्धमुक्त इत्युच्यते ॥ ५१ ॥

इति श्रीपातञ्जले सांख्यप्रवचने वैयासिके समाधिपादः प्रथमः।

What else happens to such a mind ?

**By The Stoppage Of That Too (On Account Of The Elimination Of The Latent Impressions Of Samprajñāna) Objectless Concentration Takes Place Through Suppression Of All Modifications** (1). **51.**

That objectless concentration is not only antagonistic to Samprajñāta-samādhi but is also opposed to the formation of latent impressions of that Samādhi, because latent impressions of Nirodha, which is complete stoppage of modification, or those of supreme detachment destroy the latent impressions of Samprajñāta-samādhi. From the knowledge of the duration of the time during which the mind had stopped its functioning, the existence of the latent impression of that arrested state can be inferred. In that state the mind merges in its constituent cause, the ever present Prakṛti, along with the latent impressions of Samprajñāta-samādhi as well as with such latent impressions as lead to Kaivalya or the state of liberation (2). That is why the latent impressions of such knowledge destroy the disposition to mutation and do not contribute to the continuance of the mind, because with the termination of such predilection the mind ceases to act as the latent impressions leading to salvation gather force. When the mind ceases to function, Puruṣa gets isolated in Himself, and that is why He is then called pure and liberated.

(Here concludes the Chapter on Concentration being the first part of the Comments of Vyāsa known as Sāṁkhya-pravachana on the Yoga-philosophy of Patañjali.)

(1) The latent impressions acquired in Samprajñāta-samādhi, *i.e.* the latent impressions of knowledge obtained through Samprajñāta relate to principles or Tattvas. When knowledge is acquired of the true character of the principles and the difference between Puruṣa and the knowables and when the unworthiness of the knowables is completely realised then their knowledge as well as their latent impressions are considered worth renouncing. That is how the latent impression of Nirodha-samādhi or complete restraint is opposed to, *i.e.* shuts out, knowledge as well as the latent impressions acquirable in Samprajñāna. It might be

argued that as stoppage of cognition is not a form of knowledge, how can there be latent impression thereof. In reply it may be explained that Nirodha is nothing but a break in fluctuation, and its latent impression is of that break in fluctuation. The impressions of a broken line can be called the broken parts of a line or the broken parts of no-line. Complete renunciation can give rise to latent impressions, which only bring stoppage of mutation and thus stop the mind from fluctuating. There is always a break between the appearance and disappearance of modifications of the mind, which break is only lengthened in Nirodha-samādhi. Then the sentient, mutative and static principles do not die out but only the activity due to their non-equilibrium that was taking place on being overseen by Puruṣa ceases on account of the cessation of the cause (Avidyā or nescience) which brought about the contact with Puruṣa.

Asamprajñāta-nirodha or cessation of modifications, once it takes place, does not last for ever, but such Nirodha is prolonged by practice. Consequently there is latent impression thereof. Cessation of modifications of the mind through force of such latent impressions is called Nirodha-kṣaṇa, *i.e.* moment of arrested state. It is the state of inactivity of the mind based on Para-vairāgya or supreme detachment. When apathy towards knowables is fully established and when the mind is arrested with the determination never again to receive impressions, it does not reappear. Even when such power of arresting the mind is acquired, the Yogin who wants to do good to humanity with a Nirmāṇa-chitta (constructed mind), arrests the mind for a specified time, and his mind rises after that period as a constructed mind. It has been stated before that in the opinion of the Yoga school, Īśvara arrests the mind for a cycle and at the end of it favours His devotees with supreme knowledge and thus liberates them.

(2) The concentration which brings about the stoppage of fluctuations is Samprajñāta-samādhi. The latent impressions thereof have been referred to here. Latent impressions leading to the Kaivalya state are the latent impressions of the arrested state of the mind. The mind continues to be interested in objects as long as it has a disposition to enjoyment or is trying to achieve salvation. On the attainment of discriminative knowledge, the mind ceases to have any interest in objects.

The latent impressions of Samprajñāta destroy the latent impressions of the fluctuating state. Even when the latter is totally eliminated, the mind still retains discriminative enlightenment acquired in Samprajñāta-samādhi. On the attainment of the highest state of knowledge (vide Sūtra II.27), there being nothing further to know, knowledge acquired in

Samprajñāta-samādhi and its latent impressions cease. Elimination of knowledge gained in Samprajñāta-samādhi is Nirvīja (*i.e.* objectless) concentration. When, in this way, fluctuations of the mind are totally arrested, the mind ceases to exist and this state is Kaivalya or liberation.

Thus supreme knowledge and latent impression of an arrested state are inimical to the inclination of the mind to reception of objects. And in the process the mind is eventually totally arrested—the fully arrested state of the mind being tantamount to the mind merging for ever into its constituent cause.

Although the Seer is beyond pleasure and pain and is immutable, still when the mind ceases functioning, the Seer is regarded as pure. That state being free from sorrow, the Seer is regarded as liberated. In fact, these epithets, pure and liberated, are used in reference to the state in which the mind is. The Seer is always a Seer. The mind is witnessed by Him when it is in a fluctuating state ; when it ceases to function naturally it is not witnessed by Him any more. From this empirical standpoint Puruṣa is said to be either in bondage or liberated.

BOOK II

# ON PRACTICE

भाष्यम्—उद्दिष्टः समाहितचित्तस्य योगः, कथं व्युत्थितचित्तोऽपि योगयुक्तः स्यादित्येतदारभ्यते—

तपःस्वाध्यायेश्वरप्रणिधानानि क्रियायोगः ॥ १ ॥

नातपस्विनो योगः सिध्यति। अनादिकर्मक्लेशवासनाचित्रा प्रत्युपस्थितविषयजाला चाशुद्धिर्नान्तरेण तपः सम्भेदमापद्यत इति तपस उपादानम्, तच्च चित्तप्रसादनमबाधमानमनेनासेव्यमिति मन्यते। स्वाध्यायः प्रणवादिपवित्राणां जपः, मोक्षशास्त्राध्ययनं वा। ईश्वरप्रणिधानं सर्वक्रियाणां परमगुरावर्पणं तत्फलसंन्यासो वा ॥ १ ॥

The Yoga attained by a Yogin with an engrossed mind has been stated. This Sūtra introduces how a devotee with a distracted mind can also attain Yoga.

**Tapas (Austerity Or Sturdy Self-Discipline—Mental, Moral And Physical), Svādhyāya (Repetition Of Sacred Mantras Or Study Of Sacred Literature) And Īśvara-Praṇidhāna (Complete Surrender To God) Are Kriyā-Yoga (Yoga In The Form Of Action)** (1). **1.**

A man without self-discipline cannot attain perfection in Yoga. The impurities or the dross in the mind arising out of the snares of worldly objects which are harmful to Yoga, are coloured by the Vāsanās of actions and afflictions from beginningless time, and they cannot be got rid of or dissipated without the practice of austerities. That is why austerities have to be practised. It has been recommended that an undisturbed course of self-purificatory conduct should be practised by Yogins since this leads to the cleanliness and purity of the mind.

Svādhyāya—Repetition of a sacred Mantra, *e.g.* the sacred syllable OM, or study of scriptures relating to Mokṣa or freedom from bondage.

Īśvara-praṇidhāna—Surrender of all actions to the great Master God, *i.e.* abandonment of all hankering after the fruits of action.

(1) Actions (physical) performed with the object of attainment of Yoga *i.e.* stability of mind, or actions which indirectly lead to Yoga are Kriyā-yoga. Such actions are principally of three kinds, *viz.* Tapas, Svādhyāya and Īśvara-praṇidhāna.

Tapas = Renunciation of sensuous pleasures, *i.e.* attempt to desist from actions which might bring momentary pleasures and putting up with the resulting hardship. That form of austerity which does not cause any pathological disturbance and which results in the non-performance of actions based on attachment and antipathy, is favourable to Yoga.

The descriptions of Tapas etc. are to be found in Sūtra II.32. (*)

Yoga in the form of action = Kriyā-yoga. In other words, action for the purpose of attaining Yoga is Kriyā-yoga. In fact, Tapas etc. like practice of silence, breath-control, surrender of the fruits of action to God are attempts to restrain natural afflictive actions. Svādhyāya is verbal and Īśvara-praṇidhāna is mental Kriyā-yoga. Ahiṁsā or non-injury etc. are not exactly actions but non-performance of action. The hardship involved therein comes within the category of Tapasyā.

———

भाष्यम्—स हि क्रियायोगः—

समाधिभावनार्थः क्लेशतनूकरणार्थश्च ॥ २ ॥

स ह्यासेव्यमानस्समाधिम्भावयति क्लेशांश्च प्रतनूकरोति। प्रतनूकृतान् क्लेशान्प्रसंख्यानाग्निना दग्धवीजकल्पानप्रसवधर्मिणः करिष्यतीति, तेषान्तनू-

*See appendix on Tapas.

Tapas involves correct thinking, full control over one's turbid emotions, clear understanding of moral values and consequent purification of one's character.

करणात्पुनः क्लेशैरपरामृष्टा सत्त्वपुरुषान्यताख्यातिः सूक्ष्मा प्रज्ञा समाप्ताधिकारा प्रतिप्रसवाय कल्पिष्यत इति ॥ २ ॥

That Kriyā-yoga (should be practised)

**For Bringing About Samādhi And Minimising The Kleśas. 2.**

When Kriyā-yoga is properly (1) performed, it conduces to the state of Samādhi and considerably attenuates all the Kleśas. The fire of Prasaṁkhyāna or discriminative knowledge sterilises the attenuated Kleśas like roasted seeds. When they are attenuated, they cannot obscure the realisation of the distinction between Buddhi and Puruṣa. Such realisation then lapses in the absence of the manifestation of the Guṇas.

(1) Impurities are destroyed by Kriyā-yoga. The impurities are the restlessness and the dullness of the senses, born respectively of Rajas and Tamas inherent in them. Therefore, with the elimination of impurities, Chitta turns towards Samādhi. Moreover, impurity is only an aggravated form of Kleśa ; hence through its decrease, Kleśas are also attenuated.

When Kleśas become thin they become ready for extinction. Properly attenuated Kleśas are rendered unproductive by discriminative knowledge which goes by the names of Prasaṁkhyāna or Samprajñāna or Viveka. Just as a fried seed does not sprout, so Kleśa reduced by Samprajñāna to an unproductive state does not give rise to modifications of the mind. For example :—'I am the body' is an erroneous afflictive belief based on nescience. When through the force of Samādhi Mahat-tattva (pure I-sense) is realised, it is correctly seen that 'I am not the body.' In the engrossed state the mind remains always established in that knowledge and the afflictive modification, *viz.* 'I am the body' becomes like a roasted seed ; from the latent impression of the belief 'I am the body' another such modification does not arise and all feelings based on such a belief get extinguished for all time. The impression of the notion 'I am the body' is one born of Kleśa, while the impression of the notion 'I am not the body' is one born of true knowledge and is thus non-afflictive. The latter is also called Prajñā-saṁskāra. When with the knowledge of the distinction between Buddhi and Puruṣa the mind becomes inactive through supreme detachment, the latencies of Prajñā, which are but the sterilised states of the Kleśas, also disappear (vide Sūtras I.50 and II.10). While the attenuated state of Kleśas is obtained by Kriyā-yoga, their unproductive or subtle state is attained by Samprajñāna or true knowledge.

In the above example the knowledge 'I am not the body' is derived from Samādhi or concentration. The attenuation of Kleśas is a help in the process. The means of Samādhi and of attenuation of Kleśa is Kriyā-yoga, *i.e.* calmness of body and the senses through Tapasyā, the predisposition to realisation through Svādhyāya and tranquillity of mind through Īśvara-praṇidhāna.

---

भाष्यम्—अथ के ते क्लेशाः कियन्तो वेति ?—

**अविद्याऽस्मितारागद्वेषाभिनिवेशाः पञ्च क्लेशाः ॥ ३ ॥**

क्लेशा इति पञ्चविपर्यया इत्यर्थः, ते स्यन्दमाना गुणाधिकारं द्रढयन्ति परिणाममवस्थापयन्ति कार्यकारणस्रोत उन्नमयन्ति परस्परानुग्रहतन्त्रा भूत्वा ( तन्त्रीभूत्वेति पाठान्तरम् ) कर्मविपाकं चाभिनिर्हरन्तीति ॥ ३ ॥

What are those Kleśas and how many are they ?

**Avidyā (Misapprehension About The Real Nature Of Things), Asmitā (Egoism), Rāga (Attachment), Dveṣa (Aversion) And Abhiniveśa (Fear Of Death) Are The Five Kleśas (Afflictions). 3.**

The afflictions are the five forms of wrong cognition (1). When they become active, *i.e.* become manifest, they strengthen the sway of the Guṇas, bring about change, set in motion the flow of cause and effect and in conjunction with one another bring about the fructification of action.

(1) The common feature of all the afflictions is erroneous cognition which is a source of pain. When Kleśas prevail, *i.e.* when the afflictive modifications grow, the activity of the Guṇas remains deep-rooted as the real nature of the self remains unseen. They, in their turn, set in motion the chain of mutations from Avyakta (unmanifested) to Mahat (pure I-sense) etc., *i.e.* the Guṇas change continually into Mahat, Ahaṁkāra, etc.

and the afflictions underlying the mutations bring about the fruition of actions.

———

अविद्या क्षेत्रमुत्तरेषां प्रसुप्ततनुविच्छिन्नोदाराणाम् ॥ ४ ॥

भाष्यम्—अत्राविद्या क्षेत्रं प्रसवभूमिरुत्तरेषामस्मितादीनां चतुर्विधकल्पितानां प्रसुप्ततनुविच्छिन्नोदाराणाम्। तत्र का प्रसुप्तिः? चेतसि शक्तिमात्रप्रतिष्ठानां बीजभावोपगमस्तस्य प्रबोध आलम्बने सम्मुखीभावः। प्रसंख्यानवतो दग्धक्लेशबीजस्य सम्मुखीभूतेऽप्यालम्बने नासौ पुनरस्ति, दग्धबीजस्य कुतः प्ररोह इत्यतः क्षीणक्लेशः कुशलश्चरमदेह इत्युच्यते। तत्रैव सा दग्धबीजभावा पञ्चमी क्लेशावस्था नान्यत्रेति, सतां क्लेशानां तदा बीजसामर्थ्यं दग्धमिति विषयस्य सम्मुखीभावेऽपि सति न भवत्येषां प्रबोध इत्युक्ता प्रसुप्तिर्दग्धबीजानामप्ररोहश्च। तनुत्वमुच्यते प्रतिपक्षभावनोपहताः क्लेशास्तनवो भवन्ति। तथा विच्छिद्य विच्छिद्य तेन तेनात्मना पुनः समुदाचरन्तीति विच्छिन्नाः, कथं? रागकाले क्रोधस्यादर्शनात्, न हि रागकाले क्रोधस्समुदाचरति, रागश्च क्वचिद्दृश्यमानो न विषयान्तरे नास्ति, नैकस्यां स्त्रियां चैत्रो रक्त इत्यन्यासु स्त्रीषु विरक्त इति, किन्तु तत्र रागो लब्धवृत्तिरन्यत्र भविष्यद्वृत्तिरिति, स हि तदा प्रसुप्ततनुविच्छिन्नो भवति। विषये यो लब्धवृत्तिः स उदारः।

सर्वे एवैते क्लेशविषयत्वं नातिक्रामन्ति। कस्तर्हि विच्छिन्नः प्रसुप्तस्तनुरुदारो वा क्लेश इति? उच्यते, सत्यमेवैतत्, किन्तु विशिष्टानामेवैतेषां विच्छिन्नादित्वम्। यथैव प्रतिपक्षभावनातो निवृत्तस्तथैव स्वव्यञ्जकाञ्जनेनाभिव्यक्त इति। सर्व एवामी क्लेशा अविद्याभेदाः कस्मात्? सर्वेषु अविद्यैवाभिप्लवते। यदविद्यया वस्त्वाकार्यते तदेवानुशेरते क्लेशाः, विपर्यासप्रत्ययकाले उपलभ्यन्ते, क्षीयमाणां चाविद्यामनु क्षीयन्तेति ॥ ४ ॥

**Avidyā Is The Breeding Ground For The Others Whether They Be Dormant, Attenuated, Interrupted Or Active. 4.**

In the present context, Avidyā has been referred to as the breeding ground for those (other Kleśas) mentioned later, *viz.* Asmitā etc. in their dormant, attenuated, interrupted or active condition (1). Of these, what is dormancy? It is that condition in which a Kleśa remains in the mind in a potential state. Such Kleśa awakens, *i.e.* manifests itself when it turns towards its object. In the case of one who has acquired discriminative knowledge, the seeds of affliction are singed and therefore even if the object comes before him, these do not sprout or become active. How can a roasted seed germinate? For this reason, the Yogin who has reduced his Kleśas is called proficient in the art of self-conquest and is regarded as being in his last bodily frame (2). It is in such Yogins that the afflictions reach the fifth state like burnt-up seeds, and not in others. In that state the seeds of Kleśa do indeed exist, but these lose their power of producing action and fail to germinate even when brought in proximity to appropriate objects (*i.e.* exciting causes). This is the account of dormancy or the absence of germination of a Kleśa on account of its parched condition.

Now attenuation is being spoken of. Kleśas get thin when these are overpowered by the contemplation of their opposites. When Kleśas occasionally get suppressed but come back again these are known as interrupted Kleśas. For example, when anger is not manifest at the time of attachment, it is not active. Again, when attachment is directed to one object it cannot be said to be non-existent in respect to another object. Chaitra being attached to one woman may not bear hatred to another. In such cases attachment is active for the present towards one and it can be active in the future in respect to others. In respect of the latter it is then either dormant, tenuous or interrupted. That which is manifest with reference to an object is called active. All these do not fall beyond the category of afflictions or Kleśas. Then why is Kleśa divided into dormant, attenuated, interrupted and active? That is true no doubt, but the division is based on the peculiarities of the different states. As these are held in check by contrary contemplation, so are these manifested by favouring causes. All Kleśas are but varieties of nescience, because all of them are permeated by delusion. When an object is coloured by nescience, it is followed by the other Kleśas (3). These are experienced whenever there is nescience and they dwindle away when nescience is attenuated.

(1) The four forms of Kleśa like Asmitā etc. are really variations of Avidyā. They have four states *viz.* dormant, attenuated, interrupted and active. 'Prasupti' or dormancy is existence in the form of germ or latent power. A dormant affliction awakens with an appropriate stimulus. A Tanu or attenuated Kleśa is one that is thinned by Kriyā-yoga. A Vicchinna or interrupted Kleśa is that which is suppressed by other Kleśas. Udāra means active. At the time of anger, aversion is in operation and attachment is in abeyance. When by the practice of detachment, attachment is controlled then it is called attenuated. Existence in a latent state is dormancy. Untraceable or unseen latencies though not bearing fruit at present may become fruitful later. Hence these are regarded as dormant. The state of Kleśa means a state when an afflictive mental modification is in operation.

A dormant Kleśa is somewhat like a Kleśa which has become like a parched seed, because both are unnoticeable. The dormant Kleśa, however, shows itself whenever there is an occasion while the Kleśa which has become like a parched seed will not appear even when the occasion is there. That is why the commentator has called the latter the fifth state of affliction. It is in reality entirely different from the four states mentioned before. As a burnt seed does not sprout again, so the Kleśas burnt in the fire of knowledge cannot affect the Ātman again.

(2) When the Kleśa becomes like a parched seed, then a Yogin becomes Jīvan-mukta (*i.e.* liberated though alive). Such a Yogin becomes free by subjugating the Chitta and that is why his present body becomes his last one as he is not born again.

(3) How attachment etc. are based on Avidyā will be shown later.

---

भाष्यम्—तत्राविद्यास्वरूपमुच्यते—

अनित्याशुचिदुःखानात्मसु नित्यशुचिसुखात्मख्यातिरविद्या ॥ ५ ॥

अनित्ये कार्ये नित्यख्यातिस्तद्यथा, ध्रुवा पृथिवी, ध्रुवा सचन्द्रतारका

द्यौः, अमृता दिवौकस इति। तथाऽशुचौ परमबीभत्से काये शुचिख्यातिरुक्तञ्च 'स्थानाद्बीजादुपष्टम्भान्निस्यन्दान्निधनादपि। कायमाधेयशौचत्वात्पण्डिता ह्यशुचिं विदुः' इत्यशुचौ शुचिख्यातिर्दृश्यते नवेव शशाङ्कलेखा कमनीयेयं कन्या मध्वमृतावयवनिर्मितेव चन्द्रं भित्त्वा निःसृतेव ज्ञायते, नीलोत्पलपत्रायताक्षी हावगर्भाभ्यां लोचनाभ्यां जीवलोकमाश्वासयन्तीवेति, कस्य केनाभिसम्बन्धो भवति चैवमशुचौ शुचिविपर्यय-( यांस ) प्रत्यय इति। एतेनापुण्ये पुण्यप्रत्ययस्तथैवानर्थे चार्थप्रत्ययो व्याख्यातः।

तथा दुःखे सुखख्यातिं वक्ष्यति 'परिणामतापसंस्कारदुःखैर्गुणवृत्तिविरोधाच्च दुःखमेव सर्वं विवेकिनः' इति, तत्र सुखख्यातिरविद्या। तथाऽनात्मन्यात्मख्याति-र्बाह्योपकरणेषु चेतनाचेतनेषु भोगाधिष्ठाने वा शरीरे, पुरुषोपकरणे वा मनसि अनात्मन्यात्मख्यातिरिति। तथैतदत्रोक्तं 'व्यक्तमव्यक्तं वा सत्त्वमात्मत्वेनाभि-प्रतीत्य तस्य सम्पदमनुनन्दति आत्मसम्पदं मन्वानस्तस्य व्यापदमनुशोचति आत्मव्यापदं मन्यमानः स सर्वोऽप्रतिबुद्ध' इति। एषा चतुष्पदा भवत्यविद्या मूलमस्य क्लेशसन्तानस्य कर्माशयस्य च सविपाकस्येति। तस्याश्चामित्रागोष्पद-वद् वस्तुसतत्त्वं विज्ञेयं, यथा नामित्रो मित्राभावो न मित्रमात्रं किन्तु तद्विरुद्धः सपत्नस्तथाऽगोष्पदं न गोष्पदाभावो न गोष्पदमात्रं किन्तु देश एव ताभ्यामन्यद्-वस्त्वन्तरमेवमविद्या न प्रमाणं न प्रमाणाभावः किन्तु विद्याविपरीतं ज्ञानान्तरम-विद्येति ॥ ५ ॥

Of these, the nature of Avidyā is being described—

**Avidyā Consists In Regarding A Transient Object As Everlasting, An Impure Object As Pure, Misery As Happiness And The Not-Self As Self. 5.**

To consider as permanent what is impermanent is Avidyā, *e.g.* to take the world or the sky with the moon and the stars as permanent, or again, the heavenly beings as immortal. Because of its place (of origin), of its germinal source (1), of its constituent factors, of its secretions, of its disintegration and of its adventitious purity, the body has been declared by the sages as something impure. Such a loathsome and unclean body is, however, regarded as pure ; for example, in the description 'This maiden, charming and tender as a new moon, with her body appearing to be formed of honey or nectar, has emanated, as it were, from the moon, and with her lotus-like eyes, she is refreshing living beings with her alluring glances.' What is here being compared to what? This is how a false sense of purity comes to invest that which is impure. This also illustrates the false cognition of the sacred in what is profane, and of the beneficial in what is really not so.

The false cognition of pain as pleasure will be described later in aphorism II.15, 'The discriminating persons apprehend (by analysis and anticipation) all worldly objects as sorrowful because they cause suffering in consequence, in their afflictive experiences and in their latent tendencies and also because of the contrary nature of the Guṇas (which produces changes all the time).' Looking upon misery as happiness is Avidyā. So also it is Avidyā when one looks upon things as one's own, when these are not so. For instance, people look upon external objects, other persons, animals, even one's own body and mind, which are the seat and instrument of experience, as constituting one's own Self or Puruṣa, while in reality these are not so. In this connection Āchārya (Pañchaśikha) has said: "Those who regard animate and inanimate objects as part of their own self and rejoice at their prosperity and bemoan their decay are all victims of delusion." Thus Avidyā has four divisions. It is the source from which all Kleśas flow and corresponding latent impressions are produced. It is to be noted that like 'Amitra' (not friend) and 'Agoṣpada' (not a cow's footprint), Avidyā has a positive entity. As Amitra does not mean either the mere non-existence of a friend or a friend but a positive thing opposite to a friend, *i.e.* an enemy, and as A-goṣpada does not imply either the mere absence of Goṣpada or a Goṣpada but a large place different from either, so A-vidyā is neither right cognition nor the mere absence of cognition but cognition that is contrary to correct cognition (2). (Goṣpada = land coverable by a cow's foot, *i.e.* of a very small size ; A-goṣpada = a large piece of land).

(1) The place of origin of the body is the womb ; the germ is the semen ; assimilation of food eaten is its constitution ; secretions are excretions like perspiration etc., while death makes all bodies unclean. The body also requires constant cleansing. For these reasons the body is considered as unclean. To consider any such body to be clean, pleasing, desirable and companionable is false knowledge.

(2) Of the four symptoms of Avidyā, the sense of permanence in transient things is the chief one in the kind of Kleśa called Abhiniveśa or fear (of death) ; in attachment the chief one is a sense of purity in impure things ; feeling pleasure in affliction is predominant in hatred, because although hatred is a form of misery, it appears to be pleasant or desirable; while considering things not pertaining to the self as one's own is dominant in the sense of the ego (Asmitā).

Avidyā has been variously defined by different schools of thought. Most of these definitions do not conform to logic and philosophy. That the definition given in the Yoga philosophy is incontrovertibly true will be understood by every reader. Whatever might be the reason for mistaking a piece of rope as a snake, nobody can deny that it is taking one thing for another—a kind of wrong cognition. That cognition is contray to correct cognition and is consequently false. The contradiction that exists between the true and the false is the contradiction between Vidyā and Avidyā. That does not, however, prove the contrariness of the objects themselves ; *i.e.* the snake and the rope are different but not opposed to one another. The cause of this erroneous knowledge, or the modification due to Avidyā, is the latent impression of such knowledge. Therefore the common name for false cognition and the corresponding sub-conscious impressions is Avidyā. Avidyā as false cognition is without any beginning. So also is Vidyā beginningless ; because living beings have correct as well as incorrect cognitions. Normally there is a preponderance of wrong cognition and paucity of right cognition, while in discriminative knowledge true cognition predominates and wrong cognition is negligible. There is no separate thing called Avidyā over and above the modification of the mind. Avidyā is only a form (unreal) of modification of the mind. Thus when it is said that Avidyā is eternal, it means that the flow of such modifications of the mind is eternal.

As light and darkness are relative, light where darkness is less and darkness where there is less light, so every modification of the mind is really a mixture of Vidyā and Avidyā—the former having less of Avidyā and the latter less of Vidyā. This is the difference between the two. The acme of Vidyā is discriminative knowledge, though even in that there is a trace of Asmitā, while in Avidyā there is also a subtle awareness of the Seer in the form of 'I. am', 'I know', etc. In reality all knowledge is partly real and partly unreal ; when there is preponderance of truth it is called Vidyā and in the context of preponderance of delusion it is called Avidyā. Taking an oyster for a piece of silver does not come within the category of Avidyā. It is an error. All errors are misconceptions while Avidyā is that wrong cognition which is opposed to liberation and should be removed ; that is how it is related to the practice of Yoga. This distinction must be noted.

———

दृग्दर्शनशक्त्योरेकात्मतेवाऽस्मिता ॥ ६ ॥

भाष्यम्—पुरुषो दृक्शक्तिर्बुद्धिर्दर्शनशक्तिरित्येतयोरेकस्वरूपापत्तिरिवाऽस्मिता-क्लेश उच्यते। भोक्तृभोग्यशक्त्योरत्यन्तविभक्तयोरत्यन्तासंकीर्णयोरविभागप्राप्ताविव सत्यां भोगः कल्पते, स्वरूपप्रतिलम्भे तु तयोः कैवल्यमेव भवति कुतो भोग इति। तथा चोक्तम् 'बुद्धितः परं पुरुषमाकारशीलविद्यादिभिर्विभक्तमपश्यन्कुर्य्यात्तत्रात्म-बुद्धिम्मोहेन' इति ॥ ६ ॥

**Asmitā Is Tantamount To The Identification Of Puruṣa Or Pure Consciousness With Buddhi. 6.**

Puruṣa is absolute Awareness while Buddhi or the cognitive principle is the instrument of knowing. Looking upon these two as the same is the affliction known as Asmitā. When the two utterly different entities like the experiencer and the experienced, appear united (1) that is called experience. When the real nature of the two is known it leads to liberation or the Self-in-itself and there is then no experience. So it has been said (by Āchārya Pañchaśikha) : "When one fails to see that Puruṣa is different from Buddhi by virtue of his immaculateness, immutability and metapsychic consciousness, one regards Buddhi as the true self through delusion (2)."

(1) The state of experience is of the nature of (mental) knowledge while the experiencer is of the nature of metapsychic consciousness; therefore their sameness is in the context of cognition. The sameness of the Knower and the known, is not to be imagined as like that of salt and water, *i.e.* of tangible objects. It is just the absence of distinction between Puruṣa and Prakṛti in the awareness. 'Experience (of pleasure and pain) arises from the cognition of Buddhi and Puruṣa as identical' (Sūtra III.35)—by such statement the author of the Sūtra has described the relation between Buddhi and Puruṣa. Happiness and misery are objects of experience. The inner organs are the means of experiencing happiness and misery, and therefore they are also included in the content of experience.

Identification of the organs of cognition with self is Asmitā. Buddhi or the individual cognitive principle is the primary instrument of cognition; it is, therefore, primarily pure I-sense. Considering the various sense-organs to be the self results from Asmitā. 'I am possessed of the power of seeing etc.'—this sort of imputation of the idea of self to something which is not-self, is also an example of Asmitā. This sort of imputation of self to other things may be of various kinds.

(2) The words used in the quotation from Pañchaśikha have meanings different from the current ones. As this is from a text which was prepared before technical philosophical terms were coined, many of the words used here convey ideas different from their ordinary import. Ākāra = Perpetual purity, immaculateness. Vidyā = metapsychic consciousness. Śīla = Indifference, or the attitude of an onlooker who is not affected or changed by anything he sees. Not having true knowledge about these characteristics of Puruṣa and their difference from Buddhi, deluded people under the influence of Avidyā take Buddhi as the Self, *i.e.* they form the erroneous idea that Buddhi or the pure I-sense and the absolute Knower or pure Consciousness are one and the same.

---

सुखानुशयी रागः ॥ ७ ॥

भाष्यम्—सुखाभिज्ञस्य सुखानुस्मृतिपूर्वः सुखे तत्साधने वा यो गर्द्धस्तृष्णा लोभः स राग इति ॥ ७ ॥

### Attachment Is That (Modification) Which Follows Remembrance Of Pleasure. 7.

The desire or thirst for, or hankering after pleasure or the means leading to it, which is entertained by one who has experienced pleasure and has an inclination to it, is called Rāga or attachment*(1).

(1) Desire born of the latent impressions of pleasure enjoyed is what is meant by 'that which results from remembrance of pleasure'. Thirst implies a feeling of want for the pleasure enjoyed, as one feels the need of water when thirsty. Hankering after a thing or greed is that state which brings about a longing to obtain it. In greed the sense of right and wrong is generally vitiated. The word Anuśayī or 'following' implies that it exists as a latent impression in the mind. In attachment, desire and senses are drawn involuntarily and unconsciously towards objects, and the power to consciously restrain desire disappears. That is why attachment is regarded as a kind of misapprehension. By this the Self gets linked up with the senses and their objects. Here the misapprehension is to regard the detached Self as bound up with the latent impressions of pleasure pertaining to the senses which really do not belong to the Self. Besides, to regard evil as good is also a characteristic of attachment.

———

दुःखानुशयी द्वेषः ॥ ८ ॥

भाष्यम्—दुःखाभिज्ञस्य दुःखानुस्मृतिपूर्वो दुःखे तत्साधने वा यः प्रतिघो मन्युर्जिघांसा क्रोधः स द्वेष इति ॥ ८ ॥

* Rāga or attachment is a form of Kleśa. There are, however, different forms of attachment, like reverence for saintly persons (Śraddhā), love of friends, conjugal love where attachment is most pronounced, affection for youngsters and compassion for those in distress. All these are not equally harmful. It may be noted that unlike love or affection, reverence and compassion are concerned more with the mental or physical state of the persons rather than with the individuals themselves. Besides, the element of attachment is quantitatively less and qualitatively it is more refined in both reverence and compassion, which is why they help one to progress on the path of Yoga.

**Aversion Is That (Modification) Which Results From Misery. 8.**

Aversion is the feeling of opposition, mental disinclination, propensity to hurt and anger towards misery or objects producing misery, arising out of recollection of the misery experienced before (1).

(1) Pratigha = Desire to retaliate, or to resist. To one who has no aversion there is nothing to oppose, but to one who has aversion, opposition comes at every step. Manyu = Malice. Jighāṅsā (lit. desire to kill) = Vindictiveness.

As in attachment so in aversion, the latencies of misery which do not belong to the Self are attributed to it and the inactive Self is regarded as the doer. This is also false cognition.

———

स्वरसवाही विदुषोऽपि तथारूढ़ोऽभिनिवेशः ॥ ९ ॥

भाष्यम्—सर्वस्य प्राणिन इयमात्माशीर्नित्या भवति 'मा न भूवं भूयासम्' इति। न चाननुभूतमरणधर्मकस्यैषा भवत्यात्माशीः, एतया च पूर्वजन्मानुभवः प्रतीयते। स चायमभिनिवेशः क्लेशः स्वरसवाही कृमेरपि जातमात्रस्य। प्रत्यक्षानुमानागमैरसम्भावितो मरणत्रास उच्छेददृष्ट्यात्मकः पूर्वजन्मानुभूतं मरणदुःखमनुमापयति। यथा चायमत्यन्तमूढ़ेषु दृश्यते क्लेशस्तथा विदुषोऽपि विज्ञातपूर्वापरान्तस्य रूढ़ः कस्मात्, समाना हि तयोः कुशलाकुशलयोर्मरणदुःखानुभवादियं वासनेति ॥ ९ ॥

**As In The Ignorant So In The Learned The Firmly Established Inborn Fear Of Annihilation Is The Affliction Called Abhiniveśa (1). 9.**

Every creature always has this craving 'Let me never be non-existent ; let me be alive.' One who has not felt the dread of death before cannot have this kind of craving. This demonstrates the experience of a previous birth. This afflictive anxiety is spontaneous. It is seen even in worms from their birth. Unestablished by (direct) perception or by inference or from statement of authoritative persons, this fear of extinction leads to the conclusion that fear of death had been experienced in previous births (2). As in a confirmed idiot, so in a learned man possessed of knowledge regarding previous life and the subsequent life (*i.e.* regarding whence one came and whither one will go), this fear is found to exist, because, devoid of true knowledge, both the learned and the fool have the same Vāsanā arising out of the experience of the pain of death.

(1) Svarasavāhī = with which one is born or that which springs naturally from the accumulated latent impressions. Tathārūḍha = that which is possessed by the ignorant as well as by the learned, this well-established affliction.

Attachment is rooted in pleasure. Aversion is rooted in misery. Similarly, fear of extinction is born of the torpid or benumbed feeling devoid of pleasure, pain or discrimination. Such benumbed feeling arises out of the natural (involuntary) functions of the body and the senses. In that, the identification of the body with the Self is ever present. The fear that arises out of loss or a threat of loss of that stupefied sense of identification of the body with the Self is Abhiniveśa-kleśa. It causes affliction in the shape of fear.

Although the Self is really immortal, the fear of its extinction which is the fear of death, arising out of ignorance, is the main Abhiniveśa-kleśa, the affliction caused by the fear of extinction. The commentator has shown how a previous life can be inferred from that. Other fears are also Abhiniveśa-kleśa. This Abhiniveśa is an affliction, a feeling inimical to spiritiual practice. Abhiniveśa has other meanings as well.

(2) There can be remembrance only of things felt before. When anything is felt, it is stored in the mind. Its recollection is memory. Memory of the fear of death is found in all creatures. Death has not been experienced in this life. Therefore it must be concluded that it was experienced in a previous life. In this way, the existence of a previous life is established by Abhiniveśa.

It might be urged that as fear of death is inherent, there is no need of a previous experience therein. If recollection of death is called inherent, then every memory may be said to be natural. But memory is not inherent; it arises from some cause, and past experience is that cause. When recollections always arise out of a cause, then a part of it (pertaining to fear of death etc.) cannot reasonably be called inherent. An inherent thing does not arise out of a cause. An inherent characteristic never leaves the thing to which it belongs. Fear of death is found to disappear with acquisition of true knowledge. Therefore acquisition of wrong knowledge (repeated experience of fear of death through misapprehension ) must be its cause. In this way a person's fear of death and allied distresses establish his previous experience of it and thus his previous birth.

Again, it may be asked 'What is the proof that fear of death is a form of remembrance ?' In reply, it may be said that memory is the perception of something internal without coming into contact with any external object. Remembrance arises from some form of idea analogous to it. Fear of death also arises from within through a similar process, that is why it is a form of memory.

In fact, the time of origin of the mind cannot be traced by any logical exercise. Matter is considered to be without a beginning, or else something would be presumed to be coming out of nothing. Similar is the case with the mind.

Nobody can advance any ground for holding that the mind originates with birth. In fact it is entirely wrong to say so. Those who hold that fear of death is an instinct, *i.e.* untaught ability, only speak of this life but cannot explain how instinct arises. Two answers are generally given to the question as to how instinct arises. The first is that it has been made by God, and the other (which is no answer) is that it is not knowable. Apart from the blind faith of some sects there is not an iota of evidence to show that the mind has been made by God. According to the philosophy of the Ṛṣis the mind has not been made by God but it is without a beginning. If those who hold that the origin of the mind is unknowable, admit that they do not know it, then there is an end of it. If on the other hand, they say that men cannot know it, the mind will be held to be either with or without a beginning. If the cause of mind is said to be entirely unknowable, it is indirectly saying that the mind is without a cause. What is without a cause is eternal. If a thing arises out of an antecedent cause, then it is generally said to have a beginning. Therefore a thing without a cause is without a beginning. The use of the term 'unknowable' would thus really mean that the cause exists but is not clearly knowable. It has been said that Chitta or the mind is characterised by a series of modifications. These modifications are appearing and disappearing. The three Guṇas constitute the basic ingredients of these fluctuations. Each mental modification is a change caused by the combination of the three Guṇas. The three Guṇas being without a cause are without a beginning. Therefore, the flow of fluctuations resulting from their mutations must also be without a beginning. This is the most reasonable answer to the question when and wherefrom has the mind come [vide IV.10 (1)].

———

ते प्रतिप्रसवहेयाः सूक्ष्माः ॥ १० ॥

भाष्यम्—ते पञ्च क्लेशा दग्धबीजकल्पा योगिनश्चरिताधिकारे चेतसि प्रलीने सह तेनैवास्तं गच्छन्ति ॥ १० ॥

**The Subtle Kleśas Are Forsaken (i.e. Destroyed) By The Cessation Of Productivity (i.e. Disappearance) (1) Of The Mind. 10.**

Those five Kleśas become like parched seeds and disappear with the mind of the Yogin, which having fulfilled the purpose of its existence becomes defunct.

(1) Pratiprasava = opposed to Prasava or production, *i.e.* disappearance by resolving into the cause. Subtle Kleśa implies Kleśa which has become like parched seed through Prasaṁkhyāna or discriminative knowledge. The cognition of 'I' in one's own body can be completely removed on the realisation of the principle which is beyond the body and the senses. From such realisation comes the knowledge that 'I am neither the body nor the senses.' Then no disorder in the body or of the senses affects the Yogin's mind. When the latency of such knowledge is always present in a habitually one-pointed mind then it is called discriminative knowledge opposed to Asmitā-kleśa. On account of its being established in the mind no false notion of identification of the body with the Self can rise therein, and therefore Asmitā becomes like parched seed incapable of sprouting. In other words, there cannot then arise any spontaneous cognition of the 'I' as the self associated with the body and the senses and thereby produce any distraction in the mind This sort of parched state is the subtle form of Asmitā-kleśa.

As the thought of renunciation becomes steadfast, an insight into the nature of true Self is acquired and attachment to worldly objects becomes thin or ineffective as a parched seed. So does aversion become ineffective when a person gains an insight into the purity of the mind free from malice or hatred. Likewise fear of death is attenuated with the cessation of the sense of identifying oneself with the body.

Thus by means of the latent impressions acquired through Samprajñāna (vide I.50) Kleśas are thinned. Though attenuated they are still manifest. Just as the idea 'I am the body' indicates a manifest condition of the mind, so the idea 'I am not the body' (*i.e.*the knowledge that Puruṣa is the Seer of 'I') is also a form of manifest condition. There is further similarity with the parched seed. The parched seed looks like an ordinary seed but has no power of sprouting; similarly Kleśa in a subtle state exists but produces no modification, *i.e.* no afflictive fluctuation arises in the mind wherein only perfect knowledge prevails. At the root of modification based on knowledge also there exists Asmitā-kleśa in a subtle form.

The Kleśa so reduced disappears with the disappearance of the mind. When through Para-vairāgya or supreme renunciation the mind merges into its constituent cause, the subtle Kleśas also disappear along with it. Pralaya or Vilaya implies disappearance without chance of re-emergence. In ordinary circumstances afflictive modifications taking place in the mind determine the birth, span of life and the experience of pleasure and pain. Kleśas are attenuated by Kriyā-yoga. Although in Samprajñāta-yoga relationship with the body no doubt continues, that relationship is based on such knowledge as 'I am not the body' etc. This is the subtle state of Kleśa. It is needless to say that it stops birth, span of life and further experience. In Asamprajñāta-yoga that subtle relationship with the body also ceases, *i.e.* the modifications being merged in their natural causes, Kleśas are completely destroyed.

———

भाष्यम्—स्थितानान्तु वीजभावोपगतानाम्—

ध्यानहेयास्तद्वृत्तयः ॥ ११ ॥

क्लेशानां या वृत्तयः स्थूलास्ताः क्रियायोगेन तनूकृताः सत्यः प्रसंख्यानेन ध्यानेन हातव्याः, यावत् सूक्ष्मीकृता यावद्दग्धवीजकल्पा इति। यथा च वस्त्राणां स्थूलो मलः पूर्वं निर्धूयते पश्चात् सूक्ष्मो यत्नेनोपायेन चापनीयते तथा स्वल्पप्रतिपक्षाः स्थूला वृत्तयः क्लेशानां, सूक्ष्मास्तु महाप्रतिपक्षा इति ॥ ११ ॥

Moreover, of Kleśas remaining as germs,

**Their Means Of Subsistence Or Their Gross States Are Avoidable By Meditation. 11.**

The gross manifestations of Kleśas (1) having been attenuated by Kriyā-yoga are to be destroyed through meditation on Prasaṁkhyāna or discriminative knowledge until they become reduced to the state of the parched seed. As gross dirt is first washed away from a piece of cloth and then its finer impurities are removed by care and effort, so the gross Kleśas are weak obstacles while the subtle ones are more difficult to overcome.

(1) Gross manifestations of Kleśas are those afflictive modifications of the mind based on misapprehension, Asmitā etc.

Dhyāna-heya = to be abandoned through knowledge born of meditation on discriminative knowledge. Kleśa is a kind of wrong knowledge ; hence it has to be dissipated by true knowledge. Discriminative knowledge is the best form of knowledge ; that is why afflictive modifications have to be removed by meditation on self-discernment. How thereby the Kleśas are reduced to the position of parched seeds has been stated before. The three stages in the process of destruction of Kleśas have to be carefully noted, *viz.* thinning by Kriyā-yoga, reduction to an unproductive state by meditative insight and total disappearance by the dissolution of the mind.

———

क्लेशमूलः कर्माशयो दृष्टादृष्टजन्मवेदनीयः ॥ १२ ॥

भाष्यम्—तत्र पुण्यापुण्यकर्माशयः कामलोभमोहक्रोधप्रसवः। स दृष्टजन्मवेदनीयश्चादृष्टजन्मवेदनीयश्च। तत्र तीव्रसंवेगेन मन्त्रतपःसमाधिभिर्निर्वर्त्तित ईश्वर-देवतामहर्षिमहानुभावानामाराधनाद्वा यः परिनिष्पन्नः स सद्यः परिपच्यते पुण्य-कर्माशय इति। तथा तीव्रक्लेशेन भीत-व्याधित-कृपणेषु विश्वासोपगतेषु वा महानुभावेषु वा तपस्विषु कृतः पुनः पुनरपकारः स चापि पापकर्माशयः सद्य एव परिपच्यते। यथा नन्दीश्वरः कुमारो मनुष्यपरिणामं हित्वा देवत्वेन परिणतः, तथा नहुषोऽपि देवानामिन्द्रः स्वकं परिणामं हित्वा तिर्य्यक्त्वेन परिणत इतिक्त्वु।

तत्र नारकाणां नास्ति दृष्टजन्मवेदनीयः कर्माशयः, क्षीणक्लेशानामपि नास्ति अदृष्टजन्मवेदनीयः कर्माशय इति ॥ १२ ॥

**Karmāśaya Or Latent Impression of Action Based On Afflictions, Becomes Active In This Life Or In A Life To Come (1). 12.**

Merit and demerit in latent impressions of action arise from desire, greed, delusion or anger. They become operative in the present life or in a future life. Out of these the impressions of pious actions gathered from repetition of Mantras, observation of Tapas or attainment of Samādhi—all performed with deep detachment or through worship of God, the Devas, Maharṣis or saints, fructify quickly. Similarly the impressions of vicious actions repeatedly performed with excessive Kleśas, in regard to creatures who are frightened, diseased or pitiable or to those who have come for refuge, or are noble-minded or engaged in austerities, bear fruit immediately. For example, young Nandīśvara was transferred from the human form into a Deva ; while Nahuṣa, a ruler in heaven, was transferred from the divine form into a reptile. Amongst these, those who are in purgatory do not gather any such merit or demerit to be experienced in that life, while those who have thinned their afflictions (*e.g.* Jīvanmuktas, *i.e.* freed while alive) do not carry with them any such latent impressions which might fructify in a future life (2).

(1) Karmāśaya—latent impressions of actions. The latent impressions of virtuous and vicious actions are Karmāśayas. Any manifest state of the mind leaves a like imprint on it and this is its latent impression. Saṁskāra or latent impression may be either Savīja, *i.e.* potent or Nirvīja, *i.e.* impotent. Potent Saṁskāras are of two kinds—those which are born of afflictions and those which are their opposites ; in other words, Saṁskāras based on wrong knowledge, and those based on true knowledge. The potent Saṁskāras based on Kleśas are called Karmāśayas. They are classed as white, black, and black-and-white, or divided into two classes, virtuous and vicious, or white and black only. Saṁskāras based on

knowledge realised through concentration are known as neither black nor white.

Karmāśaya brings about three consequences, *viz.* birth, span of life and experience (of pleasure or pain) in that life. In other words, the Saṁskāra which brings about such results is Karmaśaya. When the consequences take place, the Saṁskāra based on the feeling experienced thereby is called Vāsanā or subconscious latency. Vāsanā does not of itself produce any consequence or result, but for any Karmāśaya to produce result the appropriate Vāsanā is necessary. Karmāśaya is like a seed, Vāsanā is like a field, the birth or embodiment is like a tree and experience (of pleasure or pain) is like its fruits. For the convenience of the reader, Saṁskāra is being shown below in a tabular form :—

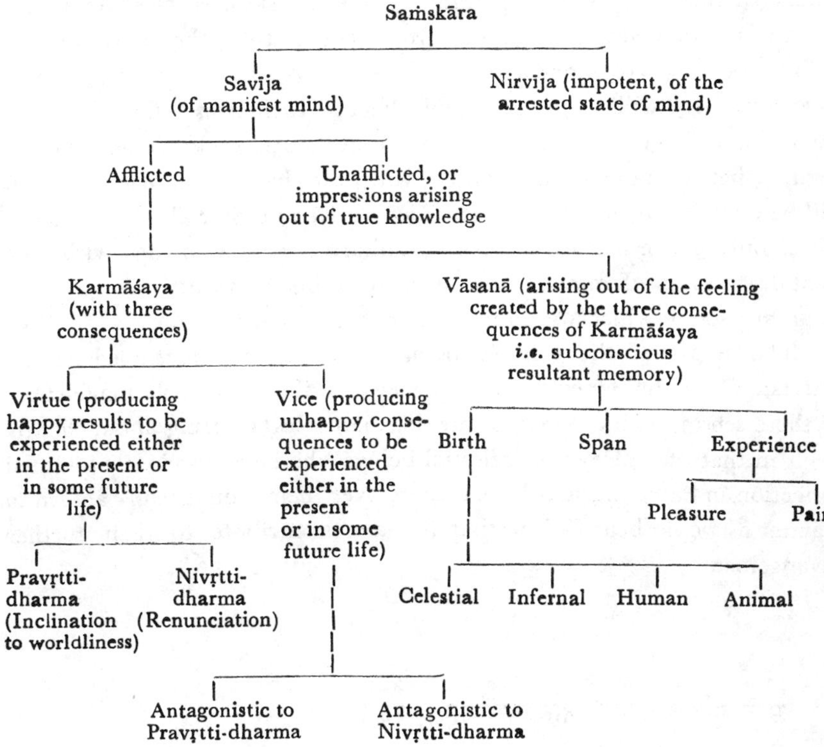


**How to effect destruction of latent impressions**

1. By Nivṛtti-dharma (the spirit of renunciation) Pravṛtti-dharma (spirit of inclination to worldliness) is weakened.

2. Thereby Karmāśaya is weakened and consequently Vāsanā no longer serves any purpose.

3. Afflictive Saṁskāras are thereby reduced, and this is what is known as the attenuated state.

4. From latencies of true knowledge, the afflictive Saṁskāras become weak and unproductive like parched seed.

5. The thinned or subtle afflictive Saṁskāras are annihilated by the latency of the arrested state of the mind.

(2) Deeds performed with Kleśas like Avidyā etc., produce afflictive latent impressions which bear fruit in this life, or in some future life. The time for fruition becomes imminent or otherwise according to the intensity of the impression. The commentator has explained by citing examples. In purgatory creatures suffer from the effects of their past actions and on termination of their sufferings they pass into another state. In purgatory their (involuntary) mental state is most dominant and because they are then suffering from great distress, they have not the ability to do any voluntary actions. Therefore it is impossible for them to exercise free-will to produce any effect in their lives. On the other hand, having only obscured organs, they continue to suffer mental anguish, being unable to do anything with the help of latencies which will be effective in that life. That is why their purgatorial life is called a life of only oppressive experience. Similarly, celestial beings with the mental states predominant and steeped in bliss have little free-will for voluntary action which would produce result in that very life.

The senses of the celestial beings, however, are developed on the Sāttvika, *i.e.* enlightened basis, and they can, if they so wish, make effort by those senses, with the help of previous latencies, to bring about happy result in that life. Devas or celestial beings who have previously attained perfection in Samādhi, and have control over their minds can act in a manner as would bear fruit in that life and contribute to their further advancement.

———

सति मूले तद्विपाको जात्यायुर्भोगाः ॥ १३ ॥

भाष्यम्—सत्सु क्लेशेषु कर्माशयो विपाकारम्भी भवति, नोच्छिन्नक्लेशमूलः। यथा तुषावनद्धाः शालितण्डुला: अदग्धवीजभावाः प्ररोहसमर्था भवन्ति नापनीत-तुषा दग्धवीजभावा वा, तथा क्लेशावनद्धः कर्माशयो विपाकप्ररोही भवति, नापनीतक्लेशो न प्रसंख्यानदग्धक्लेशवीजभावो वेति। स च विपाकस्त्रिविधो जातिरायुर्भोग इति।

तत्रेदं विचार्यते किमेकं कर्मैकस्य जन्मनः कारणम्, अथैकं कर्मानेकं जन्माक्षिपतीति। द्वितीया विचारणा किमनेकं कर्मानेकं जन्म निर्वर्तयति, अथानेकं कर्मैकं जन्म निर्वर्तयतीति। न तावदेकं कर्मैकस्य जन्मनः कारणम्, कस्मात्, अनादिकालप्रचितस्यासंख्येयस्यावशिष्टकर्मणः साम्प्रतिकस्य च फलक्रमानियमादनाश्वासो लोकस्य प्रसक्तः स चानिष्ट इति। न चैकं कर्मानेकस्य जन्मनः कारणम्, कस्मात्, अनेकेषु कर्मस्वेकैकमेव कर्मानेकस्य जन्मनः कारणमित्यवशिष्टस्य विपाककालाभावः प्रसक्तः, स चाप्यनिष्ट इति। न चानेकं कर्मानेकस्य जन्मनः कारणम्, कस्मात्, तदनेकं जन्म युगपन्न सम्भवतीति, क्रमेण वाच्यम्? तथा च पूर्वदोषानुषङ्गः। तस्माज्जन्म-प्रायणान्तरे कृतः पुण्यापुण्यकर्माशयप्रचयो विचित्रः प्रधानोपसर्जनभावेनावस्थितः प्रायणाभिव्यक्त एकप्रघट्टकेन मिलित्वा मरणं प्रसाध्य संमूर्च्छित एकमेव जन्म करोति। तच्च जन्म तेनैव कर्मणा लब्धायुष्कं भवति, तस्मिन्नायुषि तेनैव कर्मणा भोगः सम्पद्यत इति। असौ कर्माशयो जन्मायुर्भोगहेतुत्वात् त्रिविपाकोऽभिधीयत इति। अत एकभविकः कर्माशय उक्त इति।

दृष्टजन्मवेदनीयस्त्वेकविपाकारम्भी भोगहेतुत्वात्, द्विविपाकारम्भी वा आयुर्भोगहेतुत्वान्नन्दीश्वरवन्नहुषवद्वा इति। क्लेशकर्मविपाकानुभवनिमित्ताभिस्तु वासनाभिरनादिकालसम्मूर्च्छितमिदं चित्तं चित्रीकृतमिव सर्वतो मत्स्यजालं ग्रन्थिभिरिवाततमित्येता अनेकभवपूर्विका वासनाः। यस्त्वयं कर्माशय एष एवैकभविक उक्त इति। ये संस्काराः स्मृतिहेतवस्ता वासनास्ताश्चानादिकालीना इति।

यस्त्वसावेकभविकः कर्माशयः स नियतविपाकश्चानियतविपाकश्च। तत्र दृष्टजन्मवेदनीयस्य नियतविपाकस्यैवायं नियमः, न त्वदृष्टजन्मवेदनीयस्यानियतविपाकस्य, कस्मात्, यो ह्यदृष्टजन्मवेदनीयोऽनियतविपाकस्तस्य त्रयी गतिः कृतस्याविपक्वस्य नाशः, प्रधानकर्मण्यावापगमनं वा, नियतविपाकप्रधानकर्मणाऽभिभूतस्य वा चिरमवस्थानमिति। तत्र कृतस्याऽविपक्वस्य नाशो यथा शुक्लकर्मोदयादिहैव नाशः कृष्णस्य, यत्रेदमुक्तम्, 'द्वे द्वे ह वै कर्मणी वेदितव्ये पापकस्यैको राशिः पुण्यकृतोऽपहन्ति। तदिच्छस्व कर्माणि सुकृतानि कर्तुमिहैव ते कर्म कवयो वेदयन्ते'।

प्रधानकर्मण्यावापगमनम्, यत्रेदमुक्तम्, 'स्यात्स्वल्पस्संकरः सपरिहारस्सप्रत्यवमर्षः, कुशलस्य नापकर्षायालं कस्मात्, कुशलं हि मे बह्वन्यदस्ति यत्रायमावापं गतस्स्वर्गेऽप्यपकर्षमल्पं करिष्यति' इति।

नियतविपाकप्रधानकर्मणाभिभूतस्य वा चिरमवस्थानम्, कथमिति, अदृष्ट-जन्मवेदनीयस्यैव नियतविपाकस्य कर्मणः समानं मरणमभिव्यक्तिकारणमुक्तम्, नत्वदृष्टजन्मवेदनीयस्यानियतविपाकस्य। यस्त्वदृष्टजन्मवेदनीयं कर्मानियतविपाकं तन्नश्येदावापं वा गच्छेदभिभूतं वा चिरमप्युपासीत यावत्समानं कर्माभिव्यञ्जकं निमित्तमस्य न विपाकाभिमुखं करोतीति। तद्विपाकस्यैव देशकालनिमित्तानव-धारणादियं कर्मगतिर्विचित्रा दुर्विज्ञाना चेति न चोत्सर्गस्यापवादान्निवृत्तिरिति एकभविकः कर्माशयोऽनुज्ञायत इति ॥ १३ ॥

**As Long As Kleśa Remains At The Root, Karmāśaya Produces Three Consequences In The Form Of Birth, Span Of Life And Experience (1). 13.**

Karmāśaya begins to fructify when there is Kleśa at its root ; but it does not do so when Kleśa is uprooted. As rice when in the husk and not reduced to the burnt condition, can germinate but does not do so when the chaff is removed or reduced to a parched state, so Karmāśaya when based on Kleśa, is capable of producing consequences, but it does not produce any consequence when Kleśa is removed or is reduced to a burnt state through acquisition of knowledge. The consequence is of three kinds : birth, span of life and experience of pleasure or pain in life.

In this respect (2) it is to be considered :—whether one action is responsible for one birth or one action brings about many births. The second point is :—do many actions bring about many births or do they bring about only one birth ? Now, a single action can never be the cause of one birth ; because in that case, there being no regularity of succession in the fruition of present actions and of innumerable actions that have been stored up as Karmāśaya from time without beginning—some of which still remain unfructified—people would lose faith in the performance of actions. This is therefore untenable. Again, a single action cannot account for many births. Because in that case if one out of many actions brings about many births then the remaining actions would have no time to bear fruit. This view, therefore, is also untenable. Again, many actions are not responsible for many births ; because the many births cannot take place at the same time, and if it is said that they take place gradually, then also the difficulty mentioned before arises. For these reasons the accumulation of diverse latencies of actions, whether of merit or demerit, done between birth and death, whether dominant or in a subordinate state, is brought into action through death and massed together in one effort which simultaneously effecting death causes a single birth. That birth gets its span of life from the accumulated Karmāśaya and in that span the experiences are felt as a result of that Karmāśaya. Karmāśaya, being the cause of birth, of the span of life and of affective experience, is called 'Trivipāka' or that which has three consequences. For the same reason Karmāśaya has been called 'Eka-bhavika' or gathered in one birth (life) only.

When Karmāśaya becomes operative in the present life and is responsible for affective experience only it is said to be 'of single consequence' ; while if it is responsible for the span of life as well as for experience, it is 'of double consequence'—as in the cases of Nandīśvara and Nahuṣa (of double effect and of a single effect). Mind nourished from time immemorial on latencies (Vāsanā) of Kleśas and the execution of actions, is like a variegated picture or like a fishing net with knots all over. That is why Vāsanā is derived from many previous births, while Karmāśaya is derived from one birth or life. Those subconscious latent impressions, which give rise to memory only, are known as Vāsanās and they are without beginning.

Karmāśaya, which is of one life only, has either certain fruition or uncertain fruition. Of these two classes, the rule that Karmāśaya is active in one life only, is (fully) applicable to Karmāśaya of certain fruition ; while those of uncertain fruition which can bear fruit in some future life cannot be held to be active only in one life. This is because Karmāśaya of uncertain fruition, to be operative in a future life, has three kinds of outcome :—first, unfructified Karmāśaya may be destroyed through atonement before it becomes operative ; secondly, it may be mixed up with the dominant Karmāśaya as a subordinate element ; thirdly, it may be overshadowed by the dominant Karmāśaya and may remain for a long time in a dormant state. Of these, the first is illustrated by the extinction in this life of dark deeds by the performance of pious ones. In this connection it has been said : "Know the action to be of two kinds of which a series of virtuous actions nullifies one of vicious actions. Therefore resolve to do good deeds. Those good deeds are to be done in this life ; so have the sages demonstrated to you."

Regarding fruition of minor Karmāśayas as subsidiary to dominant Karmāśayas it has been said by Pañchaśikha : "In sacrificial rites, along with the principal Karmāśaya of virtue is also produced the Karmāśaya of sin. In the principal Karmāśaya of virtue that sin is small, mixed with virtue, and removable by atonement. But if no atonement is done it brings a touch of suffering as in the midst of profuse enjoyment a man feels the pangs of hunger if he goes without food. That sin is, however, unable to reduce the Karmāśaya of virtue, because it might be said : 'I have many virtuous deeds to my credit, which will overwhelm the sinful Karmāśayas and will greatly reduce their effectiveness in causing distress in heaven.' " How it remains dormant for a long time overpowered by the chief unrestricted Karmāśayas is being explained here. Death has been said to be the general cause of manifestation of the unrestricted Karmāśaya operative in future life ; but this rule does not always hold good, because death is not always the cause of complete manifestation of limited Karma operative in future life. Karmas which are to be operative in a future life and which have not yet become mature enough to bear fruits can be destroyed ; or they may get mixed up or stand overpowered and may not fructify for a long time, until similar actions favourable to their manifestation incline them towards fruition. Since the time, the place and the cause of such manifestation cannot be determined, the course of Karma is regarded as variegated and undiscernible. But (in such a case) this being an exception the general rule is not broken. Therefore, it has been held that Karmāśaya is uni-genital, *i.e.* of one birth (life) only.

(1) Fluctuations due to nescience are the general states of the manifested mind. When through knowledge, nescience is destroyed, the 'me-mine' feeling, from which springs the identification of the self with the body, is destroyed completely and consequently the fluctuations of the mind also cease. When the mind remains completely arrested there can be no birth, nor span of life nor experience of pleasure or pain as they are co-existent with fluctuations only. Therefore when there is Kleśa at the root, *i.e.* a deed is done under Kleśa and latency thereof is stored in the mind, it produces birth, span of life and experience, unless it is nullified by insight which can counteract that latency. Jāti = Form assumed at birth of various species, *e.g.* man, cattle, etc., Āyus = Period of existence of that body, Bhoga = Pleasure or pain experienced in the life. Karmāśaya is the cause of all these three. Nothing takes place without a cause. When an action conducive to longevity or its opposite is done, the span of life is found to be increased or diminished in this very life. Pleasure or pain is also experienced as a result of action done in this very life. There are many instances of human babies, stolen and reared by wild animals, having been changed almost into animals, imitating their ways of life.

Thus it is seen that the cumulative latencies of actions done in this very life change the nature of the mundane body and yield results in the shape of longevity and experience. Therefore, actions are the cause of birth in a particular species, of span of life and of experience therein. The birth, span of life and experience which are not the result of action in this life must, therefore, have been caused by some action done in a previous life which had not fructified in that life.

What are the reasons for birth, span of life and experience therein ? Men have so far discovered three answers to that question : first, ordained by God ; secondly, the reason is not known to man, *i.e.* man has no means of knowing it ; and thirdly, Karma or action is their cause.

There is no proof that these have been ordained by God. Those who hold this view say that it is a matter of faith and not of reason. In their view, God is unknowable and as a corollary, the reason for birth etc. must also be unknowable. If such people say that the matter is 'unknown to us' then that would be reasonable. But when they say that it is unknown to all men, they cannot offer adequate justification for that statement. The doctrine of Karma therefore appears to be more rational than the other two theories.

(2) The commentator has explained some general rules relating to the principle of Karma. The commentary can be better followed if those rules are clearly understood. They are :—

A. One Karmāśaya is not responsible for many births. If it were so, there would be no chance for the fruition of all Karmas. In every birth many Karmāśayas are accumulated and it would then be difficult to find time for the fruition of all these. Therefore such statements as 'killing of one animal will involve millions of birth as animal' etc. are untenable.

B. For the same reason the proposition that one Karma brings about one birth cannot also be correct.

C. Many Karmas do not cause many births simultaneously, because many births at the same time is an impossibility.

D. That many Karmāśayas go to bring about one birth appears to be the correct rule. In fact it is seen that in one life the fruits of many actions are experienced. Therefore many Karmas would appear to be the cause of one birth.

E. The Karmāśayas responsible for a birth also determine its span of life, and the experience of pleasure and pain therein.

F. Karmāśaya is Eka-bhavika, *i.e.* is mainly accumulated in one life. Take X = previous birth and Y = the subsequent birth. The Karmāśayas responsible for Y have been mainly collected in X. Therefore Karmāśaya is Eka-bhavika or of one birth. This is the general rule. The exception to this will be mentioned later. How Karmāśaya gathered in one life causes a subsequent life can be seen in the commentary.

G. The outcome of Karmāśaya which will bear fruit in a future life is threefold, *viz.* birth, duration of existence, and experience of pleasure and pain. But as the outcome of Karma, which becomes operative in that very life, does not entail another birth (*i.e.* its fruits are experienced in that life), it involves only Bhoga or Bhoga and Āyus. Therefore Karmāśaya which is operative in the same life brings about either one or two results.

H. Karmāśaya is mainly of one birth but Vāsanā [Matrix latency—see II.12(1)] is of many births. The three consequences experienced in the chain of births coming down from time without a beginning, have produced latencies in the shape of Vāsanās, which are thus eternal, *i.e.* of various births.

I. Karmāśayas are of two kinds—those which must mature and those which may not. Those which must produce results are called Niyata-vipāka, while those which being influenced by others cannot produce complete results are called Aniyata-vipāka.

J. Uni-genital birth (life) is the general rule for Karmāśayas but there are exceptions.

K. In respect of Niyata-vipāka Karmāśayas which are operative in that birth, the rule being operative in one life, holds good fully. They are fully gathered in that life. Therefore they are Eka-bhavika.

L. In respect of Aniyata-vipāka Karmāśayas which are to bear fruit in some future life, that rule does not apply, for there are three courses which such Karmas may take :—

(a) The unfructified Karma may be nullified, *e.g.* virtue destroyed by vice and vice versa. The vicious Karmāśaya born of latency of sin arising out of anger, is neutralized by the constant practice of non-anger. Therefore it cannot be said that there is no exception to the rule that when a Karma is done its result must be borne. Karma, however, inevitably bears fruit unless it is destroyed by a contrary action or by proper insight.

The uni-genital rule does not fully apply to Karmāśaya, due to be operative in some future life because Karmāśaya gathered in one life can, to some extent, be destroyed in that very life.

(b) When a minor Karmāśaya matures with a chief Karmāśaya it is manifested feebly ; hence the rule that it would fructify in the following birth, does not apply in this case.

Dominant or chief Karmāśaya = that which is capable of bearing fruit independently.

Minor Karmāśaya = that which is slow in action or is there in a secondary position.

The latency of Karma done under intense lust, anger, spirit of forgiveness, charity, etc. is dominant Karmāśaya. It is always ready to fructify. Its opposite, the minor Karmāśaya, does not become operative independently ; it acts as secondary to the chief Karmāśaya. The Karmāśaya responsible for future births, is thus an aggregate of primary and secondary ones. The minor Karmāśayas do not fructify completely ; so the rule that 'the result of all actions in this life will come about in the following life' is not fully applicable in the case of minor ones.

(c) When a very strong or primary Karmāśaya bears fruit, the opposite secondary one remains subdued. It does not bear fruit at the time, but it can fructify at some future time if roused by some kindred Karmāśaya. Here also as some minor Karmas of one life remain suppressed the uni-genital rule does not apply. An example of this is as follows :—A man performs pious deeds in his boyhood. Then in his youth he commits many beastly acts through greed. At the time of his death, the fully mature latencies of sin form the appropriate Karmāśayas. As a result, the life of a beast that he gets, does not show the result of the pious actions done previously ; but such of the pious deeds as are enjoyable in a human life, remain stored up, and they will become operative when he is again born as a man. These will be helpful when he does pious acts in his subsequent human life. In this illustration the pious and vicious actions should be understood to be not mutually antagonistic. If they had been so, the vice would have destroyed the effect of the virtuous deeds. Suppose, forgiveness is a virtue and stealing a vice. Larceny does not destroy forgiveness, but only anger or non-forgiveness will do it.

———

ते ह्लादपरितापफलाः पुण्यापुण्यहेतुत्वात् ॥ १४ ॥

भाष्यम्—ते जन्मायुर्भोगाः पुण्यहेतुकाः सुखफलाः, अपुण्यहेतुकाः दुःखफला इति। यथा चेदं दुःखं प्रतिकूलात्मकमेवं विषयसुखकालेऽपि दुःखमस्त्येव प्रतिकूलात्मकं योगिनः ॥ १४ ॥

**Because Of Virtue And Vice These (Birth, Span And Experience) Produce Pleasurable And Painful Experiences. 14.**

These, *i.e.* the species in which birth takes place, the span of life and the experience therein, produce happiness if caused by virtue and misery if caused by vice (1). Just as misery is undesirable (to ordinary beings) so to a Yogin's mind even the enjoyment of pleasant objects is undesirable since this eventually involves pain also.

(1) The causes of misery are nescience, Asmitā, attachment, aversion and fear. Consequently actions which are opposed to them or weaken them are considered virtuous, while actions which support them are vicious.

Contentment, forgiveness, self-restraint, non-covetousness, cleanliness, discipline of the senses, wisdom, discriminative learning, truth and non-anger, these ten are regarded as pious acts. Amity and kindness as well as benevolence and charity based on them, are also regarded as virtues because these are partially opposed to nescience. Actions opposed to virtue, *e.g.* anger, greed, violence based on ignorance, untruth, incontinence are sinful actions. According to Āchārya Gauḍapāda : Yama, Niyama, (*vide* II.29) compassion and charity constitute virtuous acts.

———

भाष्यम्—कथं तदुपपद्यते ?—

परिणामतापसंस्कारदुःखैर्गुणवृत्तिविरोधाच्च दुःखमेव सर्वं विवेकिनः ॥ १५ ॥

सर्वस्यायं रागानुविद्धश्चेतनाचेतनसाधनाधीनः सुखानुभव इति तत्रास्ति रागजः कर्माशयः। तथा च द्वेष्टि दुःखसाधनानि मुह्यति चेति द्वेषमोहकृतोऽप्यस्ति कर्माशयः। तथा चोक्तम्। नानुपहत्य भूतानि उपभोगः सम्भवतीति हिंसाकृतोऽप्यस्ति शारीरः कर्माशय इति, विषयसुखं चाविद्येत्युक्तम्। या भोगेष्विन्द्रियाणां तृप्तेरुपशान्तिस्तत्सुखम्, या लौल्यादनुपशान्तिस्तद्दुःखम्। न चेन्द्रियाणां भोगाभ्यासेन वैतृष्ण्यं कर्तुं शक्यं, कस्मात् ? यतो भोगाभ्यासमनु विवर्द्धन्ते रागाः कौशलानि चेन्द्रियाणामिति, तस्मादनुपायः सुखस्य भोगाभ्यास इति। स खल्वयं वृश्चिकविषभीत इवाशीविषेण दष्टो यः सुखार्थी विषयानुवासितो महति दुःखपङ्के निमग्न इति। एषा परिणामदुःखता नाम प्रतिकूला सुखावस्थायामपि योगिनमेव क्लिश्नाति।

अथ का तापदुःखता ? सर्वस्य द्वेषानुविद्धश्चेतनाचेतनसाधनाधीनस्तापानुभव इति तत्रास्ति द्वेषजः कर्माशयः। सुखसाधनानि च प्रार्थयमानः कायेन वाचा मनसा च परिस्पन्दते ततः परमनुगृह्णात्युपहन्ति च, इति परानुग्रहपीड़ाभ्यां धर्माधर्मावुपचिनोति, स कर्माशयो लोभान्मोहाच्च भवति। इत्येषा तापदुःखतोच्यते।

का पुनस्संस्कारदुःखता ? सुखानुभवात्सुखसंस्काराशयो दुःखानुभवादपि दुःखसंस्काराशय इति, एवं कर्मभ्यो विपाकेऽनुभूयमाने सुखे दुःखे वा पुनः कर्माशयप्रचय इति। एवमिदमनादि दुःखस्रोतो विप्रसृतं योगिनमेव प्रतिकूलात्मकत्वादुद्वेजयति, कस्मात् ? अक्षिपात्रकल्पो हि विद्वानिति। यथोर्णातन्तुरक्षिपात्रे न्यस्तः स्पर्शेन दुःखयति नान्येषु गात्रावयवेषु, एवमेतानि दुःखानि अक्षिपात्रकल्पं योगिनमेव

क्लिश्नन्ति नेतरं प्रतिपत्तारम्। इतरन्तु स्वकर्मोपहृतं दुःखमुपात्तमुपात्तं त्यजन्तं त्यक्तं त्यक्तमुपाददानमनादिवासनाविचित्रया चित्तवृत्त्या समन्ततोऽनुविद्धमिवाविद्यया हातव्य एवाहंकारममकारानुपातिनं जातं जातं वाह्याध्यात्मिकोभयनिमित्तास्त्रि-पर्वाणस्तापा अनुप्लवन्ते। तदेवमनादिदुःखस्रोतसा व्युह्यमानमात्मानं भूतग्रामं च दृष्ट्वा योगी सर्वदुःखक्षयकारणं सम्यग्दर्शनं शरणं प्रपद्यत इति।

गुणवृत्तिविरोधाच्च दुःखमेव सर्वं विवेकिनः। प्रख्याप्रवृत्तिस्थितिरूपा बुद्धि-गुणाः परस्परानुग्रहतन्त्रा भूत्वा शान्तं घोरं मूढं वा प्रत्ययं त्रिगुणमेवारभन्ते। चलं च गुणवृत्तमिति क्षिप्रपरिणामि चित्तमुक्तम्। 'रूपातिशया वृत्त्यतिशयाश्च परस्परेण विरुध्यन्ते सामान्यानि त्वतिशयैः सह प्रवर्त्तन्ते।' एवमेते गुणा इतरेतराश्रयेणोपार्जितसुखदुःखमोहप्रत्यया इति सर्वे सर्वरूपा भवन्ति, गुणप्रधान-भावकृतस्त्वेषां विशेष इति। तस्माद् दुःखमेव सर्वं विवेकिन इति।

तदस्य महतो दुःखसमुदायस्य प्रभववीजमविद्या, तस्याश्च सम्यग्दर्शन-मभावहेतुः। यथा चिकित्साशास्त्रं चतुर्व्यूहं रोगो रोगहेतुरारोग्यम्भैषज्य-मित्येवमिदमपि शास्त्रं चतुर्व्यूहमेव, तद्यथा संसारस्संसारहेतुर्मोक्षो मोक्षोपाय इति। तत्र दुःखबहुलः संसारो हेयः, प्रधानपुरुषयोः संयोगो हेयहेतुः, संयोग-स्यात्यन्तिकी निवृत्तिर्हानं, हानोपायः सम्यग्दर्शनम्। तत्र हातुः स्वरूपमुपादेयं हेयं वा न भवितुमर्हति इति, हाने तस्योच्छेदवादप्रसङ्गः, उपादाने च हेतुवादः, उभयप्रत्याख्याने च शाश्वतवाद इत्येतत्सम्यग्दर्शनम्॥ १५॥

How is it possible (that the Yogins do not find satisfaction even in the pleasant, enjoyable objects of the world)?

**The Discriminating Persons Apprehend (By Analysis And Anticipation) All Worldly Objects As Sorrowful Because They Cause Suffering In Consequence, In Their Afflictive Experiences And In Their Latencies And Also Because Of The Contrary Nature Of The Guṇas (Which Produces Changes All The Time). (1) 15.**

Experience of happiness is due to attachment to objects, animate (*e.g.* wife and family) or inanimate. From such feeling of happiness arises Karmāśaya based on attachment. Similarly, objects which cause suffering are hated by all and men are stupefied by them. This is how Karmāśaya is born of hatred and stupefaction. This has been explained before. No enjoyment is possible without injury to another. Thus in the enjoyment of objects, bodily Karmāśaya based on malevolence is also formed. The enjoyment of objects has, therefore, been called nescience. In other words when through gratification of the thirst for enjoyables, the senses are calmed and do not go after the objects—that is happiness ; while restlessness due to thirst for enjoyment is unhappiness (2). Through practice (or continuance) of enjoyment the senses cannot be inclined to renunciation, for enjoyment increases attachment as well as the adroitness of the senses. That is why enjoyment is not the means of attaining spiritual happiness. A seeker of happiness gets into slough of misery through enjoyment of objects and longing for them. This is similar to the suffering of a person who, unable even to stand the sting of a scorpion gets bitten by a serpent. These adverse experiences entailing misery in the end, even though pleasant for the time being, cause only unhappiness to Yogins (*i.e.* things that cause unhappiness in the long run to a non-Yogin are regarded as unhappiness by a discriminating Yogin even when they are producing pleasure).

What is afflictive misery ? Everyone is afflicted with pain when pursuing animate and inanimate objects with aversion. This gives rise to Karmāśaya of aversion. Again, when (to overcome this afflictive misery) men seek pleasure with body, mind and words, they either favour or cause pain to others, which results in accumulation of piety and impiety. This Karmāśaya is the result of greed and infatuation. This is called afflictive misery.

What is the painfulness of Saṁskāra (subconscious impressions) ? Experiences of pleasure and pain give rise to corresponding latencies. Thus from experience of pleasure and pain resulting from Karma, fresh Karmāśaya is accumulated (through corresponding Vāsanā) (3). In this way the eternal stream of misery causes distress only to a Yogin, because the mind of a wise man is as sensitive as the surface of an eye-ball. As the touch of a falling cobweb hurts only the eye-ball, but no other part of the body, so these miseries (due to the mutative nature of things) affect only a Yogin who is as sensitive as an eye-ball and not others. Others, under the influence of nescience in their mind, eternally variegated by Vāsanā and subject to the mistaken notions of 'me' and 'mine', which are to be given up eventually for obtaining correct knowledge of Self, suffer from the misery due to their own deeds. They go on giving up this misery and regaining it over and over again with the result that they are born again and again and are thus overwhelmed by three-fold sorrow produced by external and internal causes. The Yogin, however, seeing himself and others carried away by this eternal flow of misery takes refuge in right knowledge for the elimination of all sorrows.

Also on account of the mutual opposition of the modifications of the Guṇas, everything is sorrowful to a discriminating person. "The phases of Buddhi in the shape of Sattva, Rajas and Tamas, reacting on one another, give rise to tranquil, intense or stupefied experience. The products of the Guṇas are in a state of flux, *i.e.* always mutating, and that is why the mind has been called fast-changing. When any of the forms of Buddhi (these are eight in number, *viz.* merit and demerit, right and wrong apprehensions, the spirit of detachment and attachment, supremacy and its opposite) and its states (these are three in number, *viz.* tranquillity, misery and stupor) become more intense, it opposes the weaker ones, while feebler forms and states co-operate with the stronger ones." Thus by admixture the Guṇas produce experience of pleasure, pain and stupor. So all experiences have the aspects of all the Guṇas, *viz.* Sattva, Rajas and Tamas, but their specific characters, *e.g.* the Sāttvika, the Rājasika and the Tāmasika ones are caused by the preponderance of one or other of the Guṇas. For that reason (*viz.* that nothing can be purely Sāttvika or producer of pleasure only), to a discriminating person everything (even worldly pleasure) is full of misery.

Nescience is the root cause of the prevalence of extensive misery and sorrow, while true knowledge is the cause of disappearance of nescience. As medical science has four divisions : illness, cause of illness, recovery and therapeutics—so this philosophy of salvation has four parts, *viz.* cycle of births, its cause, liberation and the means of liberation. Of these the cycle of births is Heya, *i.e.* to be discarded ; the association of Puruṣa and Pradhāna (Prakṛti) is Heyahetu or the cause of Heya (which is to be discarded) ; perpetual stoppage of this association is Hāna or liberation ; and right knowledge is the means of liberation (Hānopāya). Of these the real nature of Puruṣa, who witnesses the liberation, can neither be discarded nor attained for it would entail its elimination in the former case and its generation (*i.e.* its having a cause) in the latter. Rejecting both the views we arrive at the doctrine of eternal immutability which is right knowledge (4).

(1) Worldliness entailing births is full of misery. Enlightened Yogins of pure character finding this cycle of births to be full of sorrow, try to bring about its cessation. Attachment brings about sorrow in the end. Aversion brings about direct mental distress resulting in sorrow, while out of latencies of experience of pleasure and pain arise sorrows due to those latencies. Although attachment arises from pleasure and pleasure is derived from attachment, yet in the long run much misery arises therefrom ; this has been clearly shown by the commentator.

Aversion is felt towards painful things and so a feeling of misery is inevitable where there is hatred. When pleasure and pain are experienced, they produce subconscious latencies in the shape of Vāsanā. But Vāsanā being the mould of Karmāśaya, is the source of misery, because the latencies of Vāsanā cause the accumulation of the Karmāśaya.

Aversion is a form of misapprehension, that is why it causes suffering. It might be asked : 'Does not pleasure arise from hatred towards sin ? It does not cause misery.' That is true. Hatred towards sin means hatred towards sorrow. If misery is remedied thereby, it would bring happiness. In effecting the remedy, however, there is sorrow but it is very small, while in the end happiness is greater. Hatred towards sin arises out of experience of misery in it ; so misery out of hatred and hatred out of misery are the two unmistakable signs of hatred.

The ultimate misery arising out of attachment is a future contingency, the affliction due to hatred is for the present, while the latency of sorrow relates to the past. This is the opinion of the author of Maṇiprabhā which is very much like the statement of the commentator, the purport of which is that there is pleasure in attachment, but it brings pain in the long run, while in hatred there is misery both in the present and in the future. From latencies of past experience of pleasure and pain, there is misery in the future. Thus from all the three aspects there is inevitable misery in the future, which should be avoided.

From an analysis of the character of effects it is understood that worldliness is responsible for all miseries. From an examination of the basic cause also it would appear that it is impossible to get pure, uninterrupted pleasure out of the cycle of births. The three Guṇas, Sattva, Rajas and Tamas, constitute the basic ingredient of the mind. By their nature, they work together. If in any state the preponderance of one particular Guṇa is noticed, it is called after that Guṇa, *e.g.* Sāttvika, Rājasika or Tāmasika. A Sāttvika state includes Rajas and Tamas also. Happiness, misery and stupor are respectively Sāttvika, Rājasika and Tāmasika modifications. As in every modification all the three Guṇas are present, there cannot be uninterrupted happiness free from Rajas and Tamas, and on account of the 'subversive' character of the Guṇas their modifications go on dominating one another. That is why misery and stupor are inevitable after happiness. Therefore, it is impossible to get uninterrupted pleasure in this world.

(2) Attempts to derive pleasure by sensuous enjoyment sharpen the senses and intensify attachment, which in the long run cause great unhappiness.

(3) Latency here refers to subconscious impressions of experiences in the shape of Vāsanā—not the latent impressions of pious and impious actions. These latter have been referred to in connection with consequent and afflictive miseries. Vāsanā only produces memory. That memory is of births, longevity and experience. Vāsanā does not produce pain by itself but it being the receptacle of the latent impressions of pious and vicious Karmāśaya becomes the cause of unhappiness. The case is like that of an oven which is not the direct cause of burn but which burns on account of stored burning fuel which causes the burn. Vāsanā is like that. In the oven of Vāsanā the Karmāśaya fuel is stored which causes the burn of misery.

(4) The real nature of the agent which destroys misery cannot be realised because Puruṣa, the destroyer of misery, is neither the cause nor

the effect. Otherwise, Puruṣa becomes mutable and the unalterable state of liberation becomes impossible. Nevertheless the existence of the agent cannot be eliminated altogether, *i.e.* the theory that there is no Puruṣa beyond the mind is not tenable. If that were so, there would be no inclination towards elimination of misery. Cessation of misery and dissolution of the mind are the same thing. If there were no basic entity beyond the mind, there could be no effort for its dissolution. In fact we practise for liberation with the resolution 'let me be free from misery by suspending the activities of the mind.' It is rational to think that 'I shall be free from misery when the activities of the mind are stopped,' *i.e.* there will then remain a pure 'I' free from the pangs of misery. The Self beyond the mind is the real nature of the agent. If the existence of that agent is not admitted, then the question 'for whose sake is liberation being sought ?' cannot be answered.

Therefore both the viewpoints,—that the agent is an object of attainment and that it is not existent, are untenable. The view that the agent in its real nature, *i.e.* the Self, is eternal and immutably existent, embodies right knowledge.

———

भाष्यम्—तदेतच्छास्त्रं चतुर्व्यूहमित्यभिधीयते ।

हेयं दुःखमनागतम् ॥ १६ ॥

दुःखमतीतमुपभोगेनातिवाहितं न हेयपक्षे वर्त्तते, वर्त्तमानं च स्वक्षणे भोगारूढमिति न तत् क्षणान्तरे हेयतामापद्यते । तस्माद् यदेवानागतं दुःखं तदेवाक्षिपात्रकल्पं योगिनं क्लिश्नाति, नेतरं प्रतिपत्तारं, तदेव हेयतामापद्यते ॥ १६ ॥

That is why this Śāstra has been described as consisting of four parts of which

**Pain Which Is Yet To Come Is To Be Discarded** (1). **16.**

Past suffering cannot be avoided as it has already been undergone through experience. Present suffering is operative at the present moment, and cannot therefore be forsaken in the next moment. Hence that pain alone, which has not yet been experienced, troubles the Yogin who is as sensitive as an eye-ball, and not any other perceiver. Therefore that alone is the avoidable pain.

(1) 'What is avoidable' : the most logical and clear answer to that is 'the pain that has not come yet.'

---

भाष्यम्—तस्माद् यदेव हेयमित्युच्यते तस्यैव कारणं प्रतिनिर्दिश्यते—

द्रष्टृदृश्ययोः संयोगो हेयहेतुः ॥ १७ ॥

द्रष्टा बुद्धेः प्रतिसंवेदी पुरुषः, दृश्याः बुद्धिसत्त्वोपारूढाः सर्वे धर्माः। तदेतद् दृश्यमयस्कान्तमणिकल्पं सन्निधिमात्रोपकारि दृश्यत्वेन भवति पुरुषस्य स्वं दृशिरूपस्य स्वामिनः। अनुभवकर्मविषयतामापन्नमन्यस्वरूपेण प्रतिलब्धात्मकं स्वतन्त्रमपि परार्थत्वात् परतन्त्रम्। तयोर्दृग्दर्शनशक्त्योरनादिरर्थकृतः संयोगो हेयहेतुः दुःखस्य कारणमित्यर्थः। तथा चोक्तम् 'तत्संयोगहेतुविवर्जनात् स्यादयमात्यन्तिको दुःखप्रतीकारः', कस्मात्? दुःखहेतोः परिहार्यस्य प्रतिकारदर्शनात्, तद्यथा, पादतलस्य भेद्यता, कण्टकस्य भेत्तृत्वं, परिहारः कण्टकस्य पादानधिष्ठानं, पादत्राणव्यवहितेन वाऽधिष्ठानम्। एतत्त्रयं यो वेद लोके स तत्र प्रतिकारमारभमाणो भेदजं दुःखं नाप्नोति, कस्मात्, त्रित्वोपलब्धिसामर्थ्यादिति। अत्रापि तापकस्य रजसः सत्त्वमेव तप्यं कस्मात्, तपिक्रियायाः कर्मस्थत्वात् सत्त्वे कर्मणि तपिक्रिया नापरिणामिनि निष्क्रिये क्षेत्रज्ञे। दर्शितविषयत्वात् सत्त्वे तु तप्यमाने तदाकारानुरोधी पुरुषोऽनुतप्यत इति दृश्यते ॥ १७ ॥

For that reason the cause of that which has been mentioned as avoidable is being described.

**Uniting The Seer Or The Subject With The Seen Or The Object, Is The Cause Of That Which Has To Be Avoided. 17.**

The Seer is Puruṣa who is the reflector of Buddhi (or pure I-sense) and all that are experienced by Buddhi are the objects (knowables). Like a magnet, the objects of experience act on that which is near them (1) by virtue of proximity.

By their character of being knowables they become the property of Puruṣa whose nature is Awareness ; the knowable (here knowable means Buddhi) becoming the object of experience or action is naturally revealed as something else, *i.e.* like Puruṣa (2), and though independent in itself, it becomes dependent in serving as the object of another, *i.e.* Puruṣa (3). That beginningless alliance between Consciousness and the object is the cause of the avoidable, *i.e.* misery. That is why it has been said (by Āchārya Pañchaśikha) : "By giving up the cause of correlation with Buddhi, this absolute remedy of affliction can be effected," because it is seen that the avoidable cause of trouble can be remedied. For example, the sole of the foot being susceptible to damage from thorn, the piercing power of the thorn can be avoided by not putting the foot on the thorn, or by having a shoe on. One who knows these three can avoid the trouble arising from a thorn by adopting a remedy. How ? By the ability to know the nature of these three. In spiritual experience also the afflictive Guṇa, Rajas, can disturb the Sattva. Why ? Because affliction must operate on an entity which is amenable to mutation. Sattva being amenable to mutation can be disturbed while the Self who is beyond action and mutation cannot be so affected. Since the objects presented by Buddhi are witnessed by Puruṣa, when these are fraught with pain, Puruṣa also appears to be aware of their painful nature (4).

(1) The comparison with the magnet means that although Puruṣa undergoes no change and does not come into contact with the knowable, the object (knowable) on account of its proximity to Puruṣa becomes cognisable. Proximity here does not indicate spatial nearness, but it implies the type of close relationship that exists between the knower and the known, for instance, in the proposition—'I am the knower of it.' In this proposition 'it' or a knowable, is seen or understood by experience as the object of action. The object of action and experience is of three kinds—perceptible, usable (*i.e.* property of being used), and retentive. The usable objects are those of the organs of action, that is, of tangible actions. Retentiveness lies in the action of the Prāṇas and in the latent impress-

ions. They are intangible action and indistinct feeling respectively. While perceptible objects are directly apprehended, usable and retentive objects also are experienced. It is cognised that the knower of these notions is 'I'. That cognition is Buddhi. In the sentence, 'I know also I am the knower of objects,' the self implied by the first 'I' is the pure Seer who is the reflector of Buddhi or the empiric ego (vide I.7).

The nature of the correlation between the Seer and Buddhi is being stated here. It is a fact that there exists a correlation between them which is apparent from such modifications as 'I am the body', 'I am the knower', etc. Asmitā or I-sense is the point of such contact or union.

In order to comprehend the nature and character of this union the different types of such union are to be understood first. When more than one separate thing are perceived as not separate or without any gap between them, they are said to be united. Contact or union may be of three kinds, *viz.* spatial, temporal, or one not distinguished by either time or space.

External objects situated without any intervening gap represent spatial union. It is not necessary to give an example of this. An object may exist in time only, appearing and disappearing in time, *e.g.* the mind, or it may extend over time and space. Union of notions pertaining to them is temporal, for instance the union of the feeling of pleasure etc. with the knowledge thereof. Knowledge is a state of the mind, pleasure is also a state of the mind. As it is not possible for knowledge and the feeling of happiness to be present or felt at the same time, they are really perceived one after the other (it being noted that only what is directly perceived is present) but the interval between the two is neither noticeable nor perceivable. That is why both are regarded as present and are perceived as simultaneous. The union of entities which are beyond time and space is neither in time nor in space. The only instance of such union or contact is the idea of the ultimate Knower and the ultimate knowable as one or united or identical. Like all other forms of knowledge, the knowledge of contact may be both correct and otherwise. When we use the word 'contact' with reference to an actual state of things, such use is correct, *e.g.* the contact between a tree and a bird sitting on it. When, however, through defective vision things, though separate, are regarded as being united, such knowledge of their union is incorrect. But it is true that, whether correct or incorrect, in both cases they appear to the observer as united. 'Contact' or 'union' or a form of 'proximity' is only a word while the united objects are real things. The concept conveyed by a word exists though there may not be a real object beyond it. (The concept of the words may be correct, but there may not be a real entity.)

Action is required for bringing separate things into contact. Such action might be of one, of both, or of the cogniser of the contact. This need not be illustrated, but it is to be noted that if separate things are regarded as united through the action of the cogniser then it is only an incorrect cognition.

The Seer and the primal knowable are not entities extending over time and space. Time and space are forms of knowledge ; therefore the Knower thereof is an entity beyond time and space. Also, the ingredient of that knowledge (*viz.* the three Guṇas) would be naturally something beyond time and space. For these reasons the contact of the Seer and the seen is neither spatial co-existence nor presence at the same time. More so as they are not mental characteristics or substrata thereof, their union cannot be in time. The ultimate Seer and the ultimate seen are not characteristics of anything ; nor are they the aggregates of any real characteristics. Therefore, they are not entities united in time. In Puruṣa there is no such characteristic as past or present, because such things are mutable. Primordial Prakṛti has also no characteristic as past or present. To say Puruṣa (or Prakṛti) 'was' or 'will be' will be tantamount to Viparyaya. The statement Puruṣa (or Prakṛti) 'is' is an example of Vikalpa, attributing notion of time to 'principles' which are beyond both space and time.

Sentience, activity and retention are not characteristics but basic nature of the three Guṇas. The question might be asked in this connection that if activity is mutative, then why should it not be a characteristic ? Basic activity is not mutative but only mutation (*i.e.* 'mutation in itself', not a manifest mutative phenomenon). It is always there. If it had ever been without mutation, then Rajas would have been changeable (by being mutative and non-mutative). In this way the Seer and the seen, being beyond the purview of the characteristic and the characterised, are beyond the touch of time. Thus as they are beyond time and space their contact is a peculiar union in which the two cannot be distinguished by the senses. The Seer and the seen being separate entities, to regard them as not separate is wrong cognition ; therefore misapprehension is the root cause of this (idea of) contact ; hence the aphorism : 'Its cause is nescience.'

Who is the cogniser of the contact ? It is 'I' who am its cogniser, because I think that I am the body etc. as well as that I am the knower. I am the product of that union, therefore how can I be its knower ? Why not ? I come into being or I come to know of it after the contact takes place. During each cognition the knower and the known appear united ; after that by analysis we know that there are separate entities therein as knower and knowable. That is why we say that knowledge is the union of the knower and the knowable ; or in other words, it is the inclusion of two different concepts, *viz.* the knower and the knowable in the same cognition. We think 'I know myself.' This happens because our basis being a self-expressive entity that faculty is present in the ego. That is why although my ego is the result of the contact, I understand that I am both the Seer and the seen.

From whose action does this contact arise ? From the action of the Rajas in the knowable. The sentience being roused by Rajas, *i.e.* the ego appearing as the Seer, is the I-sense or the union between the Seer and the seen. These two entities are capable of producing the idea of the owner and his property (see I.4). I-sense is a knowledge or a sort of sentience representing their union.

How is this contact perpetuated ? By the latent impression of the idea of the contact. From the latency of wrong cognition comes wrong knowledge of ego, and that is how the ego is propagated. Every perception rises and dissolves, and another perception takes place ; that is why this contact has a break and is not continuous. As the knower and the knowable exist from time without beginning, this form of intermittent union (like the I-sense) is like an eternal flow, *i.e.* momentary contact and break are going on from time without beginning (it is, however, to be noted that though it might be beginningless it need not be endless). This flow of non-discrimination having no beginning, the question cannot be asked as to when this contact began. Therefore, the idea entertained by many that once Prakṛti and Puruṣa were separate and suddenly their union took place, is very unphilosophical and irrational. The opposite idea or Viveka which is the knowledge of the Knower and the knowable as being separate would shut out the other (erroneous) knowledge. When other Vṛttis stop, discrimination also ceases like a lamp going out for want of oil. That is break of the contact between the knower and the knowable. It should, however, be noted that Puruṣa is witness equally to (*i.e.* disinterested in) both the contact and its break. This union beyond time and space of the knower and the knowable is indicative of the natural competence of both of them.

The term union or identity applied to the knower and the knowable is only a semantic expression of nearness and it is based on misapprehension. Misapprehension relates to more than one existing thing. As realities constitute its material and subject and since it is also a kind of knowledge, the united objects, *viz.* I-sense, desire, pleasure, pain, etc. arising therefrom are also realities ; liberation from sorrow by true knowledge arising out of real discriminative knowledge is also thus a reality.

The object of knowledge may be real or not, but its knowledge is a reality and it can never be non-existent.

Remaining contiguous is called spatial contact and to go near is called effecting contact. 'Remaining near' is not a thing but a particular arrangement of things. Similarly 'going near' is an action, the result of which is the meaning of the word 'contact'. When things are united or regarded as united, change might be noticed in their properties. For example, when copper and zinc get mixed they become yellow, but if minutely observed, it will be found that they retain their own individualities. Similarly, when the knower and the knowable are regarded as united, the knower appears like the knowable and the knowable like the knower : that is the I-sense and the entire creation born of that union.

Briefly, an analysis of the arguments relating to the union is as follows :

Spatial contact is existence side by side. What is union in time ? Time = flow of moments. Two moments cannot exist simultaneously. So there cannot be uninterrupted simultaneous existence or contact in a point of time. The example of contact in a point of time is the conception of past, present and future states existing at the same time. In other words, when we say that the past and the future are existing, we think that the present, past and the future are there without any break. Therefore contact in a point of time is possible only in the substratum where the threefold characteristics of past, present and future unite.

The union of the Seer and the seen is neither spatial nor in time, *i.e.* it is neither staying side by side nor a conglomeration of characteristics. Knowability is not a characteristic of the Seer, nor awareness that of the seen. They are separate, disunited entities. Their contact or identity is in the ego, because it is felt that a portion of 'I' is the Knower and a portion is the known. We, however, can realise this only later, not at the time when the ego is operative. This union becomes possible on account of their peculiar nature —the power of witnessing of one and of being seen of the other. In this case, to regard two distinct entities as one is wrong cognition, and nescience is the cause of the union. As this wrong knowledge is without beginning, the contact is also regarded as beginningless. When we speak of a seer, it implies something to be seen and when we speak of something as seen, it involves a seer ; the thought of this correlation is inescapable.

(2) The expression 'revealed as something else' means that the knowable is cognised by a nature different from its own, by one whose nature is Consciousness. In reality, the knowable is by nature unrevealed,

It is revealed by contact with pure Consciousness. The position has to be clearly understood. If the sun is partially covered by an opaque substance, the latter appears as a black spot. In fact, by that only a part of the sun is not visible. Imagine that the opaque cover is quadrangular. Then it will have to be said that a quadrangular part of the sun is not being seen. In fact, that quadrangular thing is being known by the light of the sun. The relationship between the Seer and the seen is like that. To know an object (knowable) is not to know the Seer fully.

This is being further elucidated. 'I know a blue object'—in this knowledge of an object, the Seer is also included ('I know that I am knowing'—this is knowledge relating to the Seer). Knowledge of blueness is an aggregate of many subtle actions of the mind each of which is apt to appear and disappear. In fact many actions here mean the continuous flow of their appearance and disappearance. Every disappearance is the state of the Seer staying in Himself and every appearance is the opposite of that state. So the intermediate state between two disappearances is the non-perception of the nature of the Self-in-itself. That is the characteristic of the knowable. As in the previous example the illumination of the sun shows the size of the cover, so also the successive perceptions are manifested by the consciousness of one's own Self. This is why an object is only realisable through another, *i.e.* the nature of the Self.

(3) The knowable, though distinct, is dependent on another as it serves as the object of another. The root cause of the object is the unmanifested. If not seen by the Seer, the object remains unmanifested. Due to its inherent changeability, however, it goes on mutating. In that respect it is an independent entity. But as it is seen by the Seer, it is His object—and as such is dependent. As a matter of fact, all manifest entities are either objects of experience as good or evil or else they are for bringing about liberation. Except serving as an object of Puruṣa, the object has no other purpose of being a knowable. From that point of view an object of knowledge is dependent on or has significance only for the subject or the Knower. It is similar to our everyday experience where entities like cattle etc., though of independent existence, acquire special importance when they serve the practical purpose of man and are under his control.

(4) The sentient state is Sattva. Where there is preponderance of sentience, and mutation and retention (Rajas and Tamas) are much less or at a minimum, that state is known as the sentient state. A sentient state is always pleasant or desirable, because comparative lack of action and more of sentience make a pleasant state of mind. Everyone knows that on the cessation of overactivity or when normal activity is not exceeded,

the feeing that arises therefrom is a pleasant feeling. Normal activity is that which the senses are habituated to perform. When through such action, inertness disappears, the feeling that arises is pleasure. Unless perception is developed and activity remains subdued, pleasurable sensation does not arise. Pleasure and pain, sentience and activity are comparative states. Feeling of bodily comfort means the feeling arising out of the normal working of the system, while uneasiness arises from over-stimulation through external causes. When mental action in the shape of desire is normal it gives pleasure but when it is too much it causes pain. Again, when on getting a wished-for object desire is satisfied (*i.e.* overaction of the mind ceases), pleasure is derived. In stupor, *i.e.* in a state in which there is no sensation of pleasure or pain, there is very little activity and sentience is indistinct. In comparison with that, there is more sentience in pleasure. Therefore, quieter sentient state (Sattva) is inseparable from pleasure while active state or Rajas is associated with pain—mental or physical. When Sattva is overcome by Rajas, pain is felt. That is why the commentator has spoken of Sattva as an objective essence liable to be affected or disturbed by Rajas. Puruṣa who is beyond the three Guṇas cannot be affected by them. He is the unaffected, pure (absolute Consciousness) Seer of disturbances (of the Guṇas) or the lack of these. When Sattva is affected or overcome by excess of activity (of Rajas), this gives the appearance of Puruṣa also being involved. So also when Sattva is dominant, Puruṣa has the appearance of being full of bliss. In reality no such attribute is applicable to Puruṣa who is beyond all change and modifications. These are only imputed to Him. What really happens is, Sattva (which has objective reality) undergoes changes due to the activity of Rajas. Puruṣa is merely the uninvolved onlooker of the different states. This has led to the interpretation that these states (the mutations) are made manifest by Puruṣa.

———

भाष्यम्—दृश्यस्वरूपमुच्यते—

प्रकाशक्रियास्थितिशीलं भूतेन्द्रियात्मकं भोगापवर्गार्थं दृश्यम् ॥ १८ ॥

प्रकाशशीलं सत्त्वं, क्रियाशीलं रजः, स्थितिशीलं तम इत्येते गुणाः परस्परोपरक्तप्रविभागाः संयोगविभागधर्माण इतरेतरोपाश्रयेणोपार्ज्जितमूर्त्तयः परस्पराङ्गाङ्गित्वेऽप्यसम्भिन्नशक्तिप्रविभागास्तुल्यजातीयातुल्यजातीयशक्तिभेदानुपातिनः प्रधानवेलायामुपदर्शितसन्निधाना गुणत्वेऽपि च व्यापारमात्रेण प्रधानान्त-

र्णीतानुमितास्तिताः पुरुषार्थकर्त्तव्यतया प्रयुक्तसामर्थ्याः सन्निधिमात्रोपकारिणोऽयस्कान्तमणिकल्पाः प्रत्ययमन्तरेणैकतमस्य वृत्तिमनु वर्त्तमानाः प्रधानशब्दवाच्या भवन्ति, एतद्दृश्यमित्युच्यते। तदेतद्दृश्यं भूतेन्द्रियात्मकं भूतभावेन पृथिव्यादिना सूक्ष्मस्थूलेन परिणमते, तथेन्द्रियभावेन श्रोत्रादिना सूक्ष्मस्थूलेन परिणमत इति। तत्तु नाप्रयोजनमपि तु प्रयोजनमुररीकृत्य प्रवर्त्तत इति भोगापवर्गार्थं हि तद्दृश्यं पुरुषस्येति। तत्रेष्टानिष्टगुणस्वरूपावधारणमविभागापन्नं भोगः, भोक्तुः स्वरूपावधारणमपवर्ग इति द्वयोरतिरिक्तमन्यद्दर्शनं नास्ति, तथा चोक्तम् 'अयन्तु खलु त्रिषु गुणेषु कर्त्तृषु अकर्त्तरि च पुरुषे तुल्यातुल्यजातीये चतुर्थे तत्क्रियासाक्षिणि उपनीयमानान्सर्वभावानुपपन्नाननुपश्यन्न दर्शनमन्यच्छङ्कत' इति।

तावेतौ भोगापवर्गौ बुद्धिकृतौ बुद्धावेव वर्त्तमानौ कथं पुरुषे व्यपदिश्येते इति, यथा विजयः पराजयो वा योद्धृषु वर्त्तमानः स्वामिनि व्यपदिश्येते स हि तस्य फलस्य भोक्तेति। एवं बन्धमोक्षौ बुद्धावेव वर्त्तमानौ पुरुषे व्यपदिश्येते स हि तत्फलस्य भोक्तेति। बुद्धेरेव पुरुषार्थाऽपरिसमाप्तिर्बन्धस्तदर्थावसायो मोक्ष इति। एतेन ग्रहणधारणोहापोहतत्त्वज्ञानाभिनिवेशा बुद्धौ वर्त्तमानाः पुरुषेऽध्यारोपितसद्भावाः स हि तत्फलस्य भोक्तेति ॥ १८ ॥

The nature of objects (knowables) is being described—

**The Object Or Knowable Is By Nature Sentient, Mutable And Inert. It Exists In The Form Of The Elements And The Organs, And Serves The Purpose Of Experience And Emancipation (1). 18.**

Sentience is the characteristic of Sattva, mutability of Rajas and inertia of Tamas. These three Guṇas are distinct though mutually related, are uniting and separating, and they co-operate to produce manifest forms. Although organically related, their properties do not get mixed up. But when one of them produces effects of homogeneous nature the other two though non-homogeneous operate as associate causes, and they all are always ready to produce homogeneous effects in their states of predominance (2) while when (any two are) subdued their existence can be inferred as subsidiary to the dominant one (3). Through their nature of being the object of Puruṣa and on account of their ability to produce forms they act by proximity as a lodestone or magnet does (4). They, in the absence of an appropriate cause (*i.e.* the exciting cause of merit or demerit), follow the lead of the dominant one (5). These Guṇas go by the name of Pradhāna. These are called objects or knowables, and they exist in the form of elements and are transformed as earth and other gross and subtle elements. Similarly, they exist in the form of sense-organs and are transformed as subtle or gross, auditory and other sense-organs (6). These objects do not operate without purpose. Rather, they act when there is need for serving Puruṣa as His object. Therefore, an object moves only for catering to experience or emancipation of Puruṣa. Of these, the realisation of the essentially beneficial and harmful by identifying the Seer and the seen, is experience, while realising the true nature of Puruṣa is emancipation or Apavarga. There is no other form of knowledge besides these two. That is why it has been said : "Although the three Guṇas are responsible for all actions and mutations, the person not possessing discriminating knowledge looks upon as natural all those experiences which are presented by Buddhi to the fourth principle (Puruṣa) who is really inactive, distinct from Buddhi in spite of some affinity and is only the witness of its modifications. Thus deluded persons do not suspect the existence of an unconditioned Awareness (beyond the empiric ego)."

This experience and emancipation being creations of Buddhi and belonging to Buddhi itself, how can they be attributed to Puruṣa ? As victory or defeat of actual fighters is ascribed to their commander who experiences them so bondage and emancipation being present in Buddhi are ascribed to Puruṣa, who experiences them. Non-completion of the above two objectives of the Self is bondage for Buddhi (7), while their completion is liberation. Thus perception, retention, recollection, elimination, conception and determination although present in Buddhi are assumed to be present in Puruṣa and He is regarded as experiencing them [see I.6 (1)].

(1) Sentient = knowing (in the context of subjective principles) or capable of being known (in the context of objective principles).

Mutable = subject to change.

Inert = opposed to sentience and mobility. All knowledge and all knowables are instances of sentience. All sorts of movement and action are instances of mutation. All forms of latencies and retention are instances of inertness. The sentient and the other constituents get transformed into two series, *viz.* Bhūtas (elements) and senses, *i.e.* that of the objective, physical world outside and that of knowledge, its process and different states. Knowledge involves knowing, acting and retaining impressions of cognitions, feelings and actions, while the physical objective reality stands for knowables, the actions and the retained. Indeed knowledge, action and similar modifications are the outcome of the joint functioning of Sattva, Rajas and Tamas. That is why in each of them sentience, mutability and inertia are traceable. Take, for example, the knowledge of a tree ; its knowledge or cognition aspect is sentience, the particular activity which produces it is mobility or the mutable aspect of it, while the potentialities, which being actualised become the manifest knowledge, constitute its retentiveness or inertia aspect. Thus the awareness that is noticed in the inner faculties, in the sense-organs, in the organs of action and in the Prāṇas, is sentience, the change of state that is noticed is mobility while the stored state of energy, before and after any action or mutation, is retention. This describes sentience, mutability and inertia as forming the series of knowledge. The three Guṇas are found in all knowable objects in the form of perceptible colour, sound ete., motions or actions, and the inert state which resists cognition and action.

In fact, we cannot know anything of Grahaṇa (one's instruments of reception) and Grāhya (knowables) apart from sentience, mutability and inertia. Truly speaking, there is nothing else to be known (as objects) ; sentience, mutability and inertia can be seen everywhere if only we learn to analyse what we see. The external world is introduced by the five elemental properties of light, sound, etc. In sound, for example, there is awareness, action which produces the awareness, and the stored energy which causes the action. Material objects like pot etc. are nothing but a collection of specific knowable characteristics like sound, touch, etc., of the changes involved in them and of particular forms of inertia like hardness etc. In the mind also the three properties of sentience, mutability and inertia are present in the form of cognition, conation and retention or storing of subconscious impressions.

Thus we see that the internal and external worlds are, in the final analysis, made up of only three fundamental Guṇas manifested as the sentient, the mobile and the inert. That whose nature is only sentience is called Sattva. The word Sattva means a thing, *i.e.* what is spoken of as 'it is' or 'it exists' while being known. When it is illumined or understood, it is spoken of as existing ; this is the reason for calling any manifestation, Sattva. The quality of being active is called Rajas. Rajas means dust ; as dust tarnishes so does Rajas tarnish Sattva and that is why it is so called. As action produces change of state, Sattva or steady existence becomes like non-existent or changes into a fluctuating state of appearance and disappearance. That is why action or Rajas is said to upset Sattva. Inertia is Tamas which literally means darkness. Like darkness it is thoroughly homogeneous and so goes unobserved like a covered object. Hence it is called Tamas.

Therefore, sentient Sattva, mutative Rajas and inert Tamas are the basic principles of the external and the internal worlds. There are no other basic principles to be known, *i.e.* there are none. All possible objects of thought come under these three Guṇas.

An object or knowable means anything that is capable of being revealed by Draṣṭā, *i.e.* Puruṣa. In other words, that which is manifested through association with the Knower and is otherwise unmanifested is an object or knowable. The elements and the organs, *i.e.* the knowables and the instruments of reception, constitute the world of objects ; besides these there are no manifest objects. The elements and the organs consist of the three Guṇas ; therefore, the three Guṇas are the basic objects. The difference between objects, as Dṛśya or knowables, and as Grāhya or perceptibles is this : The Dṛśyas are those which are manifested by the Puruṣa while the Grāhyas are those which are perceived by the (bodily) organs.

To the Seer the whole world of objects appears in two ways, *i.e.* all Dṛśyas serve two objectives, experience of pleasure and pain and liberation. Experience means the cognition of an object (Dṛśya) as desirable or as undesirable. Perception of an object implies non-awareness of the discrimination between the Knower and the knowable. Liberation implies realisation of the true nature of the Seer, *i.e.* the discriminative awareness, that the real 'I' or Knower is not an object or knowable, *i.e.* the Seer is different from the object seen. On attainment of this knowledge, there remains no further objective to be served and so it is called Apavarga or liberation or the attainment of the final goal. Then the function of the objective world ceases. Therefore, the characteristics of the object mentioned by the author of the Sūtra are of deep significance, flawless and based on profound knowledge of the truth.

(2) The nature of each different Guṇa is influenced by the nature of the other two Guṇas. Guṇas are perceived in objects which are manifestations of their mutations. In each manifestation, the three Guṇas are combined. When analysed, it shows Sattva on one side, Tamas on on the other, and Rajas in the middle. When we speak of Sattva, Rajas and Tamas are bound to be there. So also it is in the case of Rajas and Tamas.

Thus the Guṇas are influenced by one another. Sentience is always influenced by action and retention. So are also action and retention. Take, for example, the knowledge of sound ; its awareness aspect does not stand alone but is accompanied or tinted, so to say, by vibration and retention.

Uniting and separating refer to association and dissociation of the Guṇas with Puruṣa.

Guṇas combine to produce all objects and they act by mutual co-operation. That is, in Sattva or the Sattva-predominating state, Rajas and Tamas states also remain as auxiliaries. There is no state which is exclusively Sāttvika, Rājasika or Tāmasika. Everywhere there is dominance of one and subordination of the other two.

Just as in a rope made of red, black and white strands the three remain distinct, so do the Guṇas, *i.e.* their properties of sentience, mutability and inertia remain separate, and each retains its characteristic even under the influence of the others. Though unmixed, they are auxiliaries to one another. That is why it is said that 'they exhibit themselves in similar and dissimilar measures etc.' The different properties of the three Guṇas being innumerable, innumerable states are produced by them acting conjointly. The Guṇa that is the principal ingredient of a particular state becomes distinctly manifest in that state as the dominant Guṇa. As ancillary to it, however, other dissimilar Guṇas also become its ingredients. That is, if one Guṇa is dominant in a person, the other two Guṇas will exist in him in a subordinate state. For example, in a celestial body, which is the product of Sāttvika property, the Rājasa and Tāmasa powers are also present as subsidiaries.

During the state of dominance each produces its own effect. Though in certain states, the Guṇas except the dominant one act as auxiliaries, yet when their turn comes they assert themselves when the dominant one loses force as when the king dies, the prince nearest to him ascends the throne.

(3) Even when ancillary, their presence as subservient to the dominant Guṇa can be inferred from the effects, *e.g.* in the knowledge of

sound. The knowledge is predominantly sentient but it can be inferred that Rajas and Tamas are included in it. Activity is not directly visible but we know that no sound is possible without vibration. It can, therefore, be presumed that Rajas in the form of vibration is present in the knowledge of sound which is predominantly sentient.

(4) Nature of being the object of Puruṣa = experience and emancipation are the two states witnessed by Puruṣa. Unless there is witnessing by Puruṣa the Guṇas remain unmanifested. They have then no modifications and they cease to function. Hence their power of producing objects is dependent on Puruṣa's witnessing these, *i.e.* they act for the sake of Puruṣa. As only on account of the witnessing by Puruṣa, the proximate Guṇas provide experience or liberation, they are said to produce result by being near to Puruṣa. This nearness is no spatial proximity but inclusion in the same cognition. 'I am conscious'—in this cognition both consciousness and the insentient instruments of reception are included ; that is the proximity of the Guṇas to Puruṣa [II.17 (1)].

As a lodestone or magnet draws iron whenever it comes near, although it does not enter into the iron, even so the Guṇas without entering into Puruṣa produce effect only by nearness. The word 'Upakāra' means to act by nearness.

(5) 'In the absence of an appropriate cause etc.' = the cause in which a particular Guṇa is dominant constitutes the Pratyaya or mental state. For instance, merit is the cause of Sāttvika modification. Of the three Guṇas the two which have no cause to manifest themselves, remain subsidiary to the dominant one. The Guṇas are collectively known as Pradhāna or Prakṛti. That which is the material cause of an object is called Prakṛti. Primordial Prakṛti is known as Pradhāna. Prakṛti in the shape of the three Guṇas constitutes the material cause of the entire internal and external phenomenal world.

Without a clear idea about the three Guṇas it is very difficult to comprehend Sāṁkhya-yoga or the philosophy of emancipation. That is why they are being described in greater detail here. All objects other than the Self can be broadly divided into two classes, *viz.* Grahaṇa (lit. reception) and Grāhya (lit. cognisable or perceptible). All that are cognised constitute objects, while the instruments of reception are the senses. By these instruments objects are either known, moved or retained. Sound etc. are objects of knowledge, speech etc. are objects of action, and the body, the organs etc. are objects of retention. When sound as an object is analysed, sentient state of the nature of knowledge of sound, mutable state of the nature of vibration and inert state of the nature of potential energy of vibration are obtained. In respect of Sparśa (thermal sense) etc. three similar states are obtainable.

In respect of objects of organs of action like the organ of speech etc. also, the same three states are noticeable. Here the object is sound produced by vocal cords in the form of speech. The three states of sentience, mutability and inertia are also there. In objects where Tamas Guṇa predominates, *i.e.* in retentive objects the same rule applies.

When the organs are analysed, similar three states are found. Take, for instance, the organ of hearing. Its property is to make the sound known. That knowledge (of sound) is its sentient state. The nervous impulse which is excited by external vibration and other actions of the ear are the result of its mutative state. The energy stored in the nerves and muscles which when activated is transformed into knowledge of sound constitutes the retentive or storing function of the ear. Similar is the case with tactile or muscular sense inhering in the organ of action, *e.g.* the hand, which constitutes the sentient aspect ; the movement of the hand constitutes its mutative aspect while the energy underlying the nerves and muscles constitutes the retentive aspect.

These are external organs. When the internal organs are analysed, they similarly reveal the three states of sentience, mutation and retention. In every mental modification there are sentient, mutative and retentive parts.

Thus we know that everything external or internal is like an aggregate of the three states of sentience, mutation and retention. Besides these, there is not, nor can there be, any other fundamental material cause known. Thus Sattva, Rajas and Tamas are the three primal material causes of the world.

There is no action without potential energy and no sensation without action. So sensation must be preceded by action and action by potential energy. The Guṇas are thus inseparably linked. If there is one the other two must be there, but the Guṇa which preponderates will lend its name to the state. Such designation only indicates the relative dominance of one of them. For example, sentience being predominant in knowledge it is called Sāttvika, *i.e.* compared to action it is more sentient. Again, comparing two forms of knowledge if one is more illuminating than the other, it is called Sāttvika knowledge. If anything is called Sāttvika it must be understood that there are Rājasika and Tāmasika elements also included in it. The term Sāttvika applied to an object indicates that it is more sentient in comparison with some other object of the same category. There cannot be anything which would be purely Sāttvika. The same rule applies to Rājasika and Tāmasika.

This phenomenal world can for that reason be divided as Sāttvika or Rājasika or Tāmasika, but in regard to unreal or imaginary things there cannot be any such distinction. Take, for example, the term 'Sattā' which means a state of being or existence. A state of being is nothing but being ; so in this case there being no varieties, no scope of comparison can arise. When the idea denotes a real thing, it will be comparable according to the dominance of the Guṇas. It follows, therefore, that the Guṇas are the material cause of all mutable real things.

(6) The Guṇas constitute the basis of all knowables. Bhūtas or the gross elements and the organs or the instruments of reception are mutations of the Guṇas. Their activity, on account of which they are known, is of two kinds, *viz.* experience of pleasure and pain and emancipation of Puruṣa from the bondage of the Guṇas. The Guṇas are the essence of the objective world while Bhūtas and the organs are their evolutes. The activity of the objects is two-fold—resulting in (i) attachment and (ii) detachment, *e.g.* attachment to worldly objects and attachment to God. The result of the first is continuance of experience or the cycle of births, while that of the second is liberation or cessation of the cycle.

Objectivity is the state of relationship between the subject Draṣṭā and the object Dṛśya. When on account of nescience Draṣṭā and the object appear as of the same kind, then it is called experience. It is of two kinds—apprehension of things as (i) desirable and (ii) undesirable, *e.g.* identification of the Seer and the seen in the ideas 'I am happy' and 'I am unhappy.' When the Seer or subject and the seen or object are perceived to be separate as in 'I am free from pleasure and pain', it is called release (from bondage).

Experience is cognitive ; so is also emancipation. Puruṣa unaffectedly observes both pleasure and pain ; so also it observes liberation. Both experience and liberation are forms of knowledge and the observer of both means the Knower. As by reference to the relationship with Dṛśya (seen), the Draṣṭā (Seer) is so called, so by reference to experience the Seer is called the subject of experience. The knower and the knowable being two different entities, the knower does not change with the mutation of the knowable. That is why the Seer, Puruṣa, is the unchangeable and inseparable cause of witnessing the knowable and the object seen is the mutable cause of that seeing. The commentator has illustrated, by quoting the example of the commander and the soldiers, the unchangeability and inaction of the subject of experience.

Pleasure and pain are by themselves unconscious and characteristics of Buddhi. Pleasure is the state caused by a particular favourable action on the organ of reception. Therefore it is a particular action brought about by an unconscious thing. Only when pleasure is related to the conscious Self the feeling 'I am happy' becomes a conscious state, *i.e.* it appears as conscious. This has been called by the commentator before (I.7) as 'the Self's awareness' of the mental fluctuations. Without relationship with Puruṣa, pleasure becomes insensible, unknowable and unmanifested. Therefore the manifestation of happiness is dependent on the consciousness of Puruṣa. That is why happiness etc. are said to be the objects of experience of Puruṣa. It is because there is reflected consciousness from Puruṣa in the experience of pleasure and pain, that there is an inclination in the empirical self to seek pleasure and avoid pain. There is also an inclination in him to give up both pleasure and pain for the final emancipation.

According to Sāṁkhya philosophy the experiencer is the Knower. Therefore the view that Puruṣa is the enjoyer or knower of experience and liberation is the logical view.

(7) Non-completion of the object of the Self is the non-fulfilment of experience and non-attainment of liberation, while its completion is termination of experience and attainment of liberation. Witnessing of experience is called bondage while witnessing of liberation is called freedom. Thus bondage and freedom are not in Purusa but in Buddhi, the witnessing only is in Puruṣa.

The commentator has enumerated here the basic functions of the internal instruments of knowledge. They are reception, retention, recollection, elimination, conception and determination, and are the result of joint action of the mind and the senses.

Reception is the perception of an object by the sense-organs, organs of action and the Prāṇas. Perception of the state of the mind is also reception. The examples of reception are :—the sensations of light, sound, etc. perceived by sense-organs, the knowledge regarding the art of speech etc. through the organs of action, the feeling of the state of the body by the Prāṇas and the perception of the feelings of pleasure or pain by the mind.

Retention is the state of being retained in the mind of anything that is felt or experienced. All the latent impressions are the result of retention. Reception of retained things is memory or remembrance, it is a kind of cognition and not retention.

Recollection is the recalling of the retained ideas. Things perceived are retained, and to bring them back to mind is recollection.

Elimination is acceptance of certain recollected ideas and rejection of others.

Conception—A concept is a general idea or the idea that assimilates many notions and is formed by a process of elimination ; and conception is knowledge involving concepts. This knowledge may be secular as well as spiritual. Zoology, mineralogy, etc. deal with secular knowledge while knowledge of the principles of gross and subtle elements constitutes spiritual knowledge.

Determination—Acting towards or away from, consequent upon conception. Subsequent to conceptual awareness the decision that an object is desirable or not, takes place and this is determination. The thought-process may be resolved into these six steps. For example, the mind accepts many presentations like blue, yellow, sweet, sour, etc. Then they are retained in the mind. Subsequently in retrospection they are remembered, when by elimination of the particular features generalities are conceived. Thus, light element is the common generalised factor of all colours—blue, yellow, etc. which are its specific forms. Light element is therefore a principle or concept and its knowledge is conception or knowledge of that principle. With the emergence of knowledge of the essential nature in this way, the decision that it is desirable or otherwise is called determination or Abhiniveśa. This is an example of the knowledge about elements ; the ordinary knowledge of pots, clothes, etc. also follows this process [see I.6 (i)].

These six are present in all states of fluctuating minds including that of one-pointedness, while in minds where fluctuations have stopped, these have also stopped. In all objects, worldly or spiritual, there are reception, retention, etc. Reception is direct perception, retention is obscured reception, while effort to recall, selection from recalled things, conception on selected things and determining action thereon, are all retrospections. The knowledge of principles involving no reasoning process is simple reception.

These processes are characteristics of the mind. When Buddhi is impure, reception occurs in Buddhi. But being impure Buddhi does not discriminate between Draṣṭā (Seer) and Dṛśya (seen or knowable). This is due to Avidyā or nescience. When Buddhi is purified the knowledge of the difference between the two becomes clear ; and this is Vidyā or correct knowledge. Thus reception is only attributed to the Seer though it actually takes place in Buddhi. Puruṣa is only the experiencer of the result of reception or a Seer of what is happening in the mind.

भाष्यम्—दृश्यानान्तु गुणानां स्वरूपभेदावधारणार्थमिदमारभ्यते—

विशेषाविशेषलिङ्गमात्रालिङ्गानि गुणपर्वाणि ॥ १६ ॥

तत्राकाशवाय्वग्न्युदकभूमयो भूतानि शब्दस्पर्शरूपरसगन्धतन्मात्राणामविशेषाणां विशेषाः। तथा श्रोत्रत्वक्चक्षुर्जिह्वाघ्राणानि बुद्धीन्द्रियाणि, वाक्पाणिपादपायूपस्थानि कर्मेन्द्रियाणि, एकादशं मनः सर्वार्थमित्येतान्यस्मितालक्षणस्याविशेषस्य विशेषाः। गुणानामेष षोडशको विशेषपरिणामः। षड् अविशेषास्तद् यथा शब्दतन्मात्रं स्पर्शतन्मात्रं रूपतन्मात्रं रसतन्मात्रं गन्धतन्मात्रं च इत्येकद्वित्रिचतुष्पञ्चलक्षणाः शब्दादयः पञ्चाविशेषाः षष्ठश्चाविशेषोऽस्मितामात्र इति। एते सत्तामात्रस्यात्मनो महतः षड़विशेषपरिणामाः। यत् तत्परमविशेषेभ्यो लिङ्गमात्रं महत्तत्त्वं तस्मिन्नेते सत्तामात्रे महत्यात्मन्यवस्थाय विवृद्धिकाष्ठामनुभवन्ति, प्रतिसंसृज्यमानाश्च तस्मिन्नेव सत्तामात्रे महत्यात्मन्यवस्थाय यत्तन्निःसत्तासत्तं निःसदसद् निरसद् अव्यक्तमलिङ्गं प्रधानं तत्प्रतियन्तीति। एष तेषां लिङ्गमात्रः परिणामः, निःसत्ताऽसत्तश्चालिङ्गपरिणाम इति। अलिङ्गावस्थायां न पुरुषार्थो हेतुः, नालिङ्गावस्थायामादौ पुरुषार्थता कारणं भवतीति न तस्याः पुरुषार्थता कारणं भवतीति, नासौ पुरुषार्थकृतेति नित्याख्यायते। त्रयाणान्त्ववस्थाविशेषाणामादौ पुरुषार्थता कारणं भवति स चार्थो हेतुर्निमित्तं कारणं भवतीत्यनित्याख्यायते।

गुणास्तु सर्वधर्मानुपातिनो न प्रत्यस्तमयन्ते नोपजायन्ते। व्यक्तिभिरेवातीतानागतव्ययागमवतीभिर्गुणान्वयिनीभिरुपजनापायधर्मका इव प्रत्यवभासन्ते, यथा देवदत्तो दरिद्राति, कस्मात्? यतोऽस्य म्रियन्ते गाव इति गवामेव मरणात्तस्य दरिद्राणं, न स्वरूपहानादिति समः समाधिः। लिङ्गमात्रम् अलिङ्गस्य प्रत्यासन्नं, तत्र तत्संसृष्टं विविच्यते क्रमानतिवृत्तेः। तथा षड़विशेषा लिङ्गमात्रे संसृष्टा विविच्यन्ते। परिणामक्रमनियमात्तथा तेष्वविशेषेषु भूतेन्द्रियाणि संसृष्टानि विविच्यन्ते। तथा चोक्तं पुरस्तान्न विशेषेभ्यः परं तत्त्वान्तरमस्ति, इति विशेषाणां नास्ति तत्त्वान्तरपरिणामः, तेषान्तु धर्मलक्षणावस्थापरिणामा व्याख्यायिष्यन्ते ॥ १६ ॥

This Sūtra provides the means of knowing the real nature of, and the distinction between, the Guṇas which appear as knowables.

**Diversified (Viśeṣa), Undiversified (Aviśeṣa), Indicator-Only (Liṅga-Mātra), And That Which Is Without Any Indication (Aliṅga), Are The States Of The Guṇas (1). 19.**

Of these, Ākāśa, Vāyu, Agni, Udaka and Bhūmi are the Bhūtas (*i.e.* sound, thermal, light, taste and smell are the elements). They are the diversified varieties of the undiversified Śabda-tanmātra (sound monad), Sparśa-tanmātra (thermal monad), Rūpa-tanmātra (light monad), Rasa-tanmātra (taste monad) and Gandha-tanmātra (smell monad) (2). Similarly the five sense-organs : the auditory, thermal, visual, gustatory and olfactory, the five organs of action : the vocal, manual, locomotive, excremental and procreative, and mind or the eleventh sense which works as organ of perception as well as of sense, are the diversified mutations of the undiversified (mutative) ego. These are the sixteen diversified productions of the Guṇas. The undiversified are six in number (3), *viz.* Śabda-tanmātra, Sparśa-tanmātra, Rūpa-tanmātra, Rasa-tanmātra and Gandha-tanmātra which have respectively one, two, three, four and five characteristics, while the sixth one is (mutative) ego (4). These six are the six undiversified mutations of the pure I-sense which is just the awareness as existence (5). The indicator pure I-sense or Mahat is beyond these six. These undiversified reach the last stage of their development reaching the Liṅga-mātra (indicator-only) state of Mahat. And after having attained that state, they merge, in the reverse process of dissolution, into Pradhāna (6) (Prakṛti) which is neither existing nor non-existing, neither real nor unreal, *i.e.* not a fiction, is unmanifested and Aliṅga (*i.e.* never functions as an indicator). The mutations of the undiversified referred to before are indicator reductions, while further mutation into a state where it is but does not exist, is a change into Aliṅga, *i.e.* non-indicator type or unmanifested state. This state has not Puruṣārtha as its cause, because being an object of Puruṣa it cannot be the primal cause of the unmanifested nor has it been caused for serving the ends of

Puruṣa. It is moreover regarded as eternal (7). Serving as objects of Puruṣa is the cause of the particularised or phenomenal states (diversities, undiversified and indicator). Serving as objects of Puruṣa being the cause, those three states are regarded as non-eternal.

The Guṇas are of pervasive character. They neither disappear altogether, nor are they born (8). They, however, seem to be appearing or disappearing by their past and future individual phenomenal characteristics, and so appear to be subject to birth and death. For example, when we say 'Devadatta is in distress because his cattle are dying' we imply that death of the cattle is the cause of his indigence and not of the loss of his own nature. Such is the case with the Guṇas. The indicator-only, *i.e.* Mahat, is the immediate effect (*i.e.* the first manifestation) of the 'non-indicator' (Aliṅga noumenal Prakṛti). Liṅga-mātra (pure I-sense) existing in the noumenal state (Aliṅga) in an undifferentiated form, manifests itself without disturbing the sequence of mutation (9). The six undiversified, which remain merged in Mahat, separate from it in the same way. Similary, following the law of sequence of mutations, Bhūtas or elements and the organs become differentiated and manifest after having been inherent in the undiversified. It has been said before that the diversified do not admit of further classification from the point of view of principles. There is therefore no mutation into any other form of principles. Their mutations as characteristics, temporal characters and states will be explained later (III.13).

(1) The diversified (Viśeṣas) = which are not common in many. The undiversified (Aviśeṣas) = which are the common properties of many.

The diversified are the sixteen mutations like the Bhūtas and the organs. (These are so called because each of them has diverse characteristics, such as sound, light, perception, etc.) The undiversified are the Tanmātras (which are the causes of the Bhūtas) and Asmitā (which is the cause of the organs and the Tanmātras). These, being only units of sensation and feeling, have no diversities in them. The diversified can be pleasant, unpleasant, and stuporous. The undiversified are free from such characteristics. Things admitting of various distinctions like blue, yellow, sour, sweet, etc. are the diversified ones while those without such distinctions are the undiversified ones. The technical name of the sixteen mutations referred to above is Viśeṣa, and the six from which they have come are known as Aviśeṣa.

What is called Mahat is an indicator-only (Liṅga-mātra). Although from its nature it is an Aviśeṣa, still Liṅga or indicator is its proper enunciation. Liṅga means indicator. That which is the indicator of another is called its Liṅga. Mahat-tattva is the indicator of the Self and the unmanifested (Prakṛti). That is why it is their Liṅga. Liṅga-mātra means the real or chief indicator. The senses may be the indicator of Puruṣa and Prakṛti but they are chief indicators of their respective (immediate) causes. Mahat is the Liṅga or indicator of Puruṣa and Prakṛti. Aliṅga = Prakṛti, which is not the indicator of anything.

Diversified Liṅga, undiversified Liṅga, only Liṅga, and non-Liṅga are the four sections of the Guṇa trio. That is why they are called the sections or states of the Guṇas.

(2) Ordinary water, earth, etc. do not constitute the Bhūtas or elements. That whose characteristic feature is sound is Ākāśa. Similarly, tactile sense (thermal sense, not common touch), visual sense, gustatory sense and olfactory sense are respectively the characteristic features of Vāyu, Tejas, Ap and Kṣiti, *i.e.* gross elements From the point of view of principles, the Bhūtas known as Vāyu, Kṣiti, etc. are nothing but entities with features mentioned above. Earth, water, etc. are only mixtures of those elements, *i.e.* they are aggregates of all those principles.

From the point of view of cause it is found that Ākāśa is the cause of Vāyu, Vāyu is the cause of Tejas, Tejas of Ap and Ap of Kṣiti. Scientific investigation shows that if the vibrations of sound are stopped it produces heat, heat produces light, and from light (sun's rays) all chemicals (like vegetable products) are formed. Finest particles of the chemicals give rise to the sense of smell. In the Mahābhārata we find that before the creation of the Bhūtas, there was an all-pervading sound, which was followed by Vāyu, then heat, then water, and last of all came the hard Kṣiti or earth. Thus from the point of view of cause it will be seen, that which has the property of sound is succeeded by that which has the thermal sense, and so on. In this way an object of olfactory sense is the receptacle of five properties. That which is of the gustatory sense is the receptacle of four properties except the olfactory sense, that of visual sense is the receptacle of three properties, that of the thermal sense the receptacle of two, while the receptacle of sound has only sound. At the time of the final dissolution, the inverse process takes place and earth dissolves into water and water into heat, and so forth. Although in practice the Bhūtas evolve from Ākāśa onwards, from the point of view of principles, *i.e.* from the point of view of basic material cause, it is not so. There Śabda-tanmātra is the cause of gross sound, Sparśa-tanmātra is the cause of gross touch and so on.

Viewed from the standpoint of sensations, the perception of smell arises from contact with the particles of matter, taste arises from the chemical action caused by a liquid substance. From heat comes perception of colour, that is, a particular kind of heat and a particular colour are inseparably connected. Feeling of touch mainly arises from contact with gaseous matter. Our skin is surrounded on all sides by air. The sense of heat or cold mainly arises from the temperature of the surrounding air. With the sense of sound arises a sense of emptiness or void. Thus with the states of hardness, liquidity, etc. there is a relationship with the knowledge of the Bhūtas. Hardness, liquidity, etc. however arise from difference of temperature. They are not the Guṇa principles.

Therefore, considered theoretically, the Bhūtas are only mere entities of sound, touch, etc. In practice, however, with those principles, their attendant features, *e.g.* hardness etc., have to be recognised. That is why when realisation of the Bhūtas is attempted through Saṁyama, hardness etc. have to be felt.

The Bhūtas or gross elements like Kṣiti etc. are the Viśeṣas of the Tanmātras or monads like smell etc. The word Viśeṣa, or the diversified, has been used here in three senses, first, to indicate the diversities of the notes of the scale of octaves of sound ; heat, cold, etc. (thermal) ; blue, yellow, etc. (light) ; sweet, sour, etc. (taste) ; good and bad smell etc. (smell). Each of the Bhūtas has such diversities. The Tanmātras have no such varieties. Secondly, the three states of quietness, excitement and stupor are the diversities ; the varieties of sound etc., and the varieties like quietness etc. go together. Unless there is knowledge, *i.e.* appreciation of the diversities such as in the scale of sound, heat, cold, etc., worldly happiness, misery or infatuation cannot arise. Thirdly, the Bhūtas being the final (lowest form of) mutations, (*i.e.* not being the cause of further modifications) are called the Viśeṣas. Thus the characteristics of the Bhūtas can be summarised as follows : That which is endowed with the property of various sounds and causes pleasure, misery and stupor, is Ākāśa ; that which is endowed with the property of various kinds of touch and causes pleasure etc. is Vāyu ; similarly of Tejas etc. These are the five kinds of Bhūtas ; these are knowable and Viśeṣas.

The Viśeṣas known as the organs are generally counted as eleven. These are of two kinds, external and internal. The external organs deal with external objects. Mind, the internal sense, deals with objects like sound, sensations, etc. presented to it by the external organs and the feelings caused by internal causes, happiness and effort.

The external organs are generally divided into two classes, *viz.* the sense-organs of cognition and the organs of action. The Prāṇas or the vital forces being included in them are not counted separately but they are also external organs. The cognitive sense-organs are Sāttvika in character, organs of action are Rājasika and Prāṇas, Tāmasika. Each of them has five members. Thus there are five cognitive sense-organs, *e.g.* ear, the recipient of sound ; skin, receiver of the sense of touch in the form of heat or cold ; eye takes in colour ; tongue takes in taste and the nose takes in smell. The organs of action are tongue relating to spoken words ; the hands relating to art and craft ; the legs relating to locomotion ; anus relating to excretion ; and the reproductive organs relating to reproduction. Prāṇa, Udāna, Vyāna, Apāna and Samāna are the five Prāṇas or vital forces. The function of Prāṇa is to sustain the organs of perception of external objects ; Udāna sustains the tissues of the body ; Vyāna sustains the organs of movement of the body ; Apāna sustains the function of excrement or elimination and Samāna sustains the power of assimilation.

Mind is an internal organ. It makes resolve regarding objects. Correct supposition, *i.e.* reception, action and retention, is resolve. Voluntary use of knowable objects is resolve or volition.

The five Bhūtas, ten external organs and the mind—these sixteen are Viśeṣas or the diversified. They are not the causes of other modifications. They are the final modificatians.

(3) The undiversified or Aviśeṣas are six in number. The five Tanmātras (monads) are the causes of the five Bhūtas (elements) and Asmitā or Ahaṁkāra is the cause of the Tanmātras and the organs.

The word Tanmātra means 'that alone' or 'that only', *i.e.* sound alone, touch alone, etc., *e.g.* subtle sound (atom of sound), without the variation or diversity, is known as sound Tanmātra. Same is the case with touch and other Tanmātras. The other epithet of Tanmātra is Paramāṇu or atom. Atom does not mean minute (tangible) particles but the subtle sensations of sound, touch, etc. The subtle state into which the different varieties of sound, touch, etc. disappear, is known as Tanmātra. The atom is such a subtle state of sound and similar objects. Its spatial extent cannot be clearly perceived. As a matter of fact it is conceived as constituting the flow of time. For example, external sound appears to occupy extensive space, but when it is meditated upon as a subtle perception within the ear, it appears only as a flow of time. In realising atoms of sound, light, etc. they have to be conceived as subtle actions of the senses, and that is why they are realised like activity in a flow of time. Moreover, they are not realised as something occupying extensive space, *i.e.* as a divisible entity. A body which is not divisible is known as an atomic body. Tanmātra is such an atomic body. No material object smaller than an atom can be conceived. Such an atom has to be realised by a mind in deep concentration. No subtler external object can be realised even by such a mind (as in further concentration the connection with objects is broken). The atom, as recognised in Sāṁkhya, is not a matter of theory alone. It is an external object that can be directly experienced.

The general rule mentioned before that thermal sense evolves out of an object having the quality of sound, colour out of an object having the property of touch, taste out of an object having the property of colour, and smell out of an object having the property of taste is not applicable in respect of the Tanmātras. The Tanmātras have emanated from I-sense. The perception of smell arises with the help of minute particles. Therefore, that which produces the perception of smell Tanmātra can also produce perception of taste, colour, touch and sound. Thus sound Tanmātra has been said to have one quality, touch (thermal) two qualities, colour three qualities, taste four qualities and smell five qualities. Naturally, however, at the time of realisation, each Tanmātra is realised through its particular property.

(4) Asmitā = I-sense, *i.e.* the pretentious feeling relating to self. The word Asmitā refers also to the knowledge having 'I' as its determinandum (*i.e.* pure I-sense). Here it means I-sense. It has been said before (II.6) that identification of the organ of reception with supreme consciousness is Asmitā. From that point of view Buddhi is pure Asmitā or the subtlest form of egoism. Asmitā-mātra does not always denote Mahat. In the present context it is the common constituent of the six sense-organs, the common ego. Both Buddhi and mutative I-sense, which is the common constituent of all senses, are called Asmitā-mātra. When the term Asmīti-mātra is used it refers only to Mahat or pure I-sense.

The relationship of other sense-organs with the Self is also due to Asmitā, which produces the conception 'I am endowed with the power of hearing' etc. Thus the combination of one's ego with the organs of reception creates I-sense which is Abhimāna. In fact, the organs are only the different states or modifications of Asmitā. From external appearance the seats of the different organs appear as particular arrangements of the Bhūtas. Truly speaking, the Indriyas or the organs are the internal energies by which the Bhūtas are arranged in a peculiar manner. Internal sense energy is in fact a particular form of the I-sense or Asmitā. On account of the presence of ego, the whole body is conceived as 'I'. The sense-organs of cognition, the organs of action, the Prāṇas and Chitta or mind are different states or mutations of Abhimāna. For example, eye = I-sense inherent in the eye, *i.e.* ego taking the form of the eye. When this is activated by the action called 'light', the concept of light is formed. Knowledge of light implies the sense of identification of the Knower with the sensation of light. In other words, an external activity producing a change in the I-sense being attributed to the knower, is knowledge of light. This feeling of relationship between the knower and the known, *e.g.* 'I am the knower of light', is the ego called Asmitā. Asmitā is the common constituent of the organs and the sixth Aviśeṣa or undiversified principle.

(5) Self as cognition of unqualified existence = the awareness that 'I exist' or pure I-sense. The property of Buddhi or Mahat as a principle is the feeling of assurance. The feelings of assurance and existence are inseparable. Assurance in respect of a thing and that of self are both attributes of Buddhi. Of these, the one in respect of self is the final assurance. That is why it is the real nature of Buddhi. Assurance in respect of an object is a distracted modification of Buddhi. Therefore, 'I exist' or a convincing knowledge of self, or self as a pure entity, is the Mahat principle.

Modifications like 'I am the seer', 'I am the hearer', 'It is I who smell', 'It is I who am moving', etc. are possible if the conception of 'I' exists at the root. Such mutation or modification of 'I' is Ahaṁkāra. Thus from the feeling of self as an entity, which is Mahat, arises Ahaṁkāra, *i.e.* Mahat-tattva is the cause of Ahaṁkāra.

Analysing one's ego in this way it will be seen that Mahat is the first manifestation. Its modification is Asmitā, whose modifications are the senses. Tanmātras of sound etc. are also modifications of Asmitā.

The perceptible part of sound etc. is only a modification of our Asmitā, and the external action from which sound etc. emanate is a mutation of the ego of the great Brahma or Hiraṇyagarbha. Thus in both respects sound etc. are the modifications of Asmitā.

The commentator says that Mahat undergoes six undiversified modifications in the shape of Tanmātra and Asmitā. Sāṁkhya says that from

Mahat evolves Ahaṁkāra and from Ahaṁkāra come the five Tanmātras. Some say that this is a point of difference between the Sāṁkhya and the Yoga philosophies. There is, however, no real difference. In fact, the observation of the commentator is this—Liṅga-mātra is the cause of the six Aviśeṣas or undiversified states. Taking the latter states as one species, he has spoken of Mahat as their cause. In doing so he has not taken into consideration the fact that there exists a sequence of cause and effect in the Aviśeṣas also. For example, Mahat is not the immediate cause of Tanmātras like sound etc. but is their mediate cause. Similarly, the commentator has said that the Guṇas are the cause of the sixteen modifications. The Guṇas are really the root cause. In the commentary on Sūtra I.45 the commentator has spoken of the sequence in describing Ahaṁkāra as the cause of the Tanmātras, and Mahat-tattva as the cause of Ahaṁkāra.

(6) The Mahat principle gives rise to the six Aviśeṣas. From the Mahat comes Ahaṁkāra or I-sense, and the undiversified emerge from Asmitā in the following order—sound Tanmātra, thermal Tanmātra, light Tanmātra and the like.

Therefore, it is not quite correct to say that the six Aviśeṣas have evolved straight out of Mahat. The commentator also does not mean it. The correct order of succession is from Mahān Ātmā (lit. the great Self) or Mahat to Ahaṁkāra, from Ahaṁkāra to the five Tanmātras and from Tanmātras to the five Bhūtas. From Ākāśa (sound element) came Vāyu (thermal element), from Vāyu came Tejas (light element)—this order of sequence is only applicable to the qualities of hardness etc. which are inseparable from the perception of smell etc. This is true from the material standpoint but not so from the standpoint of Tattvas or of material causation. Sensation of sound cannot be the material cause of the thermal sensation. The material cause, Asmitā, can, however, be changed by the activity called sound to appear as a thermal sensation [see ante II.19(2)]. Thus subtle sound (monad) can be the cause of gross sound, from which it is established that from sound Tanmātra comes Ākāśa-bhūta, from thermal Tanmātra comes Vāyu-bhūta etc. Therefore, from Asmitā have come all the Tanmātras, and from them have come the appropriate Bhūtas.

The six undiversified evolve gradually from Mahat, which is the first manifestation. They attain their ultimate development in the sixteen mutations. At the time of dissolution, they disappear in a reversed manner and after reaching the state of Mahat merge in the unmanifested state. That is when on account of complete cessation of activity, Mahat merges into Prakṛti, the Viśeṣas and Aviśeṣas, which lie submerged in Mahat, also follow suit. When Mahat disappears nothing in the form of action remains manifest in that state. That state is known as Avyakta or the unmanifested. The commentator has given a few more epithets of that non-indicator Pradhāna (chief), the primary cause. They are now being explained.

Niḥsattāsatta = Neither with nor without Sattā. Sattā means a state of existence. Everything existing or manifest is an object of Puruṣa. Therefore, Sattā means 'being the object of Puruṣa'. To us, in ordinary circumstances, Sattā and being the object of Puruṣa are inseparable. In the unindicated unmanifested state, there being no objective of Puruṣa to be fulfilled, Pradhāna is Niḥsatta or without phenomenal existence. Since, however, it is not a nonentity (existing as it does as the material cause of the object of Puruṣa), it cannot be said to be non-existing. Therefore, it is neither Sattā nor devoid of Sattā.

Niḥsadasat = Neither Sat, *i.e.* existing nor Asat, *i.e.* non-existing. That which is not manifestly existing and serving as knowable like Mahat etc., and which being the cause of Mahat is not non-existent, is Niḥsadasat. The terms Niḥsattāsatta and Niḥsadasat have been used from the two preceding points of view. Nirasat (not fictitious)—The commentator has again used this term separately lest anyone should imagine Pradhāna to be some fictitious or utterly unreal thing. Unmanifested Pradhāna is knowable but not directly as manifest objects Mahat etc. are. Mahat and others are knowable by manifest activities while Pradhāna is knowable as their potential state. It is known by inference.

Hence Pradhāna is Nirasat (not unreal) or a particular existing entity. Avyakta = that which is not manifest or realisable. The state into which all manifested things merge is known as the Avyakta or unmanifested state.

(7) Although Prakṛti is their material cause, all manifested objects like Mahat etc. are manifested by being the object of Purusa through being witnessed by Him. Hence such objectiveness is the instrumental cause of the manifestation of Mahat etc. But this objectiveness is not the cause of the unmanifested state. Pradhāna is eternally present ; its manifestation on mutation as Mahat and its evolutes takes place because of their being the object of Puruṣa. They are mutating from time without beginning, but are impermanent because they cease when they cease to serve the purpose of Puruṣa. They are also impermament, because their existence is subject to appearance and disappearance.

(8) All manifested objects are products of the Gunas ; so the three

Guṇas can nowhere become extinct. The unmanifested state is a state of equilibrium of the three Guṇas. That is a state of dissolution of manifested objects no doubt but it is not a dissolution of the three Guṇas. On the manifestation and disappearance of an object, the three Guṇas look like manifested and dissolved, but in reality there is no increase or decrease in the three Guṇas nor is there any possibility thereof. When they are not manifest, the three Guṇas exist in the unmanifested state. The example cited by the commentator in this connection means that when Devadatta is without a cow he is poor, but he is not so when he has it. As Devadatta's affluence and indigence are caused by the possession of an external object or lack of it and not by his physical ailments, so from the appearance and disappearance of objects the three Guṇas seem to appear and disappear, but in reality the three Guṇas neither appear nor disappear. Because they have no antecedent cause, there is no rise (*i.e.* emergence from cause) or disappearance (submergence into cause) for them.

(9) Without disturbing the sequence = as it is not possible to transgress the progress of evolution. From the unmanifested (Prakṛti) comes Mahat ; from Mahat comes Ahaṁkāra, from Ahaṁkāra come the Tanmātras and the organs, from the Tanmātras come the Bhūtas. This sequence of evolution has been mentioned before and it is to be noted that evolution follows this sequence. Not having spoken of the sequence explicitly before, the commentator has stated it here.

The Viśeṣas do not undergo any further change in basic principle. The Ākāśa-bhūta, having the property of sound, is not changed into any other principle. Principle or Tattva means the common basis or material, *e.g.* the common ingredients of external material objects are Akāśa, Vāyu, etc. They are known by different organs of perception. The gross basic principles or elements (Bhūtas) can be fully established by cognitions obtained in concentration on such objects with the help of words (Vitarkānugata Samādhi I.42). By that Yogic knowledge the gross Bhūtas like Ākāśa etc. and the gross organs like ear etc. cannot be analysed any further. There are, no doubt, different varieties of sound, light, etc., but all of them come within the category of sound and light ; so there is no change in their basic principle. Similarly in animals there might be eyes with distinctive traits but all come within the principle of visual organ ; thus such distinctiveness does not indicate any change in the basic principle. That is why it has been said that the Viśeṣas or the diversified have no further modification as basic principles. The Viśeṣas can be realised in their causal forms as Aviśeṣas or the undiversified through a subtle form of cognition obtained in Savichāra and Nirvichāra concentrations.

---

भाष्यम्—व्याख्यातं दृश्यम्, अथ द्रष्टुः स्वरूपावधारणार्थमिदमारभ्यते—

द्रष्टा दृशिमात्रः शुद्धोऽपि प्रत्ययानुपश्यः ॥ २० ॥

दृशिमात्र इति दृक्शक्तिरेव विशेषणापरामृष्टेत्यर्थः, स पुरुषो बुद्धेः प्रतिसंवेदी, स बुद्धेर्न सरूपो नात्यन्तं विरूप इति। न तावत् सरूपः, कस्मात्? ज्ञाताज्ञातविषयत्वात् परिणामिनी हि बुद्धिस्तस्याश्च विषयो गवादिर्घटादिर्वा ज्ञातश्चाज्ञातश्चेति परिणामित्वं दर्शयति, सदाज्ञातविषयत्वन्तु पुरुषस्यापरिणामित्वं परिदीपयति, कस्मात्? न हि बुद्धिश्च नाम पुरुषविषयश्च स्याद् गृहीताऽगृहीता च, इति सिद्धं पुरुषस्य सदाज्ञातविषयत्वं, ततश्चापरिणामित्वमिति।

किञ्च परार्था बुद्धिः संहत्यकारित्वात्, स्वार्थः पुरुष इति। तथा सर्वार्थाध्यवसायकत्वात् त्रिगुणा बुद्धिस्त्रिगुणत्वादचेतनेति, गुणानां तूपद्रष्टा पुरुष इति, अतो न सरूपः। अस्तु तर्हि विरूप इति। नात्यन्तं विरूपः, कस्मात्? शुद्धोऽप्यसौ प्रत्ययानुपश्यो यतः प्रत्ययं बौद्धमनुपश्यति तमनुपश्यन्न तदात्माऽपि तदात्मक इव प्रत्यवभासते। तथा चोक्तम् 'अपरिणामिनी हि भोक्तृशक्तिरप्रतिसंक्रमा च परिणामिन्यर्थे प्रतिसंक्रान्तेव तद्वृत्तिमनुपतति तस्याश्च प्राप्तचैतन्योपग्रहरूपाया बुद्धिवृत्तेरनुकारमात्रतया बुद्धिवृत्त्यविशिष्टा हि ज्ञानवृत्तिरित्याख्यायते' ॥ २० ॥

The knowables having been described, this Sūtra is introduced to determine the real nature of the Seer.

**The Seer Is Absolute Knower*. Although Pure, Modifications (Of Buddhi) Are Witnessed By Him As An Onlooker. 20.**

The expression 'absolute knower' means unconditioned apperception (1). This Puruṣa (Seer) is the reflector of

* The use of the two words Draṣṭā and Dṛśimātra derived from the same root Dṛś (= to see) implies that Puruṣa is not the 'seer' in the usual meaniug ascribed to the term, because that would be imputing quality and action to Puruṣa who is beyond both. Dṛśimātra is a closer approximation of Puruṣa.

Buddhi. He is neither similar nor dissimilar to Buddhi. Not similar, because an object of knowledge can be known or unknown to Buddhi ; therefore Buddhi is mutative. The objects of knowledge, like cow (animate), pot (inanimate), though existing separately get known by colouring the Buddhi and become unknown when they do not do so. This character of knowing some objects and not knowing others indicates the mutative nature of Buddhi. On the other hand the fact that Puruṣa is ever aware illustrates His non-mutativeness, because Buddhi witnessed by Puruṣa cannot be sometimes apprehending and sometimes non-apprehending, *i.e.* it is always apprehending. Thus the ever present awareness of Puruṣa is established, and the immutability of Puruṣa is also proved (2).

Moreover, Buddhi serves the purpose of another since it acts in conjunction with others, while Puruṣa is the end in Himself (3). Furthermore, Buddhi being the faculty of generating assured cognition of all objects, is composed of the three Guṇas and is in itself unconscious*. Puruṣa is the witness or onlooker of the Guṇas (4). For these reasons Puruṣa is not similar to Buddhi. Is He then dissimilar ? No, not entirely dissimilar (5), because though pure in Himself, He sees or illuminates the cognitional states in Buddhi and thus, though different from these, He appears to be united with them.

That is why it has been said by Pañchaśikha : "The supreme entity to which experiences are due is not mutable nor transmissible. It appears to be transmitted to and follow the mutative modifications of Buddhi, which thereby seems to be endowed with consciousness, and thus pure Awareness appears to be identical with them (6)."

(1) Seer (Draṣṭā) = Immutable Knower. Knower (Grahītā) = mutable knower. The Seer and the knower are similar but not the same. The

* Buddhi is unconscious so long as it has no volitional exciting cause. It possesses and exhibits consciousness because of the existence of Puruṣa as witness.

Seer is always a Seer of Himself; the knower is a knower when it knows, but not so when it does not. 'I am the knower'—Buddhi taking this form, is the knower (Grahītā).

Absolute Knower is pure Consciousness. The word Dṛśi means knowing not subject to any condition, *i.e.* consciousness in itself. The idea that 'I exist' is first felt and then expressed. It is subject to a condition because it is a form of Buddhi. But the root of the idea of 'I', which is antecedent to that idea, and which we try to express in words, is not dependent on any condition. Śruti also says: "By what else can the Knower be known?" "The knowing principle of the Knower is never absent." What such conditions seek to reveal is an object, and the conditions themselves are also objects, therefore that which is the Seer is not an object that depends for its manifestation on some condition. Consciousness intrinsic to the knower, *i.e.* consciousness that is the essence of the Seer, is 'self'-consciousness. Seer = seer of self, *i.e.* the illuminer of Buddhi, which cognises itself as 'I am the knower.'

As long as there is something to be seen Puruṣa is to be called the Seer, but when the object to be seen (knowable) disappears the question may be raised, how can the Puruṣa be called a Seer? In reply it can be said: Do not use the appellation 'seer' if you like, then the proper word to use would be like 'knowing in itself', 'unconditioned consciousness' etc. If, however, the word 'seer' is used it would indicate the 'seer' of a mind dissolved in peace. It must be remembered that the use of different expressions does not change the nature of a real thing. Pure Consciousness (Chit) is not really a characteristic of the Seer, as Seer and Consciousness are one and the same. That is why the Seer is said to be Consciousness itself.

The word 'absolute' in 'absolute awareness' implies the negation of all qualifications and characteristics. Therefore, that which is free of all characteristics is the Seer. In the Sāṁkhya-sūtra we get the definition that 'on account of absence of any attribute, awareness is not a characteristic (of Puruṣa)'. It might be questioned why Puruṣa is then given the predicates 'unlimited', 'untransmissible', etc.

In fact the term 'unlimited' is not an adjunct nor a characteristic, but it denotes the absence of a particular characteristic. 'Untransmissible' is also similar. By negating the existence of limit and other characteristics which are generally described by use of adjectives, the idea of absence of all attributes is brought out. Negating limitation, mutation and other similar common characteristics of objects, the Seer is indicated.

Puruṣa is the reflector of Buddhi. This has been explained in Sūtra I.7(5).

(2) The commentator has mentioned the characteristics which distinguish Buddhi from Puruṣa. They are : (a) Buddhi is mutable, Puruṣa is immutable ; (b) Buddhi is a means, Puruṣa is an end in Himself ; (c) Buddhi is unconscious, Puruṣa is conscious or unconditioned consciousness. The difference between the two is known in this way. Although they are different there is some similarity between the two. In the absence of discriminative knowledge, Puruṣa appears like Buddhi and Buddhi like Puruṣa, and this appearance of sameness through lack of discriminative knowledge constitutes that similarity.

The arguments by which the similarity and difference between Puruṣa and Buddhi are established are being explained here. The objects of Buddhi are sometimes known and sometimes unknown, that is why Buddhi is mutable ; while the object of Puruṣa is always known, hence Puruṣa is immutable. The objects of Buddhi, *e.g.* cow, pot, etc. are sometimes known, and sometimes unknown. When the idea of the object appears in the mind and stays there, then the mind is similarly coloured, *e.g.* sometimes like a cow, sometimes like a pot. But Buddhi illumined by Puruṣa is always conscious. Puruṣa-viṣaya means 'of which Puruṣa is the object'. Buddhi, of which Puruṣa is the object, always appears like the knower, while Buddhi, of which the objects are sound etc., sometimes appears as known and sometimes as unknown. As Puruṣa makes Buddhi His object, *i.e.* manifests it, so Buddhi also makes Puruṣa its object, *i.e.* knows its basic illuminer as 'I am the seer'. Thus the expressions 'Puruṣa is the object of Buddhi' and 'Buddhi is the object of Puruṣa' mean almost the same.

In brief, since the objects of Buddhi, *i.e.* sound etc. are known at one time and not at another, what is knowledge of sound at one time becomes a knowledge of a different object later ; this indicates the mutability of Buddhi. On the other hand, the Buddhi of which Puruṣa is the object, *i.e.* which shows Puruṣa (the conception 'I know myself') never becomes 'I do not know myself'. As long as there is Buddhi it will be 'I know myself'. Buddhi indicating 'I do not know myself' is an unreal, unimaginable thing. Therefore, the awareness of Puruṣa is ever manifest and is never unmanifested or unknown. Thus He is an immutable unconditioned Awareness. When Buddhi is not there, *i.e.* when it merges in its causal substance, it will not be manifested. That also is a mutation of Buddhi. That will not affect the illuminer in the least. Buddhi is witnessed by its illuminer by virtue of its intrinsic power of activity. When that is not done, nothing happens to the illuminer, only Buddhi remains unmanifested.

Buddhi coloured by objects assumes different forms after the objects, while that relating to Puruṣa becomes like 'I know myself' but never 'I do not know myself'. That is why the real knower indicated by it is immutable. 'I am the knower'—this idea is Buddhi relating to Puruṣa. If it could be shown or even imagined that this form of Buddhi is ever 'not known' then Puruṣa would have been both knower and non-knower, *i.e.* mutable.

The idea 'I' is directly receptive, while 'I was' or 'I shall be' is reflective. Memory, wish, etc. are reflective. Reflection cannot take place without a reflector. That which in the shape of consciousness produces cognizance is the reflector. No cognition is imaginable without such a reflector, because every cognition is a reflected one. Therefore, any cognition unperceived by Buddhi, whose object is its reflector, Puruṣa, would be even more inconceivable than a sixth external sense. The receiver I-sense being always cognised, the Seer of the receiver is immutable Consciousness. Otherwise a fanciful thought like an unperceived receiver or unknown I-sense would arise. In other words, when it is impossible for the cognition of the form 'I am the knower' to be absent, then it must be always known. The knower of constant knowledge is constant. When it is always a knower and never a non-knower then it must be something like immutable consciousness.

For example, in 'I know myself', 'I' am the Seer or cogniser and 'myself', *i.e.* the rest of 'I', is the unconscious portion—Buddhi. Knowledge of objects (like colour, sound, etc.) is only supplementary to the cognition 'I know myself.' If the blue colour is looked at subtly through Samādhi, then it no longer continues as blue but becomes an atom of light which, if subtlety is carried on further, merges into an unmanifested state. Thus knowledge of an object is only a knowledge of relative truth regarding it. To know it in its unmanifested state, *i.e.* in its state of three Guṇas in equilibrium, is true knowledge. The Seer then is established in Himself. Knowing that, to realise that the Knower is the knower of self is to have complete knowledge concerning the Seer.

In the Śāstras, in the expression 'See the Self in the self,' one self refers to Buddhi and the other to Puruṣa. Puruṣa and Prakṛti being eternal, this self-evident relationship of Seer and seen exists. Taking only one of the entities, *e.g.* only Chit (conscious) or only Achit (unconscious), this relationship of seer and seen cannot be properly explained. As this part of the commentary is very difficult, so much explanation has been offered.

(3) The reason for the other point of difference between Buddhi and Purusa is that as Buddhi works in association with others it is a means to

an end, while Puruṣa is an end in Himself. Any action, which is the result of combination of many forces, is not for any one nor for all the forces combined. When many forces combine to produce an action, the action is for the one who engages them to act in unison. Buddhi and the senses with the help of many forces produce results which give pleasure or pain. The experiencer of those results, *i.e.* the ultimate Knower, is neither Buddhi nor the senses but Puruṣa who is behind them. Hence Buddhi serves the purpose of, or is the object of another, while Puruṣa exists for His own self, *i.e.* He is the enjoyer. This point will be further discussed in the fourth part of the book.

(4) The third argument on this subject is that Buddhi is in itself unconscious while Puruṣa is pure Consciousness. Buddhi is mutative. Whatever mutates has activity, manifestation and non-manifestation, and so is composed of three Guṇas. The three Guṇas are the ingredients of all objects, and objectivity is synonymous with insentience. Thus Buddhi has the three Guṇas and is insentient. Puruṣa is the Seer beyond the three Guṇas and is therefore conscious. There is no other thing besides the Seer and the seen, the conscious and the unconscious. Therefore, that which is not the 'seen' or knowable, is conscious and that which is not the Seer is unconscious. Buddhi is constituted by the three Guṇas since it has the property of manifestation and also determinate cognition due to Sattva (by way of reflection from Puruṣa) and wherever there is Sattva, Rajas and Tamas are also there. Since it has the three Guṇas as its constituents Buddhi (not overseen by Puruṣa) is itself unconscious.

(5) Puruṣa is not similar to Buddhi—this is established. Moreover, it is not altogether distinct from Buddhi, because though pure, *i.e.* beyond Buddhi, it witnesses or oversees the cognition or modifications of Buddhi. The overseeing of the modifications of Buddhi is called knowledge of self and not-self. The mutating part or ingredient of knowledge and its cause in the shape of overseeing by Puruṣa, appear as identical in the process of knowledge. The flow of knowledge is continuous, that is why the misconception that Puruṣa and cognitive Buddhi are identical, persists.

The question might then arise : 'Who is it that perceives that Buddhi and Puruṣa are identical ?' The reply is : 'The ego or the knower.' By what modification is it cognised ? 'By misapprehension and by memory of its latent impressions.' In other words, all ordinary knowledge is erroneous. When there is the erroneous idea of the sameness of Buddhi and Puruṣa, then is formed the idea 'I know.' Thus the concept 'I am knowing' is the mistaken notion of the sameness of Buddhi and Puruṣa. From the analogous latent impression of such mistaken notion, flow of recollection of that wrong notion continues and, therefore ordinarily, the difference between Buddhi and Puruṣa is not perceived. The awareness 'I know' gradually ceases on the attainment of discriminative knowledge and its latent impressions increase detachment, leading to complete cessation of all modifications of the mind. 'I know a blue object' is an item of knowledge. Of this, blueness, a knowable, is insentient and the consciousness is in the Knower indicated by 'I'. The blue colour is thereby cognised. Thus the manifestation of the knowledge of blueness by the Seer is the overseeing of modification of the mind. Knowledge of blue and its overseeing by Puruṣa are inseparable. Since such overseeing is an inseparable cause in all cognitions or modifications of Buddhi, the latter resembles Puruṣa to some extent. In other words, because the insentient knowledge of blueness becomes endowed with consciousness, that is becoming somewhat of the nature of Puruṣa.

(6) Pratisaṅkrama means transmission. If immutable it would be without transmission. By immutability is indicated absence of change of state, and by absence of transmission freedom from movement (*i.e.* not passing over into the object). From overseeing the modifications (the knowledge), *i.e.* manifesting the mutable modifications, the source of consciousness appears as mutable and transmissible. Pure Awareness appears as not separate or distinct from the knowing faculty of Buddhi because Buddhi is endowed with Consciousness which oversees its modifications.

———

तदर्थ एव दृश्यस्यात्मा ॥ २१ ॥

भाष्यम्—दृशिरूपस्य पुरुषस्य कर्मरूपतामापन्नं दृश्यमिति तदर्थ एव दृश्यस्यात्मा स्वरूपं भवतीत्यर्थः। तत्स्वरूपं तु पररूपेण प्रतिलब्धात्मकम्। भोगापवर्गार्थतायां कृतायां पुरुषेण न दृश्यत इति। स्वरूपहानादस्य नाशः प्राप्तो न तु विनश्यति ॥ २१ ॥

**To Serve As Objective Field To Puruṣa Is The Essence Or Nature Of The Knowable. 21.**

The knowable is endowed with the property of being the experience (1) of Puruṣa ; that is why being His (Puruṣa's) object is the essence or real nature of the knowable. The nature of the knowable is known through the other, *i.e.* Puruṣa (2). When experience and liberation are accomplished, Puruṣa no longer witnesses it. Therefore, being dispossessed of its real nature (of being the object of Puruṣa) it ceases to exist, but is not destroyed altogether.

(1) Karma-svarūpatā = Property of being an object of experience. Being a knowable and being of service to Puruṣa, fundamentally, mean the same thing. Thus the nature of the knowable is to be the object (for experience and liberation) of Puruṣa. All cognitions like that of colour etc., all feelings and all volitions are the objects of Puruṣa.

(2) Cognition of knowables depends on Puruṣa. Since, being cognised is the nature of the knowable, a manifested object becomes manifest only because of the nature of Puruṣa. In other words, since being experienced by Puruṣa is the nature of an object, its existence as object is dependent on Him. When there is no possibility of experience, the object ceases to exist as an object, but is not altogether destroyed. It then remains unmanifested. Its manifestation as an object to one Puruṣa disappears, but remains as an object for other Puruṣas, so the object never ceases to be. [In this connection note (2) to II.17 illustrates how an object is cognised through the nature of another with the example of an opaque glass and the sun.]

The object of Puruṣa *i.e.* Seer is the knowable. Taking the term 'Artha' to mean purpose, some regard Puruṣa as an entity seeking fulfilment of some purpose, and thus misinterpret the Sāṁkhya philosophy. The aforesaid misconception has arisen because of failure to grasp the proper import of certain similies cited in Sāṁkhya-kārikā and to realise that these are mere similies.

The word 'Artha' means objectivity and not purpose. Puruṣa is the Knower, Buddhi is known or revealed. The word revealer ordinarily means one who performs the act of revealing. We use the word revealed here to mean that something is manifested through a manifestor without ascribing any activity to the latter. Therefore the manifestor is not the active agent. An inactive thing is made to appear as active by the words used in describing it. We do the same thing in regard to inactive Puruṣa. On account of the presence of the self-illuminating Puruṣa behind 'I', such function of revealing as 'I am the revealer of self' or 'I am the knower of self' is done by 'I'. Thus imagining Puruṣa as the agent of such action we call Him the revealer or illuminer. In reality the act of revealing is a function of the I-sense. Since that happens on account of proximity of Puruṣa, He is said to be the revealer.

Experience and liberation or discrimination are only forms of Buddhi. The three Guṇas alone do not make Buddhi, but the mutated state of the three Guṇas in contact with the unit (individual) Seer constitutes Buddhi. Buddhi being an objective entity, the agent by which it is revealed is called its owner or manifestor. This is how we express it in language but it does not in any way make the manifestor active. 'Object of Puruṣa'— this relative term does not therefore indicate any action on the part of Puruṣa.

If experience and liberation are objective, *i.e.* manifestable, then by whom are they revealed and who will be the revealer ? The answer is Puruṣa, the Seer. To be thus an object of Puruṣa in the shape of experience or liberation is the real nature of the knowable.

———

भाष्यम्—कस्मात् ?—

कृतार्थं प्रति नष्टमप्यनष्टं तदन्यसाधारणत्वात् ॥ २२ ॥

कृतार्थमेकं पुरुषं प्रति दृश्यं नष्टमपि नाशं प्राप्तमपि अनष्टं तद् अन्यपुरुष-साधारणत्वात्। कुशलं पुरुषं प्रति नाशं प्राप्तमप्यकुशलान् पुरुषान् प्रत्यकृतार्थमिति। तेषां दृशेः कर्मविषयतामापन्नं लभते एवं पररूपेणात्मरूपमिति। अतश्च दृग्दर्शन-शक्त्योर्नित्यत्वादनादिः संयोगो व्याख्यात इति, तथा चोक्तं—'धर्म्मिणामनादि-संयोगाद्धर्म्ममात्राणामप्यनादिः संयोग' इति ॥ २२ ॥

Why (is it not destroyed) ?

**Although Ceasing To Exist In Relation To Him Whose Purpose Is Fulfilled The Knowable Does Not Cease To Exist On Account Of being Of Use To Others. 22.**

Even though destroyed, *i.e.* having disappeared in relation to one Puruṣa whose goal has been attained it is not really destroyed, being common to others. Even though destroyed in reference to a Puruṣa who has attained his goal, to Puruṣas who have not so attained, the objective character of the knowable remains unfulfilled. To them the knowable, remaining as the object of experience, is perceived through the reflection of another. Thus on account of the Knower and the knowable being ever present, their alliance has been called beginningless. Pañchaśikha has said in this connection: "Since the association of the primary constituent causes of the phenomenal world (with Puruṣa) has been beginningless, phenomena too have been associated with Him from time without beginning (1)."

(1) When through attainment of discriminative knowledge by a proficient person the knowable is destroyed in reference to him, it remains undestroyed in relation to others. As the knowable is undestroyed to-day, so will it continue to remain undestroyed for all time. The Sāṃkhya aphorism on this point is: "It will always remain as it now is. Its total destruction is not possible." If it be argued that when all beings attain discriminative knowledge then the knowable will cease to exist, the reply is—that is not possible because beings are innumerable. There is no end to innumerability. Innumerable divided by innumerable = innumerable. That is the law of innumerability. We find in the Śruti: "When the whole is taken away from the whole, the whole still remains." That is why the knowable has been present at all times and will remain for ever. The Puruṣa who has not attained proficiency has for the same reason remained eternally allied to the beginningless knowable. It cannot be that there was at first no alliance between the Seer and the seen and that it has taken place at a particular time. In such a case how will the cause for the alliance arise? It will be explained later that the cause of this alliance is Avidyā or wrong knowledge. Wrong cognition begets wrong knowledge. So the chain of misconception is beginningless. This has been very cogently described in the aphorism of Pañchaśikha quoted above. The primordial causes are the three Guṇas. As they have been allied with Puruṣa from time without beginning their modifications in the shape of Buddhi, the organs and their objects like sight, sound, etc. are also eternally allied to Puruṣa.

Plurality of Puruṣa and the unitary nature of Pradhāna (collective name of the three Guṇas) have been referred to in this aphorism (see II.23 and IV.16). On this point Vāchaspati Miśra says: "Puruṣa is not unitary like Pradhāna. The plurality of Puruṣa is established from the variety of individual selves, their births and deaths, enjoyment of pleasure and pain, liberation and bondage. It is logical to assume that the simultaneous knower of many things must be many in number. The Śruti which (apparently) advances the oneness of Puruṣa is contradicted by other evidences. Since no spatio-temporal distinction is applicable to the Seers who are beyond time and space, people argue that it is not proper to imagine that one Seer is present here and another Seer at another place, and that is why they say that the Seer is one." In reality the Śruti does not mention the oneness of the supreme Seer, but only refers to the oneness of the Lord of the universe—the Creator, the Protector and the Destroyer, the Saguṇa Īśvara. In Mahābhārata also it is said : "At the time of creation He creates, and at the time of destruction He eats it up again. Destroying everything and withdrawing all into Himself, the Lord of the universe lies in water, *i.e.* in homogeneous primordial cause." In Śruti this Creator has been called one. He is not pure Awareness or Ātmā. The unity of Prakṛti and the plurality of Puruṣa have been established directly by the Śruti as in the Śvetāśvatara Upaniṣad : "One Puruṣa without birth (*i.e.* eternal) enjoys or experiences another (*i.e.* Prakṛti) who is also without birth and is the embodiment of Rajas, Sattva and Tamas Guṇas and the creator of many, while another unborn (*i.e.* eternal) Puruṣa abandons Prakṛti who has provided experience and liberation."

———

भाष्यम्—संयोगस्वरूपाऽभिधित्सयेदं सूत्रं प्रववृते—

स्वस्वामिशक्त्योः स्वरूपोपलब्धिहेतुः संयोगः ॥ २३ ॥

पुरुषः स्वामी, दृश्येन स्वेन दर्शनार्थं संयुक्तः। तस्मात् संयोगाद् दृश्यस्योपलब्धिर्या स भोगः, या तु द्रष्टुः स्वरूपोपलब्धिः सोऽपवर्गः। दर्शनकार्यावसानः संयोग इति दर्शनं वियोगस्य कारणमुक्तम्। दर्शनमदर्शनस्य प्रतिद्वन्द्वीति अदर्शनं संयोगनिमित्तमुक्तम्। नात्र दर्शनं मोक्षकारणमदर्शनाभावादेव बन्धाभावः स मोक्ष इति। दर्शनस्य भावे बन्धकारणस्यादर्शनस्य नाश इत्यतो दर्शनज्ञानम् कैवल्यकारणमुक्तम्।

किञ्चेदमदर्शनं नाम किं गुणानामधिकारः।—१। आहोस्विद् दृशिरूपस्य स्वामिनो दर्शितविषयस्य प्रधानचित्तस्यानुत्पादः, स्वस्मिन्दृश्ये विद्यमाने दर्शनाभावः।—२। किमर्थवत्ता गुणानाम्।—३। अथाविद्या स्वचित्तेन सह निरुद्धा स्वचित्तस्योत्पत्तिवीजम्।—४। किं स्थितिसंस्कारक्षये गतिसंस्काराभिव्यक्तिः,

यत्रेदमुक्तं 'प्रधानं स्थित्यैव वर्त्तमानं विकाराकरणादप्रधानं स्यात्तथा गत्यैव वर्त्तमानं विकारनित्यत्वादप्रधानं स्यादुभयथा चास्य प्रवृत्तिः प्रधानव्यवहारं लभते नान्यथा, कारणान्तरेष्वपि कल्पितेष्वेष समानश्चर्च्चः' ।—५। दर्शनशक्तिरेवा-दर्शनमित्येके 'प्रधानस्यात्मख्यापनार्था प्रवृत्तिः' इति श्रुतेः। सर्व्वबोध्यबोधसमर्थः प्राक्प्रवृत्तेः पुरुषो न पश्यति, सर्वकार्यकरणसमर्थं दृश्यं तदा न दृश्यत इति ।—६। उभयस्याप्यदर्शनं धर्मं इत्येके। तत्रेदं दृश्यस्य स्वात्मभूतमपि पुरुषप्रत्ययापेक्षं दर्शनं दृश्यधर्मत्वेन भवति, तथा पुरुषस्यानात्मभूतमपि दृश्यप्रत्ययापेक्षं पुरुष-धर्मत्वेनेव दर्शनमवभासते ।—७। दर्शनज्ञानमेवादर्शनमिति केचिदभिदधति ।—८। इत्येते शास्त्रगता विकल्पाः, तत्र विकल्पबहुत्वमेतत्सर्व्वपुरुषाणां गुणसंयोगे साधारणविषयम् ॥ २३ ॥

This aphorism has been introduced for determining the nature of the alliance—

**Alliance Is the Means Of Realising The True Nature Of The Object Of the Knower And Of The Owner, The Knower (i.e. The Sort Of Alliance Which Contributes To The Realisation Of The Seer And The Seen Is This Relationship)** (1). **23.**

Puruṣa, the Self, is allied with the objects which are like His property, the result of which alliance is cognition (of objects). The cognition of objects that takes place as a result of the contact is experience, while the realisation of the nature of the Seer is liberation. Contact or alliance lasts till the right apprehension (or discrimination) which has therefore been called the cause of cessation of that alliance. Right apprehension (*i.e.* discrimination) is the opposite of misapprehension. Non-discrimination has been called the cause of alliance. But here discernment is not the direct cause of Mokṣa (liberation). Absence of non-discernment is the absence of bondage ; that is liberation. Wrong apprehension, which is the cause of bondage, is destroyed through discrimination. That is why right apprehension has been called the cause of bringing about liberation (2).

What is this misapprehension (3) ? Is it the sway of the Guṇas (ability to give rise to fluctuation) ? 1. Or, the non-production of primary mind, which presents experiences like sights and sounds as well as discriminative knowledge to the Seer, the Self, in other words, in spite of the presence within one's own self of both experience and Viveka, not knowing them ? 2. Or, the existence, in latent state, of experience and liberation in the Guṇas ? 3. Or, Avidyā (nescience) disappearing with the mind at the time of dissolution and again appearing as the seed of re-emergence of the mind ? 4. Or, the termination of the unmanifested state and the emergence or manifestation (of the Guṇas) ? It has been said in this connection : "If Pradhāna (primal constituent) were always in a state of inactivity, it would become Apradhāna (*i.e.* subsidiary and not primal) as it would not then produce any modification. Similarly, if it were always in a state of movement or modification, it would also become Apradhāna on account of not being their primal cause. When there is a tendency of both quiescence and movement, it gains its status of Pradhāna (primal), otherwise it could not be regarded as such. Whatever other reasons are thought of, this line of argument is applicable." 5. Some hold that the faculty of apprehension is misapprehension. "Pradhāna's propensity to make itself known"—this text of Śruti is their authority. Puruṣa, the Knower of all knowables, does not cognise Pradhāna before its manifestation, nor is Pradhāna, which is capable of producing all effects, then overseen by Puruṣa. 6. Others say that the characteristic of both (Puruṣa and Pradhāna) is Adarśana or misapprehension. According to this theory although knowledge is the property of Pradhāna it is dependent on being witnessed by Puruṣa when it becomes the character of the object. Similarly, although it (knowledge) is not in the nature of Puruṣa yet depending on Him as it does for illumining the object, it appears to be an attribute of Puruṣa. 7. Some designate knowledge itself as Adarśana or misapprehension. 8. These are only differences of opinion found in the Śāstras. Although there are various notions like these in respect of Adarśana or wrong conception, it is recognised by all that : "The Adarśana (in the general sense of the term) is that contact of Puruṣas with the Guṇas in which the Guṇas serve as objects of Puruṣas."

(1) Alliance is the cause which results in the realisation of the object as property and of Puruṣa as its owner. The union of Puruṣa and Prakṛti produces cognition. That knowledge is of two kinds, *viz.* misapprehension, *i.e.* experience of pleasure and pain and correct knowledge, *i.e.* liberation. Therefore, both experience and emancipation arise out of alliance, *i.e.* both the forms of awareness, *viz.* experience and liberation, are states of alliance between Puruṣa and Prakṛti. When emancipation is attained the two are separated.

(2) After the realisation of Buddhi-tattva (pure I-sense), when the cognitive faculty (*i.e.* Buddhi) is arrested for a time for getting to the Puruṣa principle, it (Buddhi) emerges again under the impulse of its latent impressions and the intense knowledge which then arises of Puruṣa as a separate principle beyond Buddhi is Darśana or true discriminative enlightenment. It is the knowledge of discrimination based on the retained impressions or the latency of the arrested state of the mind in which Puruṣa remains alone*. Therefore, the only result of such discernment is an arrested state of the mind, *i.e.* disunion of Puruṣa and Prakṛti. The modification of the mind in the shape of experience of pleasure and pain is Adarśana. Threfore when on attainment of discriminative knowledge, experience ceases, Adarśana or contrary knowledge (*i.e.* looking at Buddhi and Puruṣa as the same—though they are separate) also ceases. That is the cessation of knowables or the liberation of Puruṣa. Thus discriminatory knowledge gradually leads to Kaivalya or liberation.

(3) The commentator has collated eight different definitions of Adarśana advanced by authors of various scriptures. These represent diverse view-points, of which the fourth one is the most acceptable. These are being enumerated below :—

First : Sway of the Guṇas is Adarśana. Sway indicates proneness to fluctuations. This definition is correct only to the extent that Adarśana

* Puruṣa can neither be experienced nor recollected. The impression of the arrested state of mind (Nirodha which is once attained and is not perpetual) when Puruṣa abides in Himself can be retained. It is a state higher than memory and in it there is no possibility of any lapse or deviation normally associated with memory.

continues so long as the Guṇas are active. But it is fallacious like defining fever as the presence of warmth in the body.

Second : The non-production of the primary mind is Adarśana. Primary mind is that which ceases to function after presenting the objects of experience and discernment to the owner, the Seer. When right knowledge and aversion to objects of enjoyment through renunciation take place, the mind ceases to function. Mind so gifted is the primary mind. In the mind there are seeds both of gaining worldly experience and of acquiring discriminative knowledge. According to this view the non-germination of that seed is Adarśana. This definition is incomplete and is partly true like the statement 'to be unwell is illness'.

Third : Adarśana is the existence of experience and liberation in a latent state in the Guṇas. In Satkāryavāda, the doctrine of the pre-existence of the effect in the cause, both the cause and the effect are always existing. What will happen in future exists unmanifested in the present. The objective nature of the Guṇas is the existence in them of experience and liberation in a potential state. That objectivity is Adarśana. This definition also is partly true. Objẹctivity of the Guṇas and Adarśana are no doubt inseparable, but mention of their inseparability alone is not a complete description. 'What is a visible form ? It is that which has extension.' Though extension and the idea of form are inseparable, the mention of this inseparability alone is not sufficient for a conception of form. Such is this description.

Fourth : Latency of Avidyā or wrong knowledge is Adarśana or want of discrimination which is the cause of the alliance. When there is any modification based on wrong knowledge, it can be inferred that the subsequent modification will also be based on wrong knowledge, proving thereby that the latencies of wrong knowledge bring about the alliance of Buddhi and Puruṣa. Following the sequence, it is seen that the mind which at the time of dissolution submerges with impressions of wrong knowledge, emerges at the time of creation with that wrong knowledge and brings about a union of Buddhi and Puruṣa. This view alone is able to demonstrate clearly the alliance of Buddhi and Puruṣa and its co-existing Adarśana. It will be fully explained later.

Fifth : Pradhāna has a dual nature, *viz.* that it is static when it maintains equilibrium and it moves or fluctuates by losing the equilibrium. If fluctuation were its sole nature then modification would be perpetual and there would be no modification if inactivity were its only character. Of these two, Adarśana is the manifestation of the state of fluctuation (*i.e.* associated cognition of objects) on termination of the static (potential) state. This only indicates the nature of the basic cause but does not explain the immediate cause of the union which has specific cause and effect. What is an earthen pot ? It is a particular form of modification of mutable earth. Just as this description alone does not fully describe a pot, so is the case with the fifth alternative.

Sixth : The cognitive faculty is Adarśana. Objects become known when Pradhāna has a tendency to fluctuate. Therefore the state of Pradhāna in which that tendency is stored as potential energy is Adarśana. Adarśana is a kind of Darśana or knowledge and is a modification or a characteristic of the mind. In explaining it, if the basic principle only is mentioned it does not make it sufficiently clear. It is like describing rice by saying that it is a grain produced by sun's rays.

Seventh : Adarśana stands for a characteristic of both Pradhāna and Puruṣa and is a particular form of cognition. Knowledge, though it appertains to the knowables, is dependent on Puruṣa ; so it looks like a characteristic of Puruṣa even though it does not appertain to the latter. Thus knowledge, whether of sights and sounds, or discriminative knowledge, is a characteristic of both the object (knowable) and Puruṣa. When we say that sight is dependent on the sun, we do not fully describe sight but give only its dependence on the sun ; so is the present explanation.

Eighth : All knowledge except discriminative knowledge, *i.e.* such knowledge as of sights and sounds and the like, is Adarśana, and that is the state of alliance between Puruṣa and Prakṛti.

In the Sāṁkhya philosophy, these eight kinds of tenets are found in regard to Adarśana. Adarśana = lit. not-seeing. The negative prefix 'A' (=not) has six different meanings, *e.g.* (i) absence of, as in Apāpa (sinless), (ii) similarity, as in Abrāhmaṇa (like a Brāhmaṇa), (iii) difference, as in Amitra (not a friend, *i.e.* an enemy), (iv) diminutiveness, as in Anudari (possessed of a small narrow waist), (v) insufficient, as in Akeśi (not having sufficient hair), and (vi) opposition as in Asuras (demons opposed to Suras or heavenly beings).

Of the above, except that indicating absence, the others are expressive of some definite objects or states.

(4) Except the fourth definition the others indicate only the alliance between Puruṣa and Prakṛti. This union is not inherent because in that case there could be no separation. It is incidental. Therefore the mention of the cause completes the explanation of the union. Avidyā or nescience is that cause, from which arises this alliance.

In fact 'contact of the Guṇas with Puruṣa' is common to all, *i.e.* this has been admitted in all the definitions. Whenever there is union, there is modification of the Guṇas. This union of Puruṣa with modifications of the Guṇas is effected in the shape of manifestation at the time of creation and as latencies at the time of dissolution. Thus this alliance is in reality the alliance or union or contact between Buddhi, the object of Puruṣa, and individual Awareness. That alliance springs from nescience. Therefore the statement in the fourth alternative that Avidyā or nescience is the cause of the Adarśana or non-apprehension of discrimination which produces the union, is the correct definition. The author of the Sūtra has precisely stated that.

———

भाष्यम्—यस्तु प्रत्यक्चेतनस्य स्वबुद्धिसंयोगः,

तस्य हेतुरविद्या ॥ २४ ॥

विपर्ययज्ञानवासनेत्यर्थः। विपर्ययज्ञानवासनावासिता न कार्यनिष्ठां पुरुषख्यातिं बुद्धिः प्राप्नोति साधिकारा पुनरावर्त्तते। सा तु पुरुषख्यातिपर्यवसाना कार्यनिष्ठां प्राप्नोति चरिताधिकारा निवृत्तादर्शना बन्धकारणाभावान्न पुनरावर्त्तते। अत्र कश्चित् षण्डकोपाख्यानेनोद्घाटयति, मुग्धया भार्य्यया अभिधीयते षण्डकः, 'आर्यपुत्र! अपत्यवती मे भगिनी किमर्थं नाहमिति।' स तामाह, 'मृतस्तेऽहमपत्यमुत्पादयिष्यामी'ति, तथेदं विद्यमानं ज्ञानं चित्तनिवृत्तिं न करोति विनष्टं करिष्यतीति का प्रत्याशा। तत्राचार्यदेशीयो वक्ति ननु बुद्धिनिवृत्तिरेव मोक्षः, अदर्शनकारणाभावाद् बुद्धिनिवृत्तिः, तच्चादर्शनं बन्धकारणं दर्शनान्निवर्त्तते। तत्र चित्तनिवृत्तिरेव मोक्षः किमर्थमस्थान एवास्य मतिविभ्रमः ॥ २४ ॥

The alliance of the individual consciousness or Puruṣa (Pratyak-chetana) and the co-related (Sva) Buddhi, has

**Avidyā Or Nescience As Its Cause** (1). **24.**

Nescience is the latent subconscious impression or Vāsanā of wrong knowledge. The efforts of Buddhi laden with such latency do not develop fully into the illuminating knowledge of Puruṣa, and therefore it returns to its former function on account of its inclination to fluctuation. When the knowledge of Puruṣa is attained, the function of Buddhi ends. Then having fulfilled its function and being free from misapprehension and having no cause of bondage it does not appear again (2). Some opponents ridicule the proposition by citing the story of an impotent husband. A devoted wife thus addressed her husband : 'Oh my husband, my sister has a child, why have I not one ?' The impotent one replied : 'After death, I shall beget you a child.' Similarly, this knowledge while in existence, does not cause the mind to cease from action ; what hope is there then that it will cause cessation when suppressed ? In reply to this criticism a sage says : 'Cessation of the working of Buddhi is Mokṣa. When the cause in the shape of Adarśana (want of discriminative knowledge) is removed, the activities of Buddhi stop. That cause of bondage, *viz.* Adarśana (*i.e.* lack of discriminative knowledge) is removed by Darśana (*i.e.* discriminative knowledge).' In effect cessation of the activities of the mind is Mokṣa. There is thus no room for such confusion of thought.

(1) The comments on I.29 are to be seen for a full explanation of the expression 'Pratyak-chetana'. Individual consciousness in the shape of each Puruṣa is Pratyak-chetana.

Avidyā here means latent impressions (Vāsanā) of wrong knowledge. Reference may be made to the definition of Avidyā as taking the non-self for self, etc. given in connection with the discussion on erroneous knowledge. Generally speaking, regarding Puruṣa and Buddhi as not separate is the wrong knowledge which is the cause of bondage. The latent impression (Vāsanā) of that knowledge is the primary cause of the union. This contact is without beginning. Thus, there was no such time when there was no alliance. Therefore to arrive at the cause of the alliance one has to look not at how the alliance took place initially but rather at how the alliance ceases. Take the case of a lump of red arsenic. We may not have seen how the compound was formed but on analysing it we see that it is made up of sulphur and arsenic. Similar is the case with this alliance. When there is discriminative knowledge, Buddhi stops functioning altogether, *i.e.* there is a separation between Buddhi and Puruṣa ; therefore Avidyā, which is opposed to discriminative knowledge, is the cause of alliance. The commentator has shown this.

As long as the latencies (Vāsanā) of wrong knowledge continue, there is no break in the alliance. When discriminative enlightenment is fully attained, the function of the mind ends. Therefore wrong knowledge, which is opposed to discriminative knowledge of Puruṣa, is the cause of this alliance. Present wrong knowledge arises from latencies of such knowledge formed in the past. Going back, in this way, latencies will be found to be beginningless. Thus subliminal impressions (Vāsanā) of wrong knowledge from time without beginning are the cause of the alliance.

(2) In the state of Kaivalya (liberation), Darśana and Adarśana (seeing and non-seeing) both cease. Right and wrong knowledge are relative. The realisation by a concentrated mind (through discriminative knowledge) that Buddhi and Puruṣa are separate presupposes knowledge of Buddhi as a separate entity. That knowledge 'I have or had Buddhi' is an erroneous knowledge. Liberation in the shape of complete cessation of the mind cannot take place so long as awareness of Buddhi remains. Thus in Kaivalya there is neither discriminative knowledge nor erroneous knowledge. Wrong knowledge is destroyed by discriminative knowledge. Then there is complete stoppage of the mind or Buddhi.

Kleśas (afflictions) like Avidyā (wrong knowledge), Asmitā (egoism), Rāga (attachment), etc. are destroyed by discriminative knowledge and supreme detachment based thereon. It is clear that the attainment of the Samāpatti 'I am not the body etc. and I do not want anything out of them' will lead to stoppage of fluctuation of all knowables from Buddhi downwards. Therefore when with discrimination wrong knowledge is destroyed the mind ceases to have any modification. Discriminative knowledge destroys its own base as fire destroys its fuel.

———

भाष्यम्—हेयं दुःखं हेयकारणं च संयोगाख्यं सनिमित्तमुक्तम् अतःपरं हानं वक्तव्यम्—

तदभावात् संयोगाभावो हानं तद्दृशेः कैवल्यम् ॥ २५ ॥

तस्यादर्शनस्याभावाद् बुद्धिपुरुषसंयोगाभावः आत्यन्तिको बन्धनोपरम इत्यर्थ एतद् हानम् । तद्दृशेः कैवल्यम् पुरुषस्यामिश्रीभावः पुनरसंयोगो गुणैरित्यर्थः । दुःखकारणनिवृत्तौ दुःखोपरमो हानं तदा स्वरूपप्रतिष्ठः पुरुष इत्युक्तम् ॥ २५ ॥

The misery to be forsaken, the cause of that misery known as alliance, as well as the cause of that union have been described. After that, absolute freedom has to be described.

**The Absence Of Alliance That Arises From Lack Of It Is The Freedom And That Is The State Of Liberation Of The Seer. 25.**

When Adarśana ceases, the alliance of Buddhi and Puruṣa ceases and there is complete cessation of bondage for all time, which is isolation of the Seer, *i.e.* state of aloofness of Puruṣa and non-recurrence of future contact with the Guṇas. The cessation of misery that ensues from termination of the cause of misery is liberation from it. In that state Puruṣa remains established in Himself (1).

(1) Isolation of the Seer means that only the Seer exists. When there is alliance of the Seer and the seen, it cannot be said that the Seer is alone. It may be asked whether separation and non-separation are states appertaining to the Seer. No, it is not so. Buddhi only undergoes change in the form of cessation or disappearance from view, which does not and cannot affect the Seer. This point has been dealt with in II.20 (2) ante. The state of Puruṣa in Himself is the correct expression while liberation of Puruṣa is a description by implication.

———

भाष्यम्—अथ हानस्य कः प्राप्त्युपाय इति—

विवेकख्यातिरविप्लवा हानोपायः ॥ २६ ॥

सत्त्वपुरुषान्यताप्रत्ययो विवेकख्यातिः, सा त्वनिवृत्तमिथ्याज्ञाना प्लवते। यदा मिथ्याज्ञानं दग्धवीजभावं बन्ध्यप्रसवं संपद्यते तदा विधूतक्लेशरजसः सत्त्वस्य परे वैशारद्ये परस्यां वशीकारसंज्ञायां वर्त्तमानस्य विवेकप्रत्यय-प्रवाहो निर्म्मलो भवति। सा विवेकख्यातिरविप्लवा हानस्योपायः, ततो मिथ्याज्ञानस्य दग्धवीज-भावोपगमः पुनश्चाप्रसवः। इत्येष मोक्षस्य मार्गो हानस्योपाय इति ॥ २६ ॥

What then is the means of escape ?

**Clear And Distinct (Unimpaired) Discriminative Knowledge Is The Means Of Liberation. 26.**

The knowledge of distinction between Buddhi and Puruṣa is discriminative knowledge, which is obstructed by undestroyed nescience (1). When wrong knowledge reaches the state of a burnt seed and ceases to be productive, then through Buddhi attaining purity by the removal of afflictive impurities, the Yogin reaches the superior stage of renunciation known as Vaśīkārasaṅjñā and the flow of his conception of discrimination becomes clear. That unimpaired discriminative enlightenment is the means of liberation. From that (discriminative enlightenment) follows the parched seed state of nescience and cessation of its productivity. This is the way to Mokṣa or means of liberation.

(1) Discrimination has been explanied before. It means distinction between Puruṣa and Buddhi. The intense knowledge or conception, or clear idea thereof, is discriminative enlightenment.

Discriminative knowledge arises first from listening to the Śāstras or scriptures and becomes firmer and clearer through reasoned contemplation. It goes on developing gradually as one practises the different exercises of Yoga. When through Samprajñāta-yoga or engrossment therein, the possibility of acquiring wrong notion in respect of knowables, is eradicated then it is called the parched state of the seed of wrong knowledge. When that happens and the attachment to both worldly and heavenly enjoyments completely ceases, there arises enlightenment based on knowledge of discrimination purified through Samādhi. On that discriminative enlightenment becoming continuous, *i.e.* not broken by nescience, liberation, *i.e.* complete abandonment of knowables, is effected. Wrong knowledge then becomes like parched seed. When liberation is attained, both erroneous conceptions reduced to the state of parched seeds and discriminative knowledge disappear. That is Kaivalya or the Self-in-Itself.

How Buddhi disappears through discriminative enlightenment has been explained in the next aphorism.

---

तस्य सप्तधा प्रान्तभूमिः प्रज्ञा ॥ २७ ॥

भाष्यम्—तस्येति प्रत्युदितख्यातेः प्रत्याम्नायः, सप्तधेति। अशुद्ध्यावरणमलापगमाच्चित्तस्य प्रत्ययान्तरानुत्पादे सति सप्तप्रकारैव प्रज्ञा विवेकिनो भवति, तद्यथा—परिज्ञातं हेयं नास्य पुनः परिज्ञेयमस्ति।—१। क्षीणा हेयहेतवो न पुनरेतेषां क्षेतव्यमस्ति।—२। साक्षात्कृतं निरोधसमाधिना हानम्।—३। भावितो विवेकख्यातिरूपो हानोपायः।—४। इत्येषा चतुष्टयी कार्या विमुक्तिः प्रज्ञायाः। चित्तविमुक्तिस्तु त्रयी।—चरिताधिकारा बुद्धिः।—५। गुणा गिरिशिखरकूटच्युता इव ग्रावाणो निरवस्थानाः स्वकारणे प्रलयाभिमुखाः सह तेनास्तं गच्छन्ति, न चैषां विप्रलीनानां पुनरस्त्युत्पादः प्रयोजनाभावादिति।—६। एतस्यामवस्थायां गुणसम्बन्धातीतः स्वरूपमात्रज्योतिरमलः केवली पुरुष इति।—७। एतां सप्तविधां प्रान्तभूमिप्रज्ञामनुपश्यन्पुरुषः कुशल इत्याख्यायते, प्रतिप्रसवेऽपि चित्तस्य मुक्तः कुशल इत्येव भवति गुणातीतत्वादिति ॥ २७ ॥

**Seven Kinds Of Ultimate Insight Come To Him (The Yogin Who Has Acquired Discriminative Enlightenment)** (1). **27.**

This has been stated in the Śāstras in respect of a Yogin whose mind has become tranquil by the attainment of discriminative knowledge. When on account of cleansing of the impurities acting as veil on the mind, other kinds of (distractive) conception do not grow therein, the discriminator gets seven kinds of ultimate insight. These are :—(i) that which has to be forsaken has been known, there is nothing more to know in this direction ; (ii) the causes of growth of the things to be given up have been attenuated, they need not be further thinned ; (iii) liberation has become a matter of realisation through Nirodha-samādhi (Samādhi of the arrested mind) ; (iv) discriminative enlightenment has been recognised as the means of liberation. These four insights are liberation from action, while those relating to liberation of the mind are of three kinds, *viz.* (v) Buddhi has fulfilled its function ; (vi) the attributes of Buddhi, having been dislodged like boulders from the top of a hill, are rushing towards dissolution and getting merged into their cause, whence they will not rise again on account of absence of any reason thereof ; (vii) in the seventh state the insight reveals Puruṣa as in-Himself, pure, self-luminous and beyond any relation with the Guṇas. When these seven kinds of insight are acquired, the Yogin may be called Kuśala or proficient. When the mind disappears, the Yogin can be called a Mukta-kuśala or the liberated one, because he then transcends the Guṇas.

(1) Ultimate insight = Highest state of knowledge, beyond which there can be no knowledge on the subject, and on attainment of which all knowledge in respect thereof ends or ceases. It is clear that on the realisation of 'I know what is to be known, I have nothing more to know', knowledge will cease.

In the first insight, the miseries associated with objects having been fully realised, the mind desists completely from them.

In the second, the efforts at decreasing afflictions (not altogether disappearing) being successful, an insight appears that there is nothing more to be done in this respect. This is how efforts at restraint cease.

Third : On its having been realised, enquiry about the supreme goal ceases. Once release has been fully achieved by Nirodha-samādhi, then through its recollection this wisdom is gained.

Fourth : Having mastered the means of liberation the mind is no longer occupied with enquiry about the practices of Yoga. This brings about a cessation of the effort to attain proficiency in practice.

These four kinds of insight are known as liberation from action. As this liberation is attained through effort, or in other words, as it terminates the stage of practice, it is called liberation from action. The remaining three stages are known as freedom from mind. After attainment of liberation from action, these three forms of insight automatically appear and bring about complete cessation of the mind. This is the acme of wisdom in the shape of supreme renunciation. That is the foremost wisdom or the farthest limit of the activities of Buddhi. Beyond that is the Self-in-Itself. Those three insights are :—

Fifth : Buddhi has fulfilled its duty, *i.e.* has brought about the completion of both experience and liberation. When liberation is attained there is cessation of experience. 'There is nothing more to be served by Buddhi'—this sort of insight brings about a cessation of the operation of Buddhi.

Sixth : The nature of the sixth form of insight is the knowledge that the activities of Buddhi will cease and they will not rise again. It is then clearly perceived that on the disappearance of the afflictive and non-afflictive latencies, there will be complete cessation of the mental states. Just as a big stone falling from the top of a hill does not go back to its former place, so the attributes getting detached from Puruṣa do not come back again. The Guṇas referred to in the commentary are the attributes of Buddhi like pleasure, pain or delusion and not the three primal Guṇas, because they being basic cannot merge into anything.

Seventh : In this stage of insight it is recognised that Puruṣa is free from relationship with the Guṇas, is self-illuminated, pure and absolute. (Here the Guṇas referred to are the three primary Guṇas—the constituent principles.) This is not the state of Puruṣa being in-Himself alone but the best insight relating to final emancipation. In the ultimate liberation, the mental function completely stops ; hence insight also ceases. When after attaining the aforesaid seven insights, the mind stops functioning, the tranquil Yogin is regarded as Mukta-kuśala or liberated and proficient. That is the state of liberation attained by a person while still living. When misery does not touch him even in his lifetime, then the Yogin is regarded as Jīvan-mukta or free while living. On the attainment of discriminative enlightenment, there is just a touch of latency left, and the Yogin contemplating on the ultimate insights is Jīvan-mukta. In that state, though faced with misery, he may rise above it with discriminative knowledge. He is thus Jīvan-mukta or free in lifetime. Even if the Yogin lives with a created mind, he is Jīvan-mukta. In fact, a Yogin living after liberation, *i.e.* beyond the touch of misery, is called Jīvan-mukta when, though quite capable, he does not take to the state of perpetual liberation by getting into incorporeal emancipation (IV.30).

What is Jīvan-mukti according to some modern viewpoint, is according to Yoga only verbal knowledge acquired through hearing and inference. When discernment is established a Yogin is not worried with fear, nor does he lament over misery.

———

भाष्यम्—सिद्धा भवति विवेकख्यातिर्हानोपायः, न च सिद्धिरन्तरेण साधनमित्येतदारभ्यते—

योगाङ्गानुष्ठानादशुद्धिक्षये ज्ञानदीप्तिराविवेकख्यातेः ॥ २८ ॥

योगाङ्गानि अष्टावभिधायिष्यमाणानि, तेषामनुष्ठानात् पञ्चपर्वणो विपर्यय-स्याशुद्धिरूपस्य क्षयः नाशः। तत्क्षये सम्यग्ज्ञानस्याभिव्यक्तिः। यथा यथा च साधनान्यनुष्ठीयन्ते तथा तथा तनुत्वमशुद्धिरापद्यते। यथा यथा च क्षीयते तथा तथा क्षयक्रमानुरोधिनी ज्ञानस्यापि दीप्तिर्विवर्द्धते, सा खल्वेषा विवृद्धिः प्रकर्ष-मनुभवति आ विवेकख्यातेः—आ गुणपुरुषस्वरूपविज्ञानादित्यर्थः। योगाङ्गानुष्ठानम-शुद्धेर्वियोगकारणं यथा परशुश्छेद्यस्य, विवेकख्यातेस्तु प्राप्तिकारणं यथा धर्मः सुखस्य, नान्यथा कारणम्।

कति चैतानि कारणानि शास्त्रे भवन्ति, नवैवेत्याह, तद्यथा—'उत्पत्ति-स्थित्यभिव्यक्तिविकारप्रत्ययाप्तयः। वियोगान्यत्वधृतयः कारणन्नवधा स्मृतम्' इति। तत्रोत्पत्तिकारणं—मनो भवति विज्ञानस्य, स्थितिकारणं—मनसः पुरुषार्थता, शरीरस्येवाहार इति। अभिव्यक्तिकारणं यथा रूपस्यालोकस्तथा रूपज्ञानम्। विकारकारणं—मनसो विषयान्तरं, यथाग्निः पाक्यस्य। प्रत्ययकारणं—धूमज्ञान-मग्निज्ञानस्य। प्राप्तिकारणं—योगाङ्गानुष्ठानं विवेकख्यातेः। वियोगकारणं—तदेवाशुद्धेः। अन्यत्वकारणं यथा सुवर्णस्य सुवर्णकारः। एवमेकस्य स्त्रीप्रत्ययस्य अविद्या मूढत्वे, द्वेषो दुःखत्वे, रागः सुखत्वे, तत्त्वज्ञानं माध्यस्थ्ये। धृतिकारणं—शरीरमिन्द्रियाणां तानि च तस्य, महाभूतानि शरीराणां तानि च परस्परं सर्वेषां, तैर्यग्यौनमानुषदैवतानि च परस्परार्थत्वात्। इत्येवं नव कारणानि। तानि च यथासम्भवं पदार्थान्तरेष्वपि योज्यानि। योगाङ्गानुष्ठानन्तु द्विधैव कारणत्वं लभत इति॥ २८॥

Discriminative enlightenment as means of liberation can be attained. There can be no perfection without practice. That is why this (practice of Yoga) is now being introduced.

**Through The Practice Of The Different Accessories To Yoga* When Impurities Are Destroyed, There Arises Enlightenment Culminating In Discriminative Enlightenment** (1). **28.**

The accessories to Yoga about to be mentioned are eight in number. Through their practice, impurities in the form

* Yogāṅgas (literally limbs of Yoga) mean the integrated course of exercises conducive to Yoga as enumerated in Sūtra II.29.

of five types of nescience are reduced or destroyed. On their diminution, true knowledge manifests itself. As the practices are performed, the impurities are attenuated and correspondingly the lustre of knowledge increases until discriminative enlightenment is attained, *i.e.* the true nature of the distinction between Puruṣa and the Guṇas is known. Practice of Yogāṅgas is the means of eradicating the impurities (2) as an axe is the means of severing wood. And as virtue is the means to obtain happiness, practice of Yogāṅgas is the means of acquisition of discriminative knowledge. Practice of Yoga is not a cause in any other sense.

How many kinds of causes have been mentioned in the Śāstras? There are nine, *viz.* (cause of) origin, (cause of) sustenance, (cause of) manifestation, (cause of) mutation, (cause of) knowledge, (cause of) acquisition, (cause of) eradication, (cause of) diversity, and (cause of) retention. Origin: Mind is the origin of knowledge. Sustenance: Serving the objectives of Puruṣa sustains the mind as food sustains the body. Manifestation: Visible forms are manifested by light and cognition thereof (by reflex action, as 'I am knowing or seeing.'). Mutation: Shifting of the mind from one object to another produces mental modifications as fire transforms cooked food. Knowledge: Existence of fire is inferred from seeing smoke. Acquisition: Practice of exercises of Yoga leads to discriminative knowledge. Eradication: Discriminative knowledge results in destruction of impurities. Diversity: Goldsmith produces diverse articles of gold. Similarly there may be varied impressions of the same woman, *viz.* infatuation caused by Avidyā, misery caused by aversion, pleasure caused by attachment and indifference caused by right knowledge. Retention: Body retains the organs and the organs retain the body. Similarly the gross elements sustain the body and also sustain themselves. Each of the species, animal, man and Deva, being interrelated, each one is the cause of each other's support. These are the nine causes. These are also applicable *mutatis mutandis* to other cases. Thus practice of exercises of Yoga serves as a cause in two ways—severance and acquisition.

(1) Discriminative knowledge can be apprehended through learning and deductions therefrom even when the fivefold wrong knowledge like Avidyā etc., are dominant. And as the latencies of wrong knowledge weaken through practice of Yogāṅgas, discriminative knowledge gets clearer. Subsequently through engrossment acquired through Samādhi, full discernment dawns. Such clarity of discriminative knowledge is called lustre of knowledge. People who try to acquire and hold on to sensuous objects, knowing full well that attachment to these causes misery, have one type of knowledge. Such knowledge grows more vivid in persons who having realised it try to renounce sensuous objects. And full realisation of the knowledge that all sensuous objects bring sorrow is attained by persons who after having forsaken them completely refrain from taking to them. The same is true of discriminative knowledge also.

(2) The commentator, in reply to the criticism how such practice can be the cause of discriminative knowledge, has shown how the practice of restraints (Yama) and observances (Niyama) as accessories to Yoga can eradicate impurities.

Avidyā or nescience is wrong knowledge. Practice of restraints and observances enjoined by Yoga, means not to act under the influence of wrong knowledge. These weaken wrong knowledge and render discriminative knowledge more vivid. Aversion, for example, is a mental modification based on wrong knowledge. Inclination to inflict injury is the principal offshoot of aversion. Through practice of Ahiṁsā or spirit of harmlessness the effect of wrong knowledge, in the form of aversion, is arrested. Thereby discriminative knowledge gradually becomes established. Similarly, through practice of truth many other vices like greed etc. are destroyed. When through the practice of Āsana (Yogic postures) and Prāṇāyāma (breath control) the body becomes steady, motionless and insentient, as it were, the wrong notion 'I am the body' wanes and the condition favourable to the growth of the right knowledge 'I am not the body' increases. This is how practice of Yoga brings about true knowledge. Directly through them impurities, in the form of delusive latencies, are removed and it leads to the dawn of true knowledge.

Impurities mean not only wrong knowledge but also actions done under its influence and the latent impressions thereof. Practice of Yogāṅgas implies action, based on right knowledge, which destroys action based on wrong knowledge and leads to the development of right knowledge. Right knowledge eradicates wrong knowledge. With the total annihilation of misapprehension, Buddhi is arrested and liberation is attained. Practice of Yoga thus becomes the cause of emancipation.

Some people get upset on hearing that Yoga begets true knowledge. They hold that practice of Yoga can never be the cause of knowledge, which, according to them, can only be derived through direct perception, inference and from accredited teachers. Yogins do not dispute this proposition. It has been shown above how practice of Yoga is conducive to the acquisition of knowledge. In fact, Samādhi is the best form of direct perception. The reasoning that follows therefrom culminates in discriminative knowledge, while the knowledge concerning Mokṣa or liberation imparted by a preceptor who has attained direct perception is the purest Āgama.

Practice of Yoga is the cause of wisdom. The commentator has clearly explained before that the material cause is not the only cause. In fact, Mokṣa (liberation, emancipation) has no material cause. Bondage means union of the Guṇas and Puruṣa. The union of supra-spatial Puruṣa and Prakṛti is not like the union of two external objects which implies contiguous existence. Their contact is only the undifferentiated notion of them. That conception of union is destroyed by discrimination. Yoga is the means of removal of impurities and attainment of discrimination. Discrimination destroys misapprehension. This is how Yoga is the cause of emancipation. Just as there can be no material cause for the union (of Puruṣa and Prakṛti), so there cannot be any material cause of their dissociation *i.e.* of Mokṣa or dissociation from misery.

———

भाष्यम्—तत्र योगाङ्गान्यवधार्यन्ते—

यमनियमासनप्राणायामप्रत्याहारधारणाध्यानसमाधयोऽष्टावङ्गानि ॥ २९ ॥

यथाक्रममेतेषामनुष्ठानं स्वरूपं च वक्ष्यामः ॥ २९ ॥

The accessories to Yoga are being ascertained.

**Yama (Restraint), Niyama (Observance), Āsana (Posture), Prāṇāyāma (Regulation Of Breath), Pratyāhāra (Withholding Of Senses), Dhāraṇā (Fixity), Dhyāna (Meditation) And Samādhi (Perfect Concentration) Are The Eight (1) Means Of Attaining Yoga. 29.**

The method of their practice and their nature will be described later seriatim.

(1) Some raise the objection that the means of attaining Yoga have been mentioned in another Śāstra as six in number. Whatever might be the number of the practices by splitting them up, nobody can transgress the means as indicated in these eight forms. In the Mahābhārata it is stated : "In the Vedas, Yoga is described by the sages as endowed with eight forms."

———

भाष्यम्—तत्र—

अहिंसासत्यास्तेयब्रह्मचर्यापरिग्रहा यमाः ॥ ३० ॥

तत्राहिंसा सर्वथा सर्वदा सर्वभूतानामनभिद्रोहः। उत्तरे च यमनियमास्तन्मूलास्तत्सिद्धिपरतया तत्प्रतिपादनाय प्रतिपाद्यन्ते, तदवदातरूपकरणायैवोपादीयन्ते। तथा चोक्तं "स खल्वयं ब्राह्मणो यथा यथा व्रतानि बहूनि समादित्सते तथा तथा प्रमादकृतेभ्यो हिंसानिदानेभ्यो निवर्त्तमानस्तामेवावदातरूपामहिंसां करोतीति।" सत्यं यथार्थे वाङ्मनसे, यथा दृष्टं यथानुमितं यथा श्रुतं तथा वाङ्मनश्चेति। परत्र स्वबोधसंक्रान्तये वागुक्ता सा यदि न वञ्चिता भ्रान्ता वा प्रतिपत्तिबन्ध्या वा भवेदिति, एषा सर्वभूतोपकारार्थं प्रवृत्ता न भूतोपघाताय, यदि चैवमप्यभिधीयमाना भूतोपघातपरैव स्यान्न सत्यं भवेत् पापमेव भवेत्। तेन पुण्याभासेन पुण्यप्रतिरूपकेण कष्टं तमः प्राप्नुयात्, तस्मात् परीक्ष्य सर्वभूतहितं सत्यं ब्रूयात्। स्तेयमशास्त्रपूर्वकं द्रव्याणां परतः स्वीकरणम्, तत्प्रतिषेधः पुनरस्पृहारूपमस्तेयमिति। ब्रह्मचर्यं गुप्तेन्द्रियस्योपस्थस्य संयमः। विषयाणामर्जनरक्षणक्षयसङ्गहिंसादोषदर्शनादस्वीकरणमपरिग्रह इत्येते यमाः ॥ ३० ॥

Of these—

**Ahiṁsā (Non-Injury), Satya (Truth), Asteya (Abstention From Stealing), Brahmacharya (Continence) And Aparigraha (Abstinence From Avariciousness) Are The Five Yamas (Forms Of Restraint). 30.**

Of these Ahiṁsā (1) is to abstain from injuring any being, at any time and in any manner. Truth and other forms of restraints and observances are based on the spirit of non-injury. They, being the means of fulfilment of non-injury, have been recommended in the Śāstras for establishing Ahiṁsā. They are also the best means of making Ahiṁsā pure. That is why it has been stated in the Śāstras : "As the Brāhmaṇa advances in the cultivation of the many virtues prescribed for him, he abstains from acts of injury to others due either to misapprehension or ignorance and thus purifies within himself the virtue of non-injury (Ahiṁsā)."

Satya (truthfulness) (2) is correspondence of speech and mind to fact, *i.e.* saying and thinking of what has been seen, heard or inferred. Words uttered for the purpose of communicating one's thoughts to others are true provided they do not appear deceitful, delusive and meaningless to the listeners. The words should, however, be uttered not for inflicting harm on creatures but for their benefit ; because if they hurt others, they do not produce piety as truth would, but only sin. By using such apparently truthful words (which hurt others) one gets into painful consequences (or infernal region). Therefore, truthful words beneficial to all creatures should be uttered after careful consideration.

Steya (3) means unlawfully taking things belonging to others. Asteya is abstention from such tendencies even in one's mind.

Brahmacharya = Suppressing the urge of the sexual organ and of the activities of other organs leading to it (4).

Aparigraha means to desist from taking or coveting things, seeing that getting and keeping them involve trouble, that they are subject to decay, that association with them causes mischief and that they beget malice. These constitute Yama or restraint.

(1) The commentator has given a lucid exposition of non-injury. Śruti says: "Do not injure any creature." Non-injury is not merely refraining from injuring animals, but developing and entertaining feelings of amity towards all living beings. It is not possible to practise non-injury unless selfishness is given up in respect of all external matters. To nourish one's own body with the flesh of another is the chief form of inflicting injury. Besides, seeking one's own comfort inevitably involves causing pain to others. To frighten others, to hurt them with rude words etc. are acts of injury. Truth and other forms of restraints and observances weaken the selfish tendencies of greed and envy, and thereby make Ahiṁsā all the purer.

Since killing of living beings is unavoidable in the course of one's life, some people wonder how it can be possible to practise non-injury. This doubt arises out of ignorance of the principle of the practice of non-injury. The commentator has said that enjoyment of material objects is not possible without hurting others (vide II.15). Therefore in order to live, hurting living beings is inevitable. Knowing that, the Yogins practise Yoga to avoid being born again. This is the highest form of practice of non-injury. To refrain, as far as possible, from inflicting injury on trees and animals is the next form and the third is to avoid, as far as possible, infliction of pain on the higher animals. Briefly, the spirit of non-injury is abandonment of the evil tendencies such as malice, hatred, etc. from which arises the propensity to inflict injury on livings beings. Unless there is an underlying feeling of cruelty, one's action resulting in the death of even one's parents is not regarded as an act of violence from social or spiritual point of view. There are grades of harmful acts. Injuring one's children or parents and killing an assailant are not the same, because no one can do the former unless there is intensely vile cruelty in him. The vileness of one's injurious acts varies with the intensity of evil intention in one's heart. That is why killing a man and cutting grass do not involve the same amount of cruelty. Again hurting a man with rude words is not the same as killing him. Killing an assailant and felling trees etc. are not regarded as cruelty at all by ordinary men, since they get involved in such acts in self-defence and the like, and these do not debase them further. That is why Manu has said that for ordinary men there is nothing wrong in taking meat which they do out of natural propensity, but to desist from it produces excellent results.

So far for ordinary men. But for Yogins observance of Ahiṁsā is a supreme vow ; that is why they try their best to practise harmlessness. First, they refrain from doing harm to human beings—even to an attacker—and commit as little harm as possible to animals even to the extent of only frightening away a snake and not killing it. Next they practise harmlessness to plant life. This is how Yogins, in spite of their having to commit unavoidable harm in the mildest form, go on intensifying the spirit of non-injury and ultimately through proficiency in Yoga get liberated from embodied existence and thus make themselves non-injurious to all creatures. Cleansing of the heart is the aim of the practice of Yogāṅgas.

(2) Truthfulness. The effort to make the mind and speech correspond to the thing which has been correctly apprehended is the practice of truth. Truth which might pain others is not to be spoken or thought of, *i.e.* causing pain to others by pointing out their shortcomings, wishing destruction of those who tread the path of untruth and thoughts of a similar nature.

With regard to truth, Upaniṣad has said : "Truth triumphs, not falsehood." For cultivating truth, one should initially speak as little as possible or observe silence. To dispose the mind to truth, one should first desist from reading fiction. Then abandoning worldly truths, only spiritual principles have to be contemplated upon. Thoughts of spiritual principles do not get any foothold in the minds of ordinary men which remain preoccupied with imaginary things. Such people derive only a partial glimpse of truth from parables, analogies etc. For instance, the precept of truth becomes effective in their case through such incongruous examples as that of a father telling the son : 'I shall break your head if you do not speak the truth.' For a Yogin practising unalloyed truth, such instruction or thought is not useful. Leaving aside all imaginary or unreal things, they engage their speech and mind in matters of truth and established facts. Real practice of truth is difficult unless the luxury of imagination is given up. When speaking the truth is likely to harm another, silence is advisable. Untruth should not be spoken even with the best of motives ; half-truth is still worse, it is conveyed by erroneous expression or innuendo.

(3) Taking a thing not given by its owner or to which one is not entitled, is Steya or stealing. To forsake such a thing and not to have even a desire to possess it is Asteya. Even if a jewel or treasure-trove is found by chance it is not to be taken because it belongs to somebody else. Thus, not to take a thing which is not one's own and the effort to give up even

the desire for such a thing is the practice of non-covetousness. We find in Īśa Upaniṣad : "Do not covet anybody's wealth."

(4) Brahmacharya (continence). Suppressing the urge of sexual organs = Restraining all organs like eyes etc. from such activities as might cause sexual urge and thus suppressing the urge of the sexual organ is continence. Mere refraining from the sexual act is not continence. "Thinking of, talking about, joking, looking intently, secret talk, resolve, attempt and execution are the eight forms of sexual indulgence, say the sages. The seekers of salvation should practise their opposites." Refraining from these eight forms of indulgence is continence. Whenever incontinent thoughts arise in the mind, they have to be forthwith dispelled. They should never be indulged in. For practice of continence, frugal meal is necessary. Plenty of milk and butter may be Sāttvika (pure) food for an ordinary person but not for a Yogin. For a Brahmachārin (one practising continence) the body should be kept a little less invigorated through frugal diet and moderate sleep. Thereby giving up all forms of incontinence and making the mind free from all such desires, if the particular organ is rendered mentally insensible, then can continence be established. A non-Brahmachārin cannot attain self-realisation. It is said in the Muṇḍaka Upaniṣad : "This soul is realised only through constant practice of truth, discipline, perfect knowledge and continence."

(5) There is trouble in acquiring objects which give us pleasure and enjoyment, trouble again in trying to preserve them and unhappiness when we lose them. Besides, possessing them leaves latent impressions of longing for them and thus causes sorrow in future. Attempts to acquire things again entail further misery and cause unhappiness to others in the process. So people seeking release from this type of bondage and consequent suffering, remember all these undesirable results of longings for enjoyment and refrain from such a course. Only things necessary for maintaining one's body should be accepted. To preserve wealth without utilising it for the good of others is sheer selfishness and lack of sympathy for others' need and distress. As Yogins seek to reach the limit of unselfishness, it is inevitable for them to give up completely all objects of enjoyment. Maintenance of the body being essential for success in Yoga and consequent liberation from all that is evil, Yogins take only as much as is necessary for its sustenance. Possession of material objects of enjoyment may thus be a great hindrance to one's success in the path of Yoga.

---

भाष्यम्—ते तु—

जातिदेशकालसमयानवच्छिन्नाः सार्वभौमा महाव्रतम् ॥ ३१ ॥

तत्राऽहिंसा जात्यवच्छिन्ना—मत्स्यबन्धकस्य मत्स्येष्वेव नान्यत्र हिंसा। सैव देशावच्छिन्ना—न तीर्थे हनिष्यामीति। सैव कालावच्छिन्ना—न चतुर्दश्यां न पुण्येऽहनि हनिष्यामीति। सैव त्रिभिरुपरतस्य समयावच्छिन्ना—देवब्राह्मणार्थे नान्यथा हनिष्यामीति, यथा च क्षत्रियाणां युद्ध एव हिंसा नान्यत्रेति। एभिर्जातिदेशकालसमयैरनवच्छिन्ना अहिंसादयः सर्वथैव परिपालनीयाः, सर्वभूमिषु सर्वविषयेषु सर्वथैवाविदितव्यभिचाराः सार्वभौमा महाव्रतमित्युच्यते ॥ ३१ ॥

These (the restraints),

**However, (Become A) Great Vow When They Become Universal, Being Unrestricted By Any Consideration Of Class, Place, Time Or Concept Of Duty (1). 31.**

The example of non-injury restricted by class is the case of a fisherman's non-injury to all except to fish. Harmlessness limited to place is practising non-killing only in holy places but not elsewhere, while that limited to period is observance of non-killing on a particular sacred day. Harmlessness, though not so limited might be restricted by idea of duty, *e.g.* observance of sacrifice of animals only to propitiate deities or for feeding of Brahmins and not for any other purpose. Another instance is of Kṣatriyas (fighting class) committing violence in war as a matter of duty, and practising harmlessness at other times. Thus the restraints, harmlessness, truth, etc. should be observed universally irrespective of class, place, period or customary duty. When they are observed in every instance, on all subjects without fail in any way, they attain universality and are called great vows.

(1) Every devotee practises some form or other of harmlessness etc. but Yogins practise them in their totality. Hence in their case these are universal and called great vows.

Notion of rule of duty = fighting being the duty of a Kṣatriya, Arjuna had to fight. That is violence enjoined by customary duty. Yogins, however, practise non-injury everywhere and always.

———

शौचसन्तोषतपःस्वाध्यायेश्वरप्रणिधानानि नियमाः ॥ ३२ ॥

भाष्यम्—तत्र शौचं मृज्जलादिजनितं मेध्याभ्यवहरणादि च बाह्यम्। आभ्यन्तरं चित्तमलानामाक्षालनम्। सन्तोषः सन्निहितसाधनादधिकस्यानुपादित्सा। तपः द्वन्द्वसहनम्, द्वन्द्वश्च जिघत्सापिपासे शीतोष्णे स्थानासने काष्ठमौनाकारमौने च। व्रतानि चैव यथायोगं कृच्छ्रचान्द्रायणसान्तपनादीनि। स्वाध्यायः मोक्षशास्त्राणामध्ययनं प्रणवजपो वा। ईश्वरप्रणिधानं तस्मिन्परमगुरौ सर्वकर्मार्पणं, 'शय्यासनस्थोऽथ पथि व्रजन् वा स्वस्थः परिक्षीणवितर्कजालः। संसारबीजक्षयमीक्षमाणः स्यान्नित्यमुक्तोऽमृतभोगभागी'। यत्रेदमुक्तं 'ततः प्रत्यक्चेतनाधिगमोऽप्यन्तरायाभावश्च' इति ॥ ३२ ॥

**Cleanliness, Contentment, Austerity (Mental And Physical Discipline), Svādhyāya (Study Of Scriptures And Chanting Of Mantras) And Devotion To God Are The Niyamas (Observances). 32.**

Of these, purificatory wash and consumption of pure food etc. constitute external cleanliness. Internal cleanliness is removal of impurities of the mind (1). Contentment (2) implies absence of desire for any possession in excess of the immediate necessities for maintaining one's life. Austerities (3) mean ability to bear such pains of extremes like hunger and thirst, heat and cold, standing calmly and sitting in posture, Kāṣṭha-mauna or absence of all expressions and Ākāra-mauna or absence of speech. It also includes observances of fast and hardship in respect of various religious vows. Svādhyāya includes study of the Śāstras relating to liberation and the repetition of the symbolic OM.

Īśvara-praṇidhāna (5) means surrender of all actions to God. It has been said in this connection : "Whether resting in bed or seated or walking, the Yogin established in self, with doubts dispelled, sees the cause of wordly existence weakening and thus becomes always content and entitled to enjoy immortal bliss." The author of the aphorisms has said (in I.29) : "From that (Īśvara-praṇidhāna) comes realisation of the self and the obstacles are resolved."

(1) Practice of cleanliness helps continence etc. The smell of putrid animal products generates a sedative feeling. From that people seek excitement and under its influence take to drinking and seek titillation of their senses. That is why the mind of an unclean person becomes clouded and his body unfit for the pursuit of Yoga. Therefore it is necessary for a Yogin to keep his body and place of residence clean and take only pure food. Putrid, stinking, alcoholic or other exciting food articles are regarded as impure. Intoxicating drink never brings about steadiness of mind. In Yoga, the mind has to be controlled. With intoxicants, the mind ceases to be under control ; they are therefore harmful to Yoga. It is said by Charaka : "What is good or most coveted in this life or hereafter, can be secured by intense concentration of the mind while alcohol creates a disturbance of the mind. Those who are blinded by addiction to alcohol, lose sight of what is best for them."

Cleansing the mind of impurities like arrogance, conceit, malice, etc. is internal purification.

(2) Contentment. A spirit of contentment has to be developed by reflecting on the sense of satisfaction that comes from getting a desired object. Next, the thought 'What I have got is enough' should be cultivated and meditated upon. That is how contentment has to be practised. It is said in the Śāstras that just as to escape from thorns it is necessary only to wear shoes and not to cover the face of the earth with leather, so happiness can be derived from contentment and not from thinking that I shall be happy when I get all I wish for.

(3) Austerity—see notes on II.1 and Appendix B. Practice of austerity for getting only a desired worldly object, is not Yogic austerity. Those who get upset by small sufferings cannot aspire to practise Yoga. That is why endurance has to be practised through the observance of austerities. When the body develops the power to endure hardship and when the mind does not get easily upset by lack of physical comfort, one becomes qualified for practising Yoga.

Kāṣṭha-mauna = not to indicate anything by words, gestures or signs.

Ākāra-mauna = indicating by gesture or sign but refraining from speech. By observance of silence one acquires the power to refrain from useless talk and use of rude words; it also helps practice of truth, develops power to withstand abuses and restrains the begging propensity.

If one is able to endure hunger and thirst, one is not easily disturbed thereby during meditation. Through Āsana, *i.e.* Yogic posture, steadiness of body is acquired. Physical (penitential) hardship is to be practised only if necessary for expiating sins, not otherwise.

(4) Through study of the scriptures and repetition of devotional Mantras uniformity of speech, which helps in the steady recollection of the desired object, is acquired. Through the study of Śāstras relating to emancipation, worldly thoughts decrease and a taste for spiritual objects arises.

(5) Placing one's own mind in the tranquil mind of God is placing self in God and God in self. By thinking that all unavoidable efforts are being done by Him, as it were, one can give up all desires for fruits of action and thus be able to completely surrender all actions to God. Such a devotee considers himself as established in God in all his actions and thus is perfectly at peace and continues his physical existence in a detached manner until his senses stop their functions. By meditating on God as Consciousness within self, a Yogin realises his individual Self (see I.29). When a person does anything being forgetful of God, he does so in an egoistic manner, but when he does not consider himself the agent, but keeps God in mind as the Lord, and wishes that all his actions may lead to Yoga, *i.e.* cessation of activities, then and then only he can be said to have surrendered himself to God.

———

भाष्यम्—एतेषां यमनियमानाम्—

वितर्कबाधने प्रतिपक्षभावनम् ॥ ३३ ॥

यदास्य ब्राह्मणस्य हिंसादयो वितर्का जायेरन् हनिष्याम्यहमपकारिणम्, अनृतमपि वक्ष्यामि, द्रव्यमप्यस्य स्वीकरिष्यामि, दारेषु चास्य व्यवायी भविष्यामि, परिग्रहेषु चास्य स्वामी भविष्यामीत्येवमुन्मार्गप्रवणवितर्कज्वरेणातिदीप्तेन बाध्यमानस्तत्प्रतिपक्षान्भावयेत्—घोरेषु संसाराङ्गारेषु पच्यमानेन मया शरणमुपागतः सर्वभूताभयप्रदानेन योगधर्मः, स खल्वहं त्यक्त्वा वितर्कान्पुनस्तानाददानस्तुल्यः

श्ववृत्तेन इति भावयेत्। यथा श्वा वान्तावलेही तथा त्यक्तस्य पुनराददान इत्येवमादि सूत्रान्तरेष्वपि योज्यम्॥ ३३ ॥

In respect of Yamas and Niyamas,

**When These Restraints And Observances Are Inhibited By Perverse Thoughts The Opposites Should Be Thought Of** (1). **33.**

When the knower of Brahman experiences feelings of hatred etc. and is tortured by the agonising fiery passions which lead to wrong course of conduct, such as 'I shall kill him who hurts me, I shall speak untruth, I shall take his things, I shall commit adultery with his wife, I shall take things belonging to others,' he should encourage contrary thoughts. He should contemplate : 'Roasted on the pitiless burning coal of the cycle of births, I took refuge in the virtues of Yoga by promising security to all living beings. After having abjured such perverse thoughts I am behaving like a dog in betaking myself to them. As a dog licks his vomits, so it is for me to take up thoughts and lines of action discarded by me as evil.' This type of opposite or contrary thinking is to be practised also in respect of the methods prescribed in the other Sūtras.

(1) Vitarka = Perverse thoughts—which give rise to actions opposed to the ten Yamas and Niyamas (restraints and observances)—like non-injury etc. They are—injury, untruth, theft, incontinence, avarice ; and uncleanliness, discontent, lack of endurance, talkativeness, thinking of the character of low persons or of ungodly attributes.

———

वितर्का हिंसादयः कृतकारितानुमोदिता लोभक्रोधमोहपूर्वका मृदुमध्याधिमात्रा दुःखाज्ञानानन्तफला इति प्रतिपक्षभावनम्॥ ३४ ॥

भाष्यम्—तत्र हिंसा तावत्कृता कारिताऽनुमोदितेति त्रिधा। एकैका पुनस्त्रिधा, लोभेन—मांसचर्मार्थेन, क्रोधेन—अपकृतमनेनेति, मोहेन—धर्मो मे भविष्यतीति। लोभक्रोधमोहाः पुनस्त्रिविधाः मृदुमध्याधिमात्रा इति। एवं सप्तविंशतिभेदा भवन्ति हिंसायाः। मृदुमध्याधिमात्राः पुनस्त्रिधा, मृदुमृदुः मध्यमृदुः तीव्रमृदुरिति तथा मृदुमध्यः मध्यमध्यः तीव्रमध्य इति तथा मृदुतीव्रः मध्यतीव्रः अधिमात्रतीव्र इति एवमेकाशीतिभेदा हिंसा भवति। सा पुनर्नियमविकल्पसमुच्चयभेदादसंख्येया प्राणभृद्भेदस्यापरिसंख्येयत्वादिति। एवमनृतादिष्वपि योज्यम्।

ते खल्वमी वितर्का दुःखाज्ञानानन्तफला इति प्रतिपक्षभावनं दुःखमज्ञानञ्चानन्तफलं येषामिति प्रतिपक्षभावनम्। तथा च हिंसकः प्रथमं तावद् वध्यस्य वीर्यमाक्षिपति, ततः शस्त्रादिनिपातेन दुःखयति, ततो जीवितादपि मोचयति। ततो वीर्याक्षेपादस्य चेतनाचेतनमुपकरणं क्षीणवीर्यं भवति, दुःखोत्पादान्नरकतिर्यक्प्रेतादिषु दुःखमनुभवति, जीवितव्यपरोपणात्प्रतिक्षणं च जीवितात्यये वर्तमानो मरणमिच्छन्नपि दुःखविपाकस्य नियतविपाकवेदनीयत्वात्कथञ्चिदेवोच्छ्वसिति। यदि च कथञ्चित् पुण्यादपगता (पुण्यावापगता इति पाठान्तरम्) हिंसा भवेत् तत्र सुखप्राप्तौ भवेदल्पायुरिति। एवमनृतादिष्वपि योज्यं यथासम्भवम्। एवं वितर्काणां चामुमेवानुगतं विपाकमनिष्टं भावयन्न वितर्केषु मनः प्रणिदधीत। प्रतिपक्षभावनाद्धेतोर्हेया वितर्काः॥ ३४॥

**Actions Arising Out Of Perverse Thoughts Like Injury Etc. Are Either Performed By Oneself, Got Done By Another Or Approved (1) ; Performed Either Through Anger, Greed or Delusion ; And Can Be Mild, Moderate Or Intense. That They Are The Causes Of Infinite Misery And Unending Ignorance Is The Contrary Thought. 34.**

Of these, injury can be of three kinds, either done directly, got done by another or approved when so done by another. Each one of these is again of three kinds. Through greed (as killing an animal) for skin and meat ; through anger as 'This man has done me a harm, therefore can be harmed' ; through delusion as in animal-sacrifice for acquiring merit. Greed, anger and delusion can again be of three kinds —mild, moderate and intense. Thus injury can be of twenty-seven varieties. Mild, moderate and intense can each be of three kinds—gently mild, moderately mild and extremely mild ; gently moderate, moderately moderate and extremely moderate ; and, gently intense, moderately intense and violently intense. In this way injury can be of eighty-one varieties. This again becomes innumerable because of varieties due to customary restrictive injunctions, Vikalpa (option, *e.g.* sacrificing this or that animal) and Samuchchaya (collective, *e.g.* sacrificing every kind of animal) as living creatures are innumerable. This sort of classification is also applicable in the case of untruth, theft, etc.

To think that 'these perversities produce endless consequences of pain and ignorance' is contrary thinking. Moreover, the injurer (animal-killer) first reduces the power of the victim (*e.g.* by tying him up), then inflicts pain by weapons and finally deprives him of life. And on account of enervating the victim, the injurer loses the vigour of his body and senses ; on account of causing pain he suffers by going to infernal regions or being born an animal or being an evil spirit ; and for killing he suffers from a fatal disease on account of which he goes on suffering continuously through sin of certain fruition (2) and although he prays for death he goes on living. If somehow the spirit of harm is removed or suppressed through piety (3) he might get happiness though he will be shortlived. This line of argument is applicable to untruth, theft, etc. as far as possible. Thinking thus of the inevitable evil effects of perverse thoughts and deeds, the mind should never again be engaged in them. Perverse thoughts are to be forsaken through their contrary thoughts.

(1) Approved—to approve injurious action done by another. To inflict pain on an animal personally is injuring directly. To purchase meat is getting injury done by another ; while approval is to commend injury done by another to an enemy or to a fierce animal, by saying that

he has done well in killing that man or snake. This kind of injury is again done either in anger, or through greed or under a delusion, *e.g.* holding that God has created some animals to be eaten by men.

Yogins should take particular care to see that their actions are not in the least tainted by causing injury etc. Then only the purest form of Yogic virtue appears.

(2) Sin of certain fruition implies that the sinful act will bear fruits fully in this life ; hence one goes on living till the consequences of the act are borne in their entirety.

(3) Removed or suppressed means not becoming effective through force of virtue. On that account the result of injury does not fully manifest itself but it shortens the life of the individual. The word 'Apagata' does not mean destruction but failure to produce adequate result.

———

भाष्यम्—यदास्य स्युरप्रसवधर्माणस्तदा तत्कृतमैश्वर्यं योगिनः सिद्धिसूचकं भवति, तद्यथा—

अहिंसाप्रतिष्ठायां तत्सन्निधौ वैरत्यागः ॥ ३५ ॥

सर्वप्राणिनां भवति ॥ ३५ ॥

When (by the practice of contrary thoughts) the perverse thoughts like those of injury etc. become unproductive (1) (like roasted seeds), then the supernormal power acquired by the Yogin indicates his success—*viz.*

**As The Yogin Becomes Established In Non-Injury, All Beings Coming Near Him Cease To Be Hostile. 35.**

(1) One gets established in the restraints (Yama) and observances (Niyama) through Samādhi (perfect concentration) or meditation approximating to it. A deep state of meditation on God and Samādhi are achieved at the same time. Perverse thoughts like injury etc. are known in their subtlest forms only through meditation and are removed from the mind through force of meditation. Sublime meditation is the cause of establishment in restraints and observances. Many think that Yamas (restraints) have to be practised first, then Niyamas (observances).

That is wrong. From the very beginning Dhāraṇā (fixity) favourable to Yama, Niyama, Āsana, Prāṇāyāma and Pratyāhāra has to be practised. Dhāraṇā (fixity) when developed becomes Dhyāna (meditation) which later becomes Samādhi (concentration). The practice of restraints and observances becomes steady and faultless and postures etc. become perfect.

To be established in restraints and observances means that there is complete elimination of perverse thoughts. When the desire to do harm or retaliate even under provocation never arises in the mind only then can one be said to have been established in the virtues mentioned before.

It is a known fact that men can bring other human beings and also animals under control by mesmerism, through development of will-power. It is understandable, therefore, that living beings near the Yogin, who has developed his will-power to such an extent as to remove all thoughts of violence from his mind, will eschew violence under his influence.

———

सत्यप्रतिष्ठायां क्रियाफलाश्रयत्वम् ॥ ३६ ॥

भाष्यम्—धार्मिको भूया इति भवति धार्मिकः, स्वर्गं प्राप्नुहीति स्वर्गं प्राप्नोति, अमोघास्य वाग्भवति ॥ ३६ ॥

**When Truthfulness Is Achieved** (1) **The Words (Of The Yogin) Acquire The Power Of Making Them Fruitful. 36.**

The words of one who is established in truth become infallible, for example, if he says to somebody 'Be virtuous' he becomes virtuous, if he says 'Go to heaven' he goes to heaven.

(1) The result of being established in truth is produced also by will-power. One whose mind and speech are always occupied with truth and the thought of telling a lie does not occur even for saving one's life, then it is certain that one's will-force conveyed by one's speech will be infallible. Disease or habit of lying or timidity can be cured by hypnotic suggestions. Similarly, the strongly developed will-power of a Yogin, working through the channel of simple truth, can produce feeling in the mind of the listener in accord with his uttered words and weaken the contrary thoughts. Thus when he says 'Be virtuous' it leads to the mani-

festation of the latency of virtue and makes the hearer virtuous. Yogins, however, do not entertain fruitless resolutions beyond the reach of their power.

———

अस्तेयप्रतिष्ठायां सर्वरत्नोपस्थानम् ॥ ३७ ॥

भाष्यम्—सर्वदिक्स्थान्यस्योपतिष्ठन्ते रत्नानि ॥ ३७ ॥

**When Non-Stealing Is Established All Jewels Present Themselves. 37.**

Jewels from all directions come to him (1).

(1) On the establishment of non-stealing, *i.e.* non-covetousness, such look of indifference radiates from the devotee's face that any being looking at him regards him as greatly trustworthy and donors consider themselves fortunate in being able to make a present to him of their best things. Thus, as the Yogin roams from place to place jewels (best of things) from different quarters reach him. Fascinated by the powers of the Yogin and considering him as a source of great consolation, the best among the conscious beings appear before him personally, while inanimate precious things are brought to him by donors. The word Ratna or jewel implies the best of every class (animate or inanimate).

———

ब्रह्मचर्यप्रतिष्ठायां वीर्यलाभः ॥ ३८ ॥

भाष्यम्—यस्य लाभादप्रतिघान् गुणानुत्कर्षयति, सिद्धश्च विनेयेषु ज्ञानमाधातुं समर्थो भवतीति ॥ ३८ ॥

**When Continence Is Established, Vīrya Is Acquired. 38.**

Through the power acquired, unimpeded powers (1) like minification etc. are perfected, and being endowed with inborn faculty, he is enabled to instil knowledge in the minds of his disciples.

(1) Unimpeded power includes unobstructed knowledge, action and power like the power of minification or reducing oneself to a small particle. Incontinence deprives the nerves etc. of vital powers. Practice of continence prevents loss of vitality and increases Vīrya or energy [see I. 20 (2)], thereby gradually leading to accumulation of unhindered powers. And having attained knowledge, he is able to instil it in his disciples. The words of wisdom of an incontinent person do not go deep into the mind of a disciple.

Mere refraining from the sexual act while indulging in food and sleep, does not lead to being established in continence. Continence cannot be achieved unless the natural production of the body-seed is checked by abstaining from thoughts on objects of desire through a firm control over one's mind and controlled diet and sleep.

———

अपरिग्रहस्थैर्ये जन्मकथन्तासम्बोधः ॥ ३९ ॥

भाष्यम्—अस्य भवति। कोऽहमासं, कथमहमासं, किंस्विदिदं, कथंस्विदिदं, के वा भविष्यामः, कथं वा भविष्याम इति, एवमस्य पूर्वान्तपरान्तमध्येष्वात्मभावजिज्ञासा स्वरूपेणोपावर्त्तते। एता यमस्थैर्ये सिद्धयः ॥ ३९ ॥

**On Attaining Perfection In Non-Acceptance, Knowledge Of Past And Future Existences Arises. 39.**

Questionings regarding the past, present and future states of one's body, in the forms of 'Who was I and what was I ? What is this body ? How did it come about ? What shall I be in future ? How shall it be ?' get properly resolved in a Yogin (1). The powers mentioned before are developed on being established in Yamas, the restraints.

(1) When through development of a spirit of non-acceptance, objects of bodily enjoyment appear as insignificant, the body itself appears to be a superfluous burden. Thereby a sense of detachment towards sense-objects and the body arises. From meditation based on that idea, knowledge of the past life is derived. The delusion that exists from close attachment to one's body and objects stands in the way of knowledge of the past and the future. When the body is made completely steady and

effortless, powers of clairvoyance etc. are acquired irrespective of the body. Similarly when along with objects of enjoyment, the body also is regarded as a superfluous burden, one becomes conscious of the body as separate from the self and thus rising above bodily delusion comes to know one's past and future lives.

---

भाष्यम्—नियमेषु वक्ष्यामः—

शौचात्स्वाङ्गजुगुप्सा परैरसंसर्गः ॥ ४० ॥

स्वाङ्गे जुगुप्सायां शौचमारभमाणः कायावद्यदर्शी कायानभिष्वङ्गी यतिर्भवति। किञ्च परैरसंसर्गः कायस्वभावावलोकी स्वमपि कायं जिहासुर्मृज्जलादिभिराक्षालयन्नपि कायशुद्धिमपश्यन् कथं परकायैरत्यन्तमेवाप्रयतैः संसृज्येत ॥ ४० ॥

Speaking of Niyamas or observances—

**From The Practice Of Purification, Aversion Towards One's Own Body Is Developed And Thus Aversion Extends To Contact With Other Bodies. 40.**

When aversion to his own body arises, the Yogin practising purification, perceives the imperfections of the body and loses his love for it. Moreover, a distaste develops for the company of others, because one, who has developed aversion to his own body realising that he cannot properly clean it even by ablution etc., finds it impossible to come into contact with the unclean body of another person (1).

(1) Through the practice of purifying one's own body, an aversion to the body and a distaste for contact with other bodies are developed. An animal expresses its love for another animal through imitation of eating by licking it. Such expressions of animality in love are removed by the practices of purification. Love of a Yogin is expressed through sentiments of friendliness, compassion, etc. which are free from sensuousness. By the practice of purification, the desire for contact with women and children totally disappears.

---

भाष्यम्—किञ्च—

सत्त्वशुद्धिसौमनस्यैकाग्र्येन्द्रियजयात्मदर्शनयोग्यत्वानि च ॥ ४१ ॥

भवन्तीति वाक्यशेषः। शुचेः सत्त्वशुद्धिस्ततः सौमनस्यं तत ऐकाग्र्यं तत इन्द्रियजयस्ततश्चात्मदर्शनयोग्यत्वं बुद्धिसत्त्वस्य भवति। इत्येतच्छौचस्थैर्यादधिगम्यत इति ॥ ४१ ॥

Moreover—

**Purification Of The Mind, Pleasantness Of Feeling, One-Pointedness, Subjugation Of The Senses And Ability For Self-Realisation Are Acquired. 41.**

The Yogin, practising cleanliness gets purification of heart which leads to mental bliss, or spontaneous feeling of joy. From mental bliss develops one-pointedness which leads to subjugation of the senses. From subjugation of the organs, Buddhi (pure I-sense) develops the power of realising the Self (1). All these are attained by establishment in purification.

(1) The evils of arrogance, pride, attachment, etc. being wholly removed, a sense of cleanliness of the mind arises and a spirit of aloofness from one's own body as well as from others' grows. This state, uncontaminated by the body-sense, is called internal purification. It brings about purification of the mind, and lessening of impurities in the form of worldly obsession. This leads to the development of mental bliss or a feeling of gladness and the body acquires a Sāttvika form of easiness. Without such a feeling of gladness, one-pointedness of mind is not possible, without which it is not possible to realise the Soul beyond the senses.

———

सन्तोषादनुत्तमसुखलाभः ॥ ४२ ॥

भाष्यम्—तथा चोक्तम् 'यच्च कामसुखं लोके यच्च दिव्यं महत्सुखम्। तृष्णाक्षयसुखस्यैते नार्हतः षोड़शीं कलाम्' इति ॥ ४२ ॥

**From Contentment Unsurpassed Happiness Is Gained. 42.**

It has been said in this connection : "The happiness gained on this earth through the enjoyment of desired objects, or the supreme heavenly joy, is not even one-sixteenth of the happiness caused by the cessation of desires."

———

कायेन्द्रियसिद्धिरशुद्धिक्षयात्तपसः ॥ ४३ ॥

भाष्यम्—निर्वर्त्यमानमेव तपो हिनस्त्यशुद्ध्यावरणमलं, तदावरणमलापगमात्कायसिद्धिरणिमाद्या, तथेन्द्रियसिद्धिर्दूराच्छ्रवणदर्शनाद्येति ॥ ४३ ॥

**Through Destruction Of Impurities, Practice Of Austerities Brings About Perfection Of The Body And The Organs. 43.**

When austerities are practised, the veil of impurity is removed. Then perfection (Siddhi) of the body in the form of Aṇimā (minification) etc. and of the organs in the forms of clairaudience, clairvoyance, etc. develop (1).

(1) Austerities in the form of Prāṇāyāma etc. chiefly remove the impurity in the form of subjection to the limitations of the body. Removal of such subjection (*i.e.* not being affected by hunger and thirst, by steady Yogic postures, or by breathing etc.) leads to the removal of the resultant veil of impurities. Then, the mind, unaffected by bodily limitations, due to the unhindered growth of will-power can bring about perfections (Siddhis) of the body and the organs. Yogins, however, do not make use of Yogic austerities for the attainment of such forms of perfection (Siddhi), but they apply them for spiritual attainments.

Austerities like practice ofsle eplessness, steadiness of posture, abstention from food, suspension of vital energy, etc. are opposed to human nature and favourable to the nature of celestial beings, hence they bring about perfections (Siddhis) of the body and the senses. That is why Jñānayogins, who devote themselves only to the practice of renunciation and cultivation of discriminative knowledge, to the exclusion of such austerities, may not have these Siddhis. With the attainment of discriminative knowledge, Samādhi also can be attained ; and if a Yogin of that class so desires, he may attain the form of supernormal perfection called Vivekaja-siddhi (III.52). But it is not likely for the Yogin possessed of discriminative knowledge to have this desire. That is why Jñānayogins may attain emancipation without attaining the powers of Siddhi of the body and the senses [III. 55 (1)].

---

स्वाध्यायादिष्टदेवतासम्प्रयोगः ॥ ४४ ॥

भाष्यम्—देवा ऋषयः सिद्धाश्च स्वाध्यायशीलस्य दर्शनं गच्छन्ति, कार्ये चास्य वर्त्तन्त इति ॥ ४४ ॥

**From Study And Repetition Of The Mantras Communion With The Desired Deity Is Established. 44.**

The heavenly beings, sages and the Siddhas (celestials) become visible to the Yogin who practises Svādhyāya (1), and the Yogin's wishes are fulfilled by them.

(1) Ordinarily, during repetition (Japa) of Mantra (devotional chant, *e.g.* word symbolic of God) thought does not remain fixed on its meaning. The person performing Japa might be repeating the words aimlessly, with his mind roaming elsewhere. When Svādhyāya is established, the formula and the idea behind it remain uninterruptedly present before the mind. Deities invoked with such ardour and faith are sure to appear before the devotee. Invocation of God made sometimes earnestly, sometimes mechanically with the mind preoccupied with worldly affairs, does not produce the desired result.

---

समाधिसिद्धिरीश्वरप्रणिधानात् ॥ ४५ ॥

भाष्यम्—ईश्वरार्पितसर्वभावस्य समाधिसिद्धिर्यया सर्वमीप्सितमवितथं जानाति, देशान्तरे देहान्तरे कालान्तरे च, ततोऽस्य प्रज्ञा यथाभूतं प्रजानातीति ॥ ४५ ॥

**From Devotion To God, Samādhi Is Attained. 45.**

The Yogin who reposes all his thoughts on God, attains Samādhi (1). By the attainment of Samādhi, the Yogin knows all that is desired to be known, whatever happened in another life, in another place or at another time or even what is happening at present. Thereby his enlightenment reveals things as they are.

(1) Constant devotion to God easily leads to the attainment of Samādhi. Other Yamas and Niyamas conduce to the attainment of Samādhi by other means, but devotion to God directly leads to Samādhi, because it is a form of contemplation favourable to Samādhi. That contemplation becoming deep, makes the body motionless and restraining the organs from their objects, culminates in Dhāraṇā (fixity) and Dhyāna (meditation) and ultimately in Samādhi. Surrender of all thoughts to God means mentally merging oneself into God.

Ignorant people express the doubt that if the practice of devotion to God is the cause of attainment of Samādhi, then the other Yogāṅgas must be unnecessary. This is not correct. Samādhi cannot be attained by one who runs about without restraint, or whose mind is distracted by knowledge of worldly objects. Samādhi itself means the state of intense meditation (Dhyāna) which again means deepening of Dhāraṇā or fixity. Thus attainment of Samādhi implies the practice of all accessories of Yoga. What is meant is that instead of taking up other objects of meditation, if the aspirant takes to the practice of devotion to God from the very beginning, Samādhi is easily attained. After the attainment of Samādhi one gains emancipation through Samprajñāta and Asamprajñāta Yogas. This is what has been said by the commentator.

If there is a lapse in the observance of a single item of Yamas and Niyamas, the effect of all the disciplines is impaired. The Śāstras corroborate this.

———

भाष्यम्—उक्ताः सह सिद्धिभिर्यमनियमा आसनादीनि वक्ष्यामः। तत्र—

स्थिरसुखमासनम् ॥ ४६ ॥

तद् यथा पद्मासनम्, वीरासनम्, भद्रासनम्, स्वस्तिकम्, दण्डासनम्,

सोपाश्रयम्, पर्यङ्कम्, क्रौञ्चनिषदनम्, हस्तिनिषदनम्, उष्ट्रनिषदनम्, समसंस्थानम्, स्थिरसुखं यथासुखञ्च इत्येवमादीति ॥ ४६ ॥

The restraints (Yamas) and observances (Niyamas) along with their perfections (Siddhis) having been described, the Āsanas etc. are now being described.

**Motionless And Agreeable Form (Of Staying) Is Āsana (Yogic Posture). 46.**

They are as follows :—Padmāsana, Vīrāsana, Bhadrāsana, Svastikāsana, Daṇḍāsana, Sopāśraya, Paryaṅka, Krauñcha (heron)-niṣadana, Hasti (elephant)-niṣadana, Uṣṭra (camel)-niṣadana, and Sama-saṁsthāna. When these postures can be held comfortably, they are called (Yogic) Āsanas (1).

(1) Padmāsana is a well-known posture. Placing the right foot on the left thigh, and the left foot on the right thigh, one has to sit keeping the spine perfectly straight. Vīrāsana is half of Padmāsana, *i.e.* one foot has to be kept on the opposite thigh, and the other foot below the opposite thigh. In Bhadrāsana, placing the soles of feet on the ground before the scrotum, and close to each other, the soles have to be covered by the two palms. In Svastikāsana, one has to sit up straight, the soles of feet being stuck between the opposite thigh and knee. In Daṇḍāsana, one has to sit stretching the two legs, closely fixing together the two heels and toes. Sopāśraya is squatting tying the back and the two legs with a piece of cloth called 'Yoga-paṭṭaka' (a strong piece of cloth by which the back and the two legs are tied while squatting). In the Paryaṅka-āsana, one has to lie down stretching the thighs and hands ; it is also called Śavāsana, the posture of the dead. Krauñcha-niṣadana etc. have to be followed by observing the posture of resting adopted by the animals concerned. Contracting the two heels and toes, and pressing one sole with the other while squatting is called Sama-saṁsthāna.

In all the (Yogic) Āsanas, the spine has to be kept straight. The Śruti also says : "The breast, neck and the head have to be kept erect." Moreover, the posture has to be motionless and comfortable. The posture which causes pain or restlessness is not a Yogic posture (vide next Śūtra).

प्रयत्नशैथिल्यानन्तसमापत्तिभ्याम् ॥ ४७ ॥

भाष्यम्—भवतीति वाक्यशेषः। प्रयत्नोपरमात् सिध्यत्यासनं, येन नाङ्गमेजयो भवति। अनन्ते वा समापन्नं चित्तमासनन्निर्वर्त्तयतीति ॥ ४७ ॥

**By Relaxation Of Effort And Meditation On The Infinite (Āsanas Are Perfected). 47.**

By relaxation of the body Āsana is perfected ; this stops shaking of the limbs (which is an obstacle to Samādhi). Or, a mind fixed on the infinite brings about perfection (Siddhi) of the Āsana (1).

(1) Perfection of Āsana, *i.e.* perfect steadiness of the body and a sense of comfort, are attained by relaxation of the body and meditation on the infinite. Relaxation means making the body effortless like a corpse. After sitting, the whole body should be relaxed, taking care at the same time that the body does not bend. This brings about steadiness of the body, and the sense of pain being diminished, the posture (Āsana) becomes easy and perfect. Fixing the mind on the infinite, or on the surrounding void, also develops perfection of Āsana. Practice of Āsana cannot be perfected unless some amount of pain is borne in the beginning. When a posture is practised for some time pain will be felt in various parts of the body. This will disappear with the practice of relaxation and meditation on infinite space (and feeling the body as becoming void also). The habit of keeping the body always at rest and effortless, helps the practice of Āsana. In the course of the practice of Āsana, it will be felt as though the body has got fixed to the earth. On attaining further steadiness, it will be felt that the body is non-existent as it were. 'My body has become like void dissolving itself in infinite space and I am like the wide expanse of the sky'—this form of thought is called meditation on the infinite (Ananta-samāpatti).

———

ततो द्वन्द्वानभिघातः ॥ ४८ ॥

भाष्यम्—शीतोष्णादिभिर्द्वन्द्वैरासनजयान्नाभिभूयते ॥ ४८ ॥

**From That Arises Immunity From Dvandvas Or Opposite Conditions. 48.**

When perfection in Āsana is attained, the devotee is not affected by the opposite conditions like heat and cold etc. (1).

(1) The Yogin, who has perfected the practice of Āsana, is not affected by heat or cold, hunger or thirst. A state of anaesthesia, in which heat or cold is not felt, sets in when the body becomes like void from attaining steadiness in Āsana. A similar feeling of tranquillity applied to centres of sensation of hunger or thirst, makes one insensitive to these feelings. In fact, pain is a form of restlessness, which is subdued by the practice of calmness.

———

तस्मिन्सति श्वासप्रश्वासयोर्गतिविच्छेदः प्राणायामः ॥ ४६ ॥

भाष्यम्—सत्यासनजये वाह्यस्य वायोराचमनं श्वासः, कौष्ठ्यस्य वायोर्निःसारणं प्रश्वासः, तयोर्गतिविच्छेद उभयाभावः प्राणायामः ॥ ४६ ॥

**That (Āsana) Having Been Perfected, Regulation Of The Flow Of Inhalation And Exhalation Is Prāṇāyāma (Breath Control). 49.**

Āsana having been perfected, suspension of either of the processes of drawing in external air and exhaling internal air constitutes a Prāṇāyāma (1).

(1) The Prāṇāyāma mentioned in this Yoga is not the same as those mentioned in Haṭha-yoga as exhalation (Rechaka), inhalation (Pūraka) and suspension (Kumbhaka). Some commentators have tried to make the two correspond but that is not proper.

If the air is not expelled after inhalation, there is a cessation of the movement of breath ; this is one Prāṇāyāma. Similarly, if after expulsion of air, the movement of breath is suspended, that also is a Prāṇāyāma. It is the suspension of breath, following either inhalation or exhalation, that constitutes a Prāṇāyāma. Prāṇāyāmas have thus to be practised one after another. A description of the Prāṇāyāma as suspension after exhalation has been given in the Sūtra I.34.

Prāṇāyāma can be performed after Āsana has been perfected. Prāṇāyāma can be practised even before Āsana has been perfected if the body becomes steady in Āsana and the mind is occupied with a sense of void, or any other form of tranquil thought. Prāṇāyāma practised with a restless mind cannot be regarded as a part of Yoga. Prāṇāyāma does not become conducive to Samādhi unless steadiness of the body and one-pointedness of the mind on one subject are maintained along with suspension of breath. That is why Āsana is necessary from the beginning. Contemplation on God, or on a feeling of physical or mental void, or on a feeling of luminosity within the heart, has to be practised with each incoming and outgoing breath. In other words, the object contemplated upon should be present in the mind during each act of inhalation and exhalation which are to be looked upon as the predisposing causes of one-pointedness of the mind ; thus breathing and quietening of the mind have to be synchronized through practice. When this is mastered, the suspension of the movement (of breath) has to be practised. During this practice, the mind has also to be kept fixed on the object of contemplation. That is, the suspension of breath and the mind's fixation on the object of concentration should be made as a single effort. Or the mind has to be kept fixed on the object of meditation by the same effort by which suspension is attained with the feeling that the object itself is being held, as it were, tightly in a mental embrace. If fluctuations of the mind remain suspended as long as the suspension of breath is maintained, one real Prāṇāyāma is performed. Dhāraṇā (fixation of the mind on an object) has to be practised with the help of this form of Prāṇāyāma performed one after another. In Samādhi, however, the breath gets reduced progressively and becomes imperceptible, or is even wholly suspended.

The purport of this aphorism is : The suspension of the movement of air, incoming in inhalation and outgoing in exhalation, is Prāṇāyāma. The various ways in which this suspension can be practised will be shown in the next aphorism.

———

भाष्यम्—स तु—

वाह्याभ्यन्तरस्तम्भवृत्तिर्देशकालसंख्याभिः परिदृष्टो दीर्घसूक्ष्मः ॥ ५० ॥

यत्र प्रश्वासपूर्वको गत्यभावः स वाह्यः, यत्र श्वासपूर्वको गत्यभावः स आभ्यन्तरः। तृतीयः स्तम्भवृत्तिर्यत्रोभयाभावः सकृत्प्रयत्नाद् भवति, यथा तप्ते

न्यस्तमुपले जलं सर्वतः सङ्कोचमापद्येत तथा द्वयोर्युगपद् भवत्यभाव इति। त्रयोऽप्येते देशेन परिदृष्टाः—इयानस्य विषयो देश इति। कालेन परिदृष्टाः—क्षणानामियत्तावधारणेनावच्छिन्ना इत्यर्थः। संख्याभिः परिदृष्टाः—एतावद्भिः श्वासप्रश्वासैः प्रथम उद्घातस्तद्वन्निगृहीतस्यैतावद्भिर्द्वितीय उद्घात एवं तृतीय एवं मृदुरेवं मध्य एवं तीव्र इति संख्यापरिदृष्टः। स खल्वयमेवमभ्यस्तो दीर्घसूक्ष्मः ॥ ५० ॥

**That (Prāṇāyāma) Has External Operation (Vāhya-Vṛtti), Internal Operation (Ābhyantara-Vṛtti) And Suppression (Stambha-Vṛtti). These, Again, When Observed According To Space, Time And Number Become Long And Subtle** (1). **50.**

That which brings suspension of movement after exhalation is an external operation, or Vāhya-vṛtti Prāṇāyāma. That which brings suspension after inhalation is an internal operation, or Ābhyantara-vṛtti Prāṇāyāma. The third is suppression or Stambha-vṛtti. In this, the other two (*i.e.* external and internal operations) are absent. This is effected by one effort. Just as water dropped on a piece of hot stone shrinks simultaneously on all sides, even so (in the third, or suppression), the other two operations simultaneously disappear. These three operations, again, are regulated by (i) space, that is so much space is its scope, (ii) time, that is, according to the calculation of moments (Kṣaṇas), and (iii) number, *e.g.* so many incoming and outgoing breaths constitute the first stroke, so many numbers constitute the second stroke, similarly, the third stroke. Again, they are mild, moderate and intense. This is Prāṇāyāma regulated according to number. Prāṇāyāma becomes long and subtle after one gets habituated to it in this way.

(1) The words 'Rechaka' (expulsion of air), 'Pūraka' (drawing in of air) and 'Kumbhaka' (suspension of air) were not used in ancient times in the sense in which they are understood now. Had it been so, the author of the Sūtras would certainly have used them. They were coined later.

External operation (Vāhya-vṛtti), internal operation (Ābhyantara-vṛtti) and suppression (Stambha-vṛtti)—these three are not the same as expulsion of air (Rechaka), drawing in of breath (Pūraka) and suspension of breathing (Kumbhaka). The author of the Bhāṣya has described external operation as want of movement after exhalation. This is not the same as expulsion of air (Rechaka). Rechaka is a form of exhalation. In fact, later commentators only tried to reconcile the newer forms with the practices mentioned in this commentary. But none succeeded in reconciling them.

Interpreting the word 'Gatyabhāva' (suspension of movement) as 'suspension of natural movement', some sort of affinity between 'Rechaka-Pūraka' and external operation etc. may be found. After exhalation, keeping the air outside and not drawing in breath immediately, is an external operation ; this is both exhalation and suspension of breath. Similarly, the internal operation also is a combination of inhalation and suspension of breath. In some books it is stated that the suspension of breath after exhalation is the Vedic form of Prāṇāyāma, and suspension after inhalation is its Tāntric form. Thus, external operation etc. are not the same as merely Rechaka, Pūraka and Kumbhaka, as understood in modern times.

The ancient processes of 'Rechaka' etc., are similar to the processes described in the Yoga philosophy.

The particular form of effort, which brings about suppression, may be described as an effort at internal contraction of all the limbs of the body. When that effort becomes firm, suspension of breath can be maintained for a long time ; otherwise it cannot be maintained for more than two or three minutes. This should be clearly understood.

In the Haṭha-yoga that effort is called Mūla-bandha (contraction of the anus), Uddīyāna-bandha (contraction of the abdomen), and Jālandhara-bandha (contraction of the throat). The operation called Khecharī-mudrā is also similar. For the practice of this posture, the tongue has to be repeatedly pulled to elongate it gradually. Pressing the extended tongue into the nasopharynx and applying pressure on the nerves therein, or pulling them, it is possible to maintain suspension of breath and vital energies (state of catalepsy) for some time. As a result of these efforts at contraction, the nerves being inclined towards suspension, the breath and life energy may be suspended. By the adoption of a particular form of diet, and practices performed with a healthy body, the nerves and muscles attain a Sāttvika form of alacrity with the help of which this strong effort can be made (Buddhists describe this alacrity as gentleness and dexterity of the body). This effort cannot be made with a flabby body which is not muscular, hence there are instructions to make the body strong and perfectly healthy by the adoption of various postures and practices.

This is how Prāṇa (breathing) can be stopped with Haṭha, *i.e.* by enforced means. This, however, does not lead to stoppage of the activities of the mind, though it may help the process. After perfecting Prāṇāyāma if one practises control over the mind by means of Dhāraṇā etc., then only one can advance in the path of Yoga ; otherwise one will gain nothing, except keeping the body like a corpse for a period of time.

Apart from this, there are other methods of restraining the activities of Prāṇa. The functioning of Prāṇa may also be stopped by means of the Sāttvika form of restraint brought forth by sublime joy arising out of one-pointedness of mind of those who practise Īśvara-praṇidhāna (devotion to God) or Dhāraṇā on Consciousness for making their minds one-pointed. And once the one-pointedness becomes continuous, one can, remaining wholly absorbed in it, reduce or stop the intake of food and easily achieve Samādhi by stopping Prāṇa. The Mahābhārata says : "By reducing the diet, they conquer the fifth imperfection, *viz.* the breath" ; —this injunction is intended for such spiritual aspirants. The intense joy felt in the innermost being through devotion to God, Dhāraṇā of the Sāttvika type, etc. gives rise to a strong desire to hold on to it as if in an embrace by the heart, and produces a contraction of the nerve-centres that may stop the activities of Prāṇa. The impulse of contraction that is externally produced in Haṭha-yoga is internally induced in Prāṇāyāma.

To stop the activities of Prāṇa for a long time (as recommended in Haṭha-yoga) intestinal impurities have to be wholly removed. Otherwise putrid substances act as a hindrance and the abdomen cannot be fully contracted. Removal of intestinal impurities is not necessary if total fasting is observed, or a reduced diet (*i.e.* only water, or water mixed with milk) is taken.

Some people have an innate capacity to stop the activities of Prāṇa (breathing) . They can stop Prāṇa for a short or long period of time. We knew of a person who could remain buried for 10 or 12 days at a stretch. At that time, he did not wholly lose his consciousness but remained like an inert substance. Another person could, at will, make any particular limb of his body inert. It is needless to say that Yoga has nothing to do with these powers. Ignorant people may regard this as Samādhi. But let alone Samādhi, a person having the capacity to remain buried for even three months at a stretch, may not have even a remote conception of Yoga. It should always be clearly understood that Yoga primarily means control over the mind, and not merely control over the body. When the mind is wholly controlled, the body will certainly be brought under control. On the other hand, there may be full control over the body without the least control over the mind.

Suspension of breath after exhalation is an external operation of Prāṇāyāma, while suspension after inhalation is its internal operation. There is a third operation known as Stambha-vṛtti, in which there is no attempt at inhalation or exhalation. It involves total stoppage of breathing in one single effort, either in the process of inhalation or exhalation, with some air left in the lungs. The air thus remaining in the lungs is gradually exhausted. This operation gives rise to a feeling as though the whole body were being evacuated of air.

Just as water dropped on a piece of hot stone dries up simultaneously from all sides, even so by the operation of suppression, the function of breathing stops altogether. That is, air has not to be expelled from the body and held outside, for the purpose of stopping its flow ; conversely, the movement of breath has not to be stopped by inhaling air and holding it inside the body.

In the initial stage, either the external or the internal operation of Prāṇāyāma, should be adopted for practice. In the Sūtra (I.34) the author has shown preference for the external operation. Practising suppression once in a while, the breath has to be brought under control.

After practising either the external or internal operation for a time, one becomes able to practise suppression (Stambha). The ability to practise suppression develops automatically when, after practising either external or internal operation for some time, a few breaths are taken in the normal way. At first, the ability to practise suppression comes on after long intervals of time, later on it becomes more frequent. It is difficult to practise suppression when the lungs are either fully expanded or completely contracted. Only external and internal operations are possible under such conditions.

External operation, internal operation and suspension—these three forms of Prāṇāyāma practised according to the observations of space, time and number, gradually become long and subtle. Among them, observation of space comes first. Space has to be taken in two senses—external and internal. From the tip of the nose to the point up to which the flow of breath is extended, is the external space. The internal space is primarily the space inside one's body, up to the region of the heart, covered by the movement of air. Starting from the heart the entire body from head to foot, also constitutes the internal space.

Prāṇāyāma practised with observation of the distance covered by the exhaled air from the tip of the nose (keeping a watch that it covers as little distance as possible) is an operation regulated by observation of external space. This gradually weakens the exhalation. The internal space has to be perceived by feeling. When the inhaled air enters the lungs, it should be felt in the region of the heart. This constitutes Prāṇāyāma with the observation of internal space.

Taking the region of the heart as the centre, it has to be felt that a feeling of touch is spreading all over the body from about the heart during inhalation and the same feeling is being gathered and brought back to the region of the heart during exhalation. In this way it is necessary in the beginning to regard the whole body (specially up to the soles of the feet and the two palms) as the space under observation. This purifies the nerves, and the faculty of feeling spreading over the entire body becomes unobstructed, that is, the Sāttvika faculty of sentience is gained resulting in a feeling of ease all over the body. When Prāṇāyāma is practised with such a feeling of ease, it produces good result. Failing that it may make the body sick.

Having attained a feeling of ease, if along with it Stambha and other Vṛttis are practised, it leads to the augmentation of the Sāttvika quality of the body ; hence the function of Prāṇa or breath may be stopped for a long time, without much effort. Owing to the absence of inertness of the body the power to suppress (breath) also becomes exceedingly strong.

The carotid artery, running from the heart to the brain, is also to be counted as forming a part of the internal region. It has to be imagined as a flow of effulgence. Besides this, the feeling or idea of lustre emanating from the brain is also an internal region. In a particular form of Prāṇāyāma, it has to be observed.

Projecting the mind in these internal regions, Prāṇāyāma has to be practised with a feeling of internal touch. At the time of exhalation, it has to be felt as if that feeling from the whole body after being gathered in the heart-region is proceeding with the exhaled air up to 'Brahmarandhra' (the lower part of the cranium). During inhalation, it has to be felt that a feeling of touch proceeding from the heart-region is spreading over like a flow of air and pervading all parts of the body. This is how 'space' has to be observed. In the effort at suspension, 'space' has to be observed keeping the heart in view, along with an indistinct feeling of touch all over the body.

It is best to conceive the heart etc. as 'space' in the form of transparent sky. The concept of effulgent light is also useful. The image of one's desired deity may also be meditated on as being in the heart. When space is observed in these ways, the suspension in Prāṇāyāma becomes long, and the breathing becomes subtler. The author of the

Bhāṣya has said : 'So much space is its scope,' *i.e.* this form of observation is called observation of 'space'. Here by space is meant internal region about the heart and external space, and by scope, the space covered by inhalation and exhalation and the region where the mind rests during suspension.

Observation of 'time' is now being described. 'Kṣaṇa' = one fourth of the twinkling of an eye. The measure by 'Kṣaṇas', that is, the period of inhalation, exhalation and suspension should be of so many Kṣaṇas or moments. The observation of this means the practice of Prāṇāyāma regulated by time. Observation of time has to be practised by means of Japa (repetition of Mantra). Along with this, it is useful to have the awareness of time. It is through action (and the resultant mutation) that we come to have the idea of time. If the mind is fixed on the flow of sound, the conception of the passage of time becomes distinct. The idea of a movement or flow that is perceived when the mind is kept engaged in repeating very quickly Praṇava (sacred symbol OM) is the same as the experience of time. When this passage of time is once felt, every sound (*e.g.* in Anāhata-nāda, *i.e.* in the sense of sound automatically produced within, without outside vibration or concussion) will bring the idea of time. Even if the sounds are not similar they can produce a sense of the flow of time, *i.e.* the flow of time can be marked through the utterance of Gāyatrī-mantra (a Vedic hymn), or by mentally uttering Praṇava harmoniously during the time required for a deep inhalation and exhalation. Observation of space and observation of time, have to be simultaneously practised without any conflict between the two processes.

Prāṇāyāma can be practised for a specified period of time, or as long as it is possible to do so. The period of time has to be fixed by Japa (repetition) of a definite number of Praṇavas (sacred symbol OM) or Gāyatrī or other Mantras. Gāyatrī has to be repeated thrice. But in the beginning, inhalation, exhalation and suspension should be practised only to the extent they are easy to perform. In order to remember the number of Praṇavas repeated, Japa has to be practised in bunches. It is needless to say that mental Japa is preferable to other forms of Japa, because the use of the digits during Japa for keeping count diverts the mind. Practice of Japa in bunches is somewhat as follows :—Om-Om, Om-Om, Om-Om-Om. Thus in one bunch, seven repetitions of Praṇava are made. Repeating as many of these bunches as desired, it is easy to keep count of Japas.

There is another method of performing Prāṇāyāma by suspending both inhalation and exhalation as long as possible. In many cases, it is found to be the easier process. The time that is taken in exhaling, slowly and imperceptibly, or in practising suspension after exhalation, is the time covered by this form of Prāṇāyāma. In it there is no need to count the number of Japas. One Praṇava may be uttered lengthily and harmoniously (mainly with the 'M' in half-syllable), and this will easily give the idea of time, as stated above. This is how Prāṇāyāma is practised as regulated by time, through the sequence of Kṣaṇas.

Observation of time in terms of strokes, is called Prāṇāyāma regulated by numbers. For in it, time is determined by the number of inhalations and exhalations. The normal time taken in inhalation and exhalation by a healthy person is called a Mātrā. If it is assumed that fifteen inhalations and exhalations take place in a minute, then one Mātrā will comprise 4 seconds. Twelve similar Mātrās (or 48 seconds) will form an Udghāta (stroke). Twenty-four Mātrās will constitute the second stroke. Thirty-six Mātrās ($2\frac{2}{5}$ minutes) will form the third stroke. When the Prāṇāyāma takes place with twelve respirations (inhalation and exhalation taken together) it makes one stroke. This is the mild form of Prāṇāyāma. When there are two strokes or twenty-four respirations it is middling and when there are three strokes or thirty-six respirations it is the best.

According to another view, the time covered by a Mātrā is $1\frac{1}{3}$ second, or $\frac{1}{3}$ of the above calculation. Hence on this view the first stroke will consist of 36 Mātrās, the second stroke of 72 Mātrās and the third of 108 Mātrās. The term 'Udghāta' (stroke) has another meaning. According to this, Bhojarāja has said : "The air from the navel going up and striking the head is called one stroke." It means that when the breathing is stopped, the impulse felt for either inhalation or exhalation is called 'Udghāta'. Vijñāna-bhikṣu has interpreted the word 'Udghāta' as indicating only suspension of inhalation and exhalation.

In fact, all the three views can be reconciled. The meaning of 'Udghāta' is as follows : The extent of time up to which restraint of breath does not cause uneasiness for either releasing or inhaling air, constitutes an 'Udghāta. That time at first consists of 12 Mātrās, or 48 seconds ; therefore, time covering 12 Mātrās, constitutes the first 'Udghāta'.

As every 'Udghāta' is determined by a specified number of breaths, the Prāṇāyāma so performed is called Prāṇāyāma regulated by number. This number being fixed beforehand, it is not necessary to observe it during the practice of Prāṇāyāma. But observation of number may be necessary in order to determine how many Prāṇāyāmas should be practised and at what rate it should be increased. According to Haṭha-yoga, Prāṇāyāma should be practised four times a day up to a maximum of eighty each time. This number should be reached gradually and not all at once. It is said : "The number should be increased very slowly and carefully." The first 'Udghāta' is called Mṛdu (mild), the second Madhya (intermediate) and the third is called Tīvra (the best form of Prāṇāyāma).

Thus practised, Prāṇāyāma becomes both long and subtle. 'Long' means exhalation or the suspension of breath for a long time. 'Subtle' means attenuation of inhalation and exhalation and effortlessness during the holding of breath. When a fine cotton wool held at the tip of the nose does not move, it indicates the subtle form of exhalation.

---

वाह्याभ्यन्तरविषयाक्षेपी चतुर्थः ॥ ५१ ॥

भाष्यम्—देशकालसंख्याभिर्वाह्यविषयः परिदृष्ट आक्षिप्तः, तथाभ्यन्तरविषयः परिदृष्ट आक्षिप्तः, उभयथा दीर्घसूक्ष्मः। तत्पूर्वको भूमिजयात् क्रमेणोभयोर्गत्यभावश्चतुर्थः प्राणायामः। तृतीयस्तु विषयानालोचितो गत्यभावः सकृदारब्ध एव, देशकालसंख्याभिः परिदृष्टो दीर्घसूक्ष्मः। चतुर्थस्तु श्वासप्रश्वासयोर्विषयावधारणात् क्रमेण भूमिजयादुभयाक्षेपपूर्वको गत्यभावश्चतुर्थः प्राणायाम इत्ययं विशेषः ॥ ५१ ॥

**The Fourth Prāṇāyāma Transcends External And Internal Operations** (1). **51.**

When external operation regulated by space, time and number, is mastered it can be transcended by skill acquired through practice. Internal operation also, similarly regulated, can be transcended through practice. After proficiency is attained through practice, both these operations become long and subtle. Gradual suspension of external and internal operations, after these are mastered through practice as stated above, is the fourth Prāṇāyāma. Suppression of movement with one effort, without considering space, etc., is the third Prāṇāyāma. When regulated by space, time and number it becomes long and subtle. After acquiring proficiency in observing space etc. during inhalation and exhalation, gradual suspension of movement transcending them is the fourth Prāṇāyāma. This is the difference between the third and the fourth Prāṇāyāmas.

(1) Besides external operation, internal operation and suppression, there is another form of Prāṇāyāma. That also is a form of suppression. But it is somewhat different from the third form of Prāṇāyāma. The third Prāṇāyāma is performed all at once. But the fourth Prāṇāyāma is done after the practising of external and internal operations with the observation of space, time and number, and going beyond them all. After prolonged practice, when external and internal operations become very subtle, then going beyond them there arises a form of suspension which is the fourth and a very subtle form of suspension. The commentary will be understood better in the light of these observations.

Here, the other method of Prāṇāyāma is being explained in detail. At first, one must sit calmly in Āsana. Then, with the chest kept steady, air has to be inhaled and exhaled by moving the abdomenal muscles only. The exhalation has to be performed, as far as possible, slowly and completely. This will somewhat accelerate the movement of inhalation; care should, however, be taken to see that inhalation is done only by inflating the abdomen.

In this way, while exhaling and inhaling, a clear, transparent, luminous or white, all-pervading, infinite void should be imagined in the region of the heart at the centre of the chest. Initially it is necessary to meditate in this manner for a few days, instead of practising inhalation or exhalation. When that is mastered, exhalation and inhalation should be practised along with that meditation, feeling, as though, exhalation is being done in that void pervading the body, and that it is being filled in by inhalation. According to the Śāstras exhalation and inhalation should be carried out in a pleasant mood. At the same time, the mind has to be made vacant. The Śāstras direct that one should get one's mind engrossed in a vacant state, *i.e.* a sensation of touch should be felt by a vacant mind all over the body, which has to be conceived as a void. The heart should be regarded as the centre of that sense of void from which a sensation or feeling is to be conceived as spreading throughout the body during inhalation.

Initially slow exhalation and normal inhalation have to be practised along with meditation. When this is mastered, external operation should be practised now and then. That is, after exhalation one should not inhale. Similarly, internal operation also should be practised in which it should be felt that the inhaled air spreading all over the body has made it like a stationary pitcher filled with water and has stopped all restlessness of the body. It is needless to say that the inhaled air goes only into the lungs and not to other parts of the body. But after inhalation, when the lungs are full, it is felt as though that fullness has pervaded the entire body. This feeling is to be meditated upon. It should be borne in mind that this feeling over the whole body leads to perfection in Prāṇāyāma. This is the inner meaning of the expression : 'The body should be filled up with air.'

In the beginning, external and internal operations are to be practised once in a while. But afterwards, when they are mastered they may be practised without break. Initially suppression has to be practised in between these operations. After a few normal exhalations and inhalations the breathing should be stopped, with a small quantity of air left in the lungs, by contracting the lungs through internal effort. The practice of suppression should be undertaken after one feels, on account of the practice of external and internal operations mentioned earlier, a Sāttvika form of ease in the lungs and over the entire body, that is, when the body feels light and a pleasant sensation pervades it. For, then the organ of breathing can be firmly stopped, and one can easily remain without breath for a long time. As the breath is stopped when a pleasant sensation pervades, the state of suspension is felt as still more pleasant. Afterwards when the suspension of breath becomes unbearable the effort may be relaxed and normal breathing resumed. As only a slight quantity of air remains in the lungs, and most of it gets absorbed, inhalation becomes necessary after suppression, and not exhalation. Not only that, inhalation is then indispensable, otherwise the movement of heart will stop. Therefore, suspension should be practised with such small quantity of air in the lungs as would make inhalation necessary after suspension.

To start with, after practising suppression once, normal exhalation and inhalation should be carried out several times. When, however, the practice has been perfected, suppression can be undertaken without interruption. It is needless to say that during the practice of suppression also, it is necessary to keep the mind vacant, fixed to an internal region (preferably about the heart). Otherwise, the practice will be fruitless so far as Samādhi is concerned.

Desired result may be achieved by the practice of either the external or the internal operation. Suppression should be practised for the development of 'Udghāta'. Suppression itself is finally transformed into the fourth form of Prāṇāyāma, which marks the perfection of Prāṇāyāma. In practising the external and internal operations, care should be taken that exhalation and suspension in the case of the former and inhalation and suspension in that of the latter, take place harmoniously in one unbroken effort, that is, inhalation and exhalation should become subtle and imperceptibly get lost in the suspension.

The following points should be remembered by one in practising Prāṇāyāma :

(a) After feeling an internal sensation of touch along with inhalation and exhalation, the Sāttvika feeling of lightness and ease has to be vividly experienced. Prāṇāyāma performed with such feeling makes it perfect, not otherwise. Sattva-guṇa denotes revelation. Therefore, the effort which makes an act easy or natural, gives rise to appropriate feeling, meditation on which reveals the Sāttvika quality of ease. Just as meditation on sentience pervading the lungs during inhalation and exhalation leads to the sensations of lightness and ease there, so also over the whole body.

(b) Prāṇāyāma has to be practised by slow degrees, keeping an eye on health and physical well-being.

(c) Prāṇāyāma practised without meditation makes the mind more restless. That is why, in some cases it brings on lunacy. If the mind cannot first be made vacant through meditation in respect of an internal region, it is preferable not to take to Prāṇāyāma. Prāṇāyāma may, however, be undertaken if the mind can be fixed on an image conceived in an internal region. For the practice of Yoga, however, the state of void is more suitable.

(d) Attention should be given to diet. Too much of food, physical exercise and mental labour diminishes chances of progress in Prāṇāyāma. Light food, keeping the stomach partially empty, is frugality in meals. Moderation of diet will be found discussed in detail in books on Haṭha-yoga. Food containing carbohydrate should be taken, oil and fat should not be taken in excess.

It should be remembered that, ultimately, the Yogins have to give up consumption of fat altogether. If suspension of Prāṇa for a long period is desired, fasting also becomes necessary (it reduces the necessity for breathing). That is why the Mahābhārata says : "The Yogin acquires power, *i.e.* proficiency, by eating grains of rice, husks of sesame and barley gruel without fat and avoiding food containing fat. Drinking water mixed with milk, for a fortnight, month, season or year, or observing complete fast for a month, the Yogin acquires power." In the beginning, however, fat has to be taken in small quantities. In reducing diet it should be done gradually, by slow degrees.

Mere suspension of breathing is not Yogic Prāṇāyāma. There are some people who can naturally suspend breathing. It is such people, who remaining buried, show their magical power and earn money. This is neither Yoga nor Samādhi. That is why such people fail to achieve the spiritual excellence of Yoga.

The suspension of Prāṇa, which either arrests modifications of the mind or makes it one-pointed, constitutes Yogic Prāṇāyāma. Periods of stability of the mind during the practice of individual Prāṇāyāmas, growing gradually and continuously, develop finally into Samādhi. That is why it is said that twelve Prāṇāyāmas make one Pratyāhāra, and twelve Pratyāhāras make one Dhāraṇā etc. Therefore, unless the mind is steadied and made free from attachment to objects, it is not Yogic Prāṇāyāma. It would be only a physical feat. Mere suspension of breath is an external expression of Samādhi, not its internal or real characteristic.

---

ततः क्षीयते प्रकाशावरणम् ॥ ५२ ॥

भाष्यम्—प्राणायामानभ्यस्यतोऽस्य योगिनः क्षीयते विवेकज्ञानावरणीयं कर्म, यत्तदाचक्षते 'महामोहमयेनेन्द्रजालेन प्रकाशशीलं सत्त्वमावृत्य तदेवाकार्ये नियुङ्क्ते' इति। तदस्य प्रकाशावरणं कर्म संसारनिबन्धनं प्राणायामाभ्यासाद् दुर्बलं भवति, प्रतिक्षणं च क्षीयते। तथा चोक्तं 'तपो न परं प्राणायामात्ततो विशुद्धिर्मलानां दीप्तिश्च ज्ञानस्ये'ति ॥ ५२ ॥

**By That The Veil Over Manifestation (Of Knowledge) Is Thinned. 52.**

In the case of the Yogin engaged in practising Prāṇāyāma, the Karma which shuts out discriminative knowledge dwindles away (1). That (Karma) has been described in the following quotation : "The illusive magic of misapprehension covers the sentient Sattva (Buddhi) by a thick veil and directs it to improper deeds." The practice of Prāṇāyāma weakens and gradually attenuates that Karma of the Yogin which veils revelation and brings about the cycle of births. Thus it has been said : "There is no Tapas superior to Prāṇāyāma ; it removes impurities and makes the light of knowledge shine."

(1) The veil enveloping discriminative enlightenment which is worn away by Prāṇāyāma is not the veil of misapprehension but the veil of Karma based on misapprehension. Karma is the means of sustenance of wrong knowledge. Therefore attenuation of Karma attenuates misapprehension as well. Prāṇāyāma leads to immobility of the body and the organs. Its latency attenuates the latency of afflictive Karma just as the latency of anger is attenuated by that of non-anger. Thus it is clear that Prāṇāyāma weakens and causes the decay of the false knowledge based on Avidyā (which is identification of the body or the senses with the self) and actions and latencies derived therefrom. Some people raise the objection that since wrong knowledge can be destroyed only by right knowledge, how can (physical) act in the form of Prāṇāyāma cause its destruction ? In reply, it may be said that in this case also misapprehension is destroyed by knowledge. Prāṇāyāma is no doubt a physical act, but the knowledge gained by the act causes destruction of Avidyā. The practice of Prāṇāyāma separates one's I-sense from the body and the sense-organs. Therefore, knowledge corresponding to the act of Prāṇāyāma (every act has its corresponding knowledge) is 'I am neither the body nor the senses.'

———

भाष्यम्—किञ्च—

धारणासु च योग्यता मनसः ॥ ५३ ॥

प्राणायामाभ्यासादेव। 'प्रच्छर्दनविधारणाभ्यां वा प्राणस्य' इति वचनात्॥५३॥

Moreover—

**The Mind Acquires Fitness For Dhāraṇā (1).' 53.**

That fitness arises from the practice of Prāṇāyāma. This Sūtra confirms the former statement that by exhaling and restraining the breath, fixity of mind can be established.

(1) Fixity of mind on an internal region of the body is called Dhāraṇā. During the practice of Prāṇāyāma the mind has to be constantly fixed on the internal region. It is needless to say that this brings on the

ability to fix the mind there. In Sūtra I.34 it has been stated that stability of mind is acquired by the practice of Prāṇāyāma. Stability means fixity of the mind on a desired object.

———

भाष्यम्—अथ कः प्रत्याहारः—

स्वविषयासम्प्रयोगे चित्तस्य स्वरूपानुकार इवेन्द्रियाणां प्रत्याहारः ॥ ५४ ॥

स्वविषयसम्प्रयोगाभावे चित्तस्वरूपानुकार इवेति, चित्तनिरोधे चित्तवन्निरुद्धानीन्द्रियाणि, नेतरेन्द्रियजयवदुपायान्तरमपेक्षन्ते। यथा मधुकरराजं मक्षिका उत्पतन्तमनुत्पतन्ति, निविशमानमनु निविशन्ते, तथेन्द्रियाणि चित्तनिरोधे निरुद्धानि, इत्येष प्रत्याहारः ॥ ५४ ॥

What is Pratyāhāra ?

**When Separated From Their Corresponding Objects, The Organs Follow, As It Were, The Nature Of The Mind, That Is Called Pratyāhāra (Restraining Of The Organs). 54.**

Due to lack of contact with their corresponding objects, the senses, as it were, imitate the nature of the mind, *i.e.* like the mind which has suspended its functions, they also cease their functions, rendering unnecessary the application of other means for the control of the senses (1). Just as bees follow the course of the queen bee and rest when the latter rests, so when the mind stops the senses also stop their activities. This is Pratyāhāra.

(1) In other forms of discipline for the control of the senses the latter have to be kept away from objects, or the mind has to be consoled and soothed or some other methods have to be adopted, but in Pratyāhāra these are not required, the mental resolution suffices. To whatever direction the mind is wilfully turned, the senses follow it. When the mind is fixed on an internal region, the senses no longer perceive external objects. Similarly when the mind is fixed on an external object like

sound, it cognises that object only and the senses refrain from all activities related to other objects.

The principal methods for the practice of Pratyāhāra are (a) indifference to external objects, and (b) living in the world of thought. Pratyāhāra cannot be practised unless the habit of intently noticing objects with the eye and other senses is given up. The practice of Pratyāhāra becomes easy for those who cannot by nature observe external things minutely. Lunatics have a kind of Pratyāhāra, so have hysterics. Those who are amenable to hypnotic suggestions, attain Pratyāhāra well ; when offered salt for sugar, they get the taste of sugar in the salt.

Yogic Pratyāhāra is different from all the above types of Pratyāhāra. It is entirely self-regulated. When the Yogin does not want to know a thing, his power of perception stops immediately. Prāṇāyāma is helpful in such suspension. Through practice of Prāṇāyāma for a long time at a stretch, the tendency to suspend their activities gets stronger in the senses, hence Pratyāhāra becomes easier to practise. But there are other methods (meditation etc.) also, which may produce it. Pratyāhāra is beneficial when practised along with Yamas and Niyamas, otherwise the kind of Pratyāhāra, brought about on a person (*e.g.* by hypnotism) by somebody with a wicked motive, may cause harm.

Pratyāhāra in the form of suspension of activities of the senses is helpful to the Yogin for arresting his mind. When a swarm of bees leave their hive for the construction of a new one, the queen bee leads the way. Wherever that large bee rests, the other bees also rest and when she flies, the others closely follow her course. This is the example given in the Bhāṣyam to explain Pratyāhāra.

———

ततः परमा वश्यतेन्द्रियाणाम् ॥ ५५ ॥

भाष्यम्—शब्दादिष्वव्यसनम् इन्द्रियजय इति केचित्, सक्तिर्व्यसनं व्यस्यत्येनं श्रेयस इति। अविरुद्धा प्रतिपत्तिर्न्याय्या। शब्दादिसंप्रयोगः स्वेच्छयेत्यन्ये। रागद्वेषाभावे सुखदुःखशून्यं शब्दादिज्ञानमिन्द्रियजय इति केचित्। 'चित्तैकाग्र्यादप्रतिपत्तिरेवेति' जैगीषव्यः। ततश्च परमा त्वियं वश्यता यच्चित्तनिरोधे निरुद्धानीन्द्रियाणि, नेतरेन्द्रियजयवत् प्रयत्नकृतम् उपायान्तरमपेक्षन्ते योगिन इति ॥ ५५ ॥

इति श्रीपातञ्जले सांख्यप्रवचने वैयासिके साधनपादो द्वितीयः।

**That Brings Supreme Control Of The Organs. 55.**

Some say that A-vyasana or indifference to objects like sights and sounds etc., is control of the senses. The word 'Vyasana', used in this connection, means attachment or fondness, in other words, that which moves people away from righteousness. Others say that enjoyment of objects like sound etc. not forbidden by the Śāstras is permissible, meaning thereby that this is subjugation of the senses. There are still others who say : 'Control of the senses means application of the senses to objects like sound etc., out of one's own free will, without being a slave to them.' Again there are others who say : 'Experiences of sound etc., without feelings of happiness or misery on account of absence of attachment and aversion, is subjugation of the senses.' Jaigīṣavya says : "When the mind becomes one-pointed, the disinclination to objects of the senses or detachment from objects that arises, is control of the senses." Hence, what is stated by Jaigīṣavya constitutes the supreme form of sense-control of the Yogins in which, when the mind ceases its activities, the senses also stop theirs. Moreover when this is attained, the Yogins do not have to depend on other forms of effort for subjugation of the senses (1).

(Here concludes the chapter on Practice being the second part of the comments of Vyāsa known as Sāṁkhya-pravachana of the Yoga-philosophy of Patañjali).

(1) The various forms of control of the organs cited by the commentator except the last, are subtle sensuous attachments to the objects of enjoyment and are obstacles to spiritual attainment. If sinful objects are enjoyed 'disinterestedly' one will have to go to hell 'disinterestedly'. One who has realised the burning effect of fire will never want to touch fire, either interestedly or disinterestedly, either out of one's own free will or under the influence of another. Therefore, ignorance of spiritual truth is the cause of engaging the organs willingly in objects. Hence these forms of subjugation of the organs are all defective.

What the great Yogin Jaigīṣavya says is the one suitable to the

Yogins. If the function of the senses can be stopped along with suspension of the activities of the mind, whenever desired, that is the best form of sense-subjugation. Therefore control of the organs arising out of Pratyāhāra, constitutes the supreme mastery over the senses.

———

BOOK III

# SUPERNORMAL POWERS

भाष्यम्—उक्तानि पञ्च वहिरङ्गाणि साधनानि, धारणा वक्तव्या ।

देशबन्धश्चित्तस्य धारणा ॥ १ ॥

नाभिचक्रे हृदयपुण्डरीके मूर्द्धि, ज्योतिषि नासिकाग्रे जिह्वाग्रे, इत्येवमादिषु देशेषु वाह्ये वा विषये चित्तस्य वृत्तिमात्रेण बन्ध इति धारणा ॥ १ ॥

The five external aids to (or accessories of) Yoga have been explained ; (now) Dhāraṇā is to be explained.

**Dhāraṇā Is The Mind's (Chitta's) Fixation On A Particular Point In Space. 1.**

Dhāraṇā consists in holding or fixing the mind on the navel circle, or on the lotus of the heart, or on the effulgent centre of the head, or on the tip of the nose or of the tongue, or on such like spots in the body, or on any external object, by means of the modifications of the mind (1).

(1) In the case of internal regions, the mind is fixed directly through immediate feeling. But in the case of external objects the mind is fixed not directly but through the modifications of the senses. By external objects are meant external sounds, forms and the like. That fixation of the mind in which there is consciousness only of the region or object on which it has been fixed, and the other senses being withdrawn do not apprehend their respective objects, is Pratyāhāra-based Dhāraṇā and is an aid to Samādhi.

It should be noted that although Dhāraṇā or fixation of the mind is practised in Prāṇāyāma (breath control), yet it is not the primary Yogic Dhāraṇā. What is practised in Prāṇāyāma though generally called 'Dhyāna-Dhāraṇā' (holding the mind fixed in meditation) is really

Bhāvanā or contemplative thinking. On attaining certain maturity and refinement such Bhāvanā develops into Dhāraṇā and Dhyāna properly so called.

In ancient times the lotus, *i.e.* the core of the heart*, was the principal region or object for fixation of the mind, so also was the light upspringing therefrom called the light from Suṣumnā, the nerve within the spinal column. Later a system of keeping the mind steadfast on the six or twelve plexuses within the body came into vogue. According to the Sāṁkhya system these twelve plexuses, on which the mind can be fixed, fall under the three categories of objects. They are Grāhya—the knowable, Grahaṇa—the organs of reception and Grahītā—the receiver. Asamprajñāta-yoga can ultimately be attained after the mind attains concentration through practice of Dhāraṇā on such objects. That depends, however, on the realisation of the fundamental principles. When the knowledge of Puruṣa is gained [vide II.23(2)], then shutting out even that knowledge with Para-vairāgya or supreme renunciation, the state of liberation is reached.

Fixity of mind is of two kinds—(i) on the knowledge of the Tattvas and (ii) on other objects. The Sāṁkhyaites who follow the path of self-knowledge adopt the first. Initially fixing their minds on external objects impinging on the organs, they fix their minds on organs as belonging to the I-sense, on I-sense as based on the pure I-sense, and pure I-sense as overseen by Puruṣa. In conformity with these assumptions attempts are made to realise and rest in Self which is absolute Awareness. In this process, aid of internal location of the organs has to be taken, but the principal support of such meditation is the knowledge of the principles or Tattvas.

In the matter of fixing the mind on objects, the two principal objects are sound and effulgence. Of these, the chief method is the adoption of the effulgence in the heart as the support for fixity on the pure I-sense or Buddhi. As regards fixity on sound, one has to focus one's attention on a spontaneous unstruck sound (Anāhata-nāda) emanating within the body.

There are various forms of Dhāraṇā as aids to fixing the mind for purposes of meditation, but it should be remembered that fixity of mind alone does not bring about the desired result. After getting the mind steadied through practice and renunciation, deep meditation and concentration have to be achieved in order to gain the full benefit.

---

* About meditating on the heart see footnote to Sūtra I.28.

तत्र प्रत्ययैकतानता ध्यानम् ॥ २ ॥

भाष्यम्—तस्मिन्देशे ध्येयालम्बनस्य प्रत्ययस्यैकतानता सदृशः प्रवाहः प्रत्ययान्तरेणापरामृष्टो ध्यानम् ॥ २ ॥

**In That (Dhāraṇā) The Continuous Flow Of Similar Mental Modifications Is Called Dhyāna Or Meditation. 2.**

In that place (mentioned in the commentary on the previous Sūtra) the flow of the mental modifications relating to the same object of meditation being continuous, *i.e.* being uninterrupted by any other knowledge or thought, is known as Dhyāna or meditation (1).

(1) In Dhāraṇā or fixity, the flow of similar mental modifications on the same object is confined to the desired place. But the thought-process on the same object is intermittent and in succession. When through practice that becomes continuous, *i.e.* appears as an unbroken flow, then it is called Dhyāna. This is the Dhyāna in Yogic terminology and has nothing to do with the object meditated upon. It is a particular state of calmness of the mind and can be applied to any object of meditation. If flow of knowledge in Dhāraṇā may be compared to succession of similar drops of water, in Dhyāna the flow of knowledge is continuous like flow of oil or honey. That is the implication of the word 'continuous'. When knowledge is continuous it appears as though a single idea is present in the mind.

———

तदेवार्थमात्रनिर्भासं स्वरूपशून्यमिव समाधिः ॥ ३ ॥

भाष्यम्—ध्यानमेव ध्येयाकारनिर्भासं प्रत्ययात्मकेन स्वरूपेण शून्यमिव यदा भवति ध्येयस्वभावावेशात्तदा समाधिरित्युच्यते ॥ ३ ॥

**When The Object Of Meditation Only Shines Forth In The Mind, As Though Devoid Of The Thought Of Even The Self (Who Is Meditating), That State Is Called Samādhi Or Concentration. 3.**

When the state of meditation (Dhyāna) becomes so deep that only the object stands by itself, obliterating, as it were, all traces of reflective thought, it is known as Samādhi (1).

(1) Samādhi or concentration is the highest stage of meditation. It is the best form of calmness of the mind. There cannot be any subtler concentration than that. This refers no doubt to concentration having an object. Seedless or objectless concentration is not referred to herein.

When meditation is full of the object meditated on, *i.e.* when meditation becomes so intense that nothing but the object meditated on is present therein, it is called Samādhi or concentration. As the mind is then full of the nature of the object meditated upon, the reflective knowledge is lost sight of. In other words, the nature of the process of meditation (*e.g.* I am meditating) is lost in the nature of the object. Meditation losing consciousness of self, is Samādhi. In plain language, when in the process of meditating, consciousness of self seems to disappear and only the object meditated upon appears to exist, when the self is forgotten and the difference between the self and the object is effaced, such concentration of the mind on the object is called Samādhi.

This characteristic of Samādhi should be clearly understood and carefully remembered, otherwise nothing can be realised about Yoga. In the Bṛhad-āraṇyaka Upaniṣad, it is stated : "Refraining from unnecessary activities, restraining speech, body and mind, in a spirit of renunciation and forbearance, patiently bearing the hardships of a devotional life, one engaged in Samādhi can see the Self in oneself (that is, in one's own ego)." In the Kaṭha Upaniṣad, it is stated : "People who do not desist from evil deeds and unnecessary activities, are unmeditative, and have not controlled their minds, cannot reach the Self simply by superior knowledge." These prove that only through Samādhi, and by nothing else, can one realise the Self.

This might give rise to the question that as Samādhi is meditation forgetting oneself, how can meditation on the pure I-sense bring about Samādhi ? In reply, it can be stated that when the ideas 'I am knowing' 'I am knowing' appear in succession then undiluted knowledge or intense concentration is not achieved. When there is a continuous flow of the process of knowing alone without any reference to the knower, or the Self, then that uninterrupted state of concentration is called Samādhi. The process of cognition only is present in the mind at the time. When expressed in words, it has to be put as 'I was knowing myself.'

———

भाष्यम्—तदेतद्धारणा-ध्यान-समाधित्रयमेकत्र संयमः—

त्रयमेकत्र संयमः ॥ ४ ॥

एकविषयाणि त्रीणि साधनानि संयम इत्युच्यते, तदस्य त्रयस्य तान्त्रिकी परिभाषा संयम इति ॥ ४ ॥

These three, *viz.* Dhāraṇā (fixity), Dhyāna (meditation) and Samādhi (concentration) taken together is called Saṁyama.

**The Three Together On The Same Object Is Called Saṁyama. 4.**

The three forms of practice when directed to the same object is called Saṁyama. They go by the technical Yogic name of Saṁyama (1).

(1) The question might arise that as Samādhi or concentration implies fixity of mind and meditation, it should denote Saṁyama and it would be unnecessary to mention Dhāraṇā and Dhyāna separately. In reply, it can be said that Saṁyama is spoken of as the means of acquiring knowledge in respect of, and control over, the thing contemplated upon. If concentration is attained on only one aspect of a single object, one would not achieve the above objective. The object contemplated upon has to be thought of from all sides and in all its aspects and then should concentration take place on it. In one Saṁyama there might be several chains of Dhāraṇā, Dhyāna and Samādhi ; that is why, the three together has been called Saṁyama. For this reason it has been said by the commentator in Sūtra III.16 that the three-fold mutation is directly realised through Saṁyama. Direct realisation means sustained knowledge

acquired by repeatedly practising Dhāraṇā-Dhyāna-Samādhi on the same object.

———

तज्जयात्प्रज्ञालोकः ॥ ५ ॥

भाष्यम्—तस्य संयमस्य जयात् समाधिप्रज्ञाया भवत्यालोकः, यथा यथा संयमः स्थिरपदो भवति तथा तथा समाधिप्रज्ञा विशारदी भवति ॥ ५ ॥

**By Mastering That, The Light Of Knowledge (Prajñā) Dawns. 5.**

By mastering the art of Saṁyama, the light of knowledge emanating from concentration shines forth (1). As Saṁyama gets firmly established so does the knowledge attained in Samādhi get purer and purer.

(1) Knowledge acquired in Samādhi improves if Saṁyama is applied step by step. In other words, as Saṁyama is practised in respect of more and more subtle objects, the knowledge gets more and more clear. Acquisition of knowledge in respect of the Tattvas has been mentioned before in Book I. In this Book the method of acquisition of unrestricted powers and other kinds of knowledge by application of Saṁyama is chiefly spoken of.

Supernormal knowledge and powers are gained through concentration. If the faculty of knowing is directed to only one object to the total exclusion of other objects, ultimate knowledge of that object will certainly be gained. As the faculty of knowing fluctuates, *i.e.* moves constantly from one object to another, full knowledge of any one of them is not acquired. The faculty of knowing and the knowable come close to each other particularly in Samādhi because the two do not then appear to be separate. This is a characteristic of Samādhi.

The light of knowledge referred to here denotes the enlightenment attained in Samprajñāta-yoga—not supernormal knowledge of the cosmic world (vide III. 26) etc. It refers mainly to the ultimate knowledge of (*i.e.* Samāpatti in) the Tattvas—Grāhya, Grahaṇa and Grahītā, which is a step to the attainment of Kaivalya. Supernormal knowledge other than this, *e.g.* knowledge of minute or distant objects, is really an impediment to Kaivalya and does not go by the name of Prajñā or supreme knowledge.

———

तस्य भूमिषु विनियोगः ॥ ६ ॥

भाष्यम्—तस्य संयमस्य जितभूमेर्यानन्तरा भूमिस्तत्र विनियोगः, न ह्यजिताऽधरभूमिरनन्तरभूमिं विलङ्घ्य प्रान्तभूमिषु संयमं लभते, तदभावाच्च कुतस्तस्य प्रज्ञालोकः। ईश्वरप्रसादात् (ईश्वरप्रणिधानात्) जितोत्तरभूमिकस्य च नाधरभूमिषु परचित्तज्ञानादिषु संयमो युक्तः, कस्मात्, तदर्थस्यान्यत एवावगतत्वात्। भूमेरस्या इयमनन्तरा भूमिरित्यत्र योग एवोपाध्यायः, कथम्, एवमुक्तम् 'योगेन योगो ज्ञातव्यो योगो योगात्प्रवर्त्तते। योऽप्रमत्तस्तु योगेन स योगे रमते चिरम्' इति ॥ ६ ॥

**It (Saṁyama) Is To Be Applied To The Stages (Of Practice). 6.**

It has to be practised in respect of the stage next to the one attained (1). One who has not mastered the lower stages, cannot at once attain the higher stages of Saṁyama by skipping over the intermediate stages. Without them how can one get the full light of knowledge ? One who has attained a higher stage by the grace of God (2) need not practise Saṁyama in respect of the lower stages, *e.g.* thought-reading etc., because proficiency in respect of the lower stages would then be available through other sources (God's grace) also. 'This stage is higher than the other one'—such knowledge is attainable only by Yoga. How this is possible is explained in the following saying : "Yoga is to be known by Yoga, and Yoga itself leads to Yoga. He who remains steadfast in Yoga always delights in it."

(1) The first stage of Samprajñāta-yoga is Grāhya-samāpatti (engrossment in objects of knowledge), the sccond is Grahaṇa-samāpatti (engrossment in organs of reception) and the third is Grahītṛ-samāpatti (engrossment in the receiver) ; the highest stage is Viveka-khyāti or discriminative enlightenment. The highest stage cannot be reached all at once and can only be reached after attaining perfection in the previous stages one after another. If, however, through the grace of God (earned by special devotion to Him) enlightenment of the last stage is gained, that of the lower stages can be easily developed.

(2) 'Through the grace of God' and 'through Īśvara-praṇidhāna' (special devotion to God, vide Book I, Sūtra 23) mean the same thing. Through special devotion God's grace is earned, and from that spiritual fulfilment may come irrespective of stages. It might be questioned that God being always merciful, how can the point about His special grace arise. In reply it may be stated that in Īśvara-praṇidhāna, God has to be thought of as being present within one's own self through which the latent divinity existing in every being becomes manifest. The full manifestation of the divinity is Kaivalya or the state of liberation. On the attainment of such divinity, the attainment of other stages might be irrespective of succession. As in a piece of stone all sorts of images are always present (only waiting to be chiselled out), so in our minds there is an inherent divinity which is like the mind of God. To think of that divinity is to think of God. Although that is within us, in our present state we always think of it as a different being within us. Full realisation of that idea is Divine grace.

---

त्रयमन्तरङ्गम्पूर्वेभ्यः ।। ७ ।।

भाष्यम्—तदेतद् धारणा-ध्यान-समाधित्रयम् अन्तरङ्गं सम्प्रज्ञातस्य समाधेः पूर्वेभ्यो यमादिसाधनेभ्य इति ।। ७ ।।

**These Three Are More Intimate Practices Than The Previously Mentioned Ones. 7.**

Dhāraṇā, Dhyāna and Samādhi, these three are more internal in respect of Samprajñāta-yoga than Yama, Niyama etc. (1).

(1) Fixity, meditation and concentration are really the intimate practices conducive to Samprajñāta-yoga, because when clear knowledge of the various Tattvas is gained through intense concentration and that knowledge is retained by the one-pointed mind, it is called Samprajñāna.

---

तदपि वहिरङ्गं निर्वीजस्य ॥ ८ ॥

भाष्यम्—तदपि अन्तरङ्गं साधनत्रयं निर्वीजस्य योगस्य वहिरङ्गं, कस्मात्, तदभावे भावादिति ॥ ८ ॥

**That Also Is (To Be Regarded As) External In Respect Of Nirvīja Or Seedless Concentration. 8.**

That, *viz.* the three practices mentioned before as intimate is external as far as seedless concentration is concerned, because seedlessness is attained when these three are also absent (1).

(1) Fixity, meditation, etc. are external practices as far as Asamprajñāta-yoga is concerned. Its internal practice is only the supreme renunciation. It has been stated before that the characteristics of Samādhi are not traceable in Asamprajñāta-yoga, because the latter is—as the name implies—absence of, *i.e.* beyond Samprajñāna or supreme knowledge. As far as stoppage of fluctuations of the mind is concerned, Samprajñāta and Asamprajñāta are both Yoga or concentration, but Asamprajñāta is concentration without any external reference, *i.e.* arresting of mind without any reference even to an object of concentration.

———

भाष्यम्—अथ निरोधचित्तक्षणेषु चलं गुणवृत्तमिति कीदृशस्तदा चित्तपरिणामः—

व्युत्थाननिरोधसंस्कारयोरभिभवप्रादुर्भावौ
निरोधक्षणचित्तान्वयो निरोधपरिणामः ॥ ९ ॥

व्युत्थानसंस्काराश्चित्तधर्मा न ते प्रत्ययात्मका इति प्रत्ययनिरोधे न निरुद्धाः, निरोधसंस्कारा अपि चित्तधर्माः। तयोरभिभवप्रादुर्भावौ व्युत्थानसंस्कारा हीयन्ते, निरोधसंस्कारा आधीयन्ते ; निरोधक्षणं चित्तमन्वेति। तदेकस्य चित्तस्य प्रतिक्षणमिदं संस्कारान्यथात्वं निरोधपरिणामः। तदा संस्कारशेषं चित्तमिति निरोधसमाधौ व्याख्यातम् ॥ ९ ॥

The products of the Guṇas or the three basic constituent principles, are always mutable. What are the changes which take place in the mind (mind being made up of the Guṇas) at the moment when it is in an arrested state ?

**Suppression Of The Latencies Of Fluctuation And Appearance Of The Latencies Of Arrested State Taking Place At Every Moment Of Blankness Of The Arrested State In The Same Mind, Is The Mutation Of The Arrested State Of The Mind** (1). **9.**

Latent impressions of the fluctuations are characteristics of the mind. They are not of the nature of cognition, so on the cessation of cognition they do not disappear. Latent impressions of the arrested state of the mind are also characteristics of the mind. Their appearances and disappearances are thus attenuation of latent impressions of fluctuation and accumulation of latent impression of the arrested state respectively ; and they figure in a mind in an arrested state. This change of latent impressions taking place every moment in the same mind is called Nirodha-pariṇāma or the mutation of an arrested state of the mind. At that time the mind has nothing but subliminal impressions. This has been explained in I.18.

(1) Mutation means change from one state to another, *i.e.* modification. The change from a state of flux to an arrested state is a form of mutation. An arrested state is a characteristic of the mind. Mind is made up of three Guṇas which are always mutating. Therefore, change takes place even when the mind is in an arrested state, but there is no manifestation of that change as it cannot be perceived by the mind. What the nature of that change is, is being explained by the author of the Sūtra in this aphorism.

The appearance of one characteristic of an object and the disappearance of another is called its change of character. In the mutation of the arrested state the basic object is the arrested blank mind. In that mind the latent impressions of the true knowledge gained by concentration in a one-pointed mind decrease while the latent impressions of the arrested state of the mind increase. Both these features figure in the mind in an arrested state, just as the characteristics of both a clod and an earthen pot are latent in the same lump of clay. 'Moment of blankness' means the vacant or seemingly inactive state of mind that prevails when the mind remains arrested. Although no change is noticeable in that state, mutation goes on, because the latent impression of the arrested state goes on increasing and there is also a break in it. (However long the period of suspension may appear to an onlooker it is but a moment to the arrested mind. There can be no ideation of time when fluctuation ceases.)

Since the latent impression of Nirodha goes on increasing with practice, the increase must be taking place by suppressing mental fluctuations. In fact, in that state a tussle goes on between appearance and disappearance of latent impression of arrest on the one hand and that of fluctuations on the other, and that is also a form of unseen change.

Fluctuations are caused by latent impressions of fluctuations. So the inability of fluctuations to appear implies the overpowering of their impressions. Nirodha or the arrested state is one of only residual, *i.e.* latent impressions and is not a state of cognition. Thus the tussle is between latent impressions. That is why, the commentator has spoken of the appearance and disappearance of two sets of latent impressions. As the fight is between two sets of impressions, it is unnoticed and not cognised like knowledge, because the impression of the effort at arrest overcomes the impression of fluctuation. Although not perceptible, it is in effect mutation. It is like the struggle of a spring under the stress of weight.

Behind the struggle between the appearances and disappearances of two sets of latent impressions what undergoes change ? The reply is, the then mind. What is the mind like at that time ? It is then in a moment of blankness. This is the mutation of increasing the state of stoppage of all mental states. This statement might give rise to a further question that if concentration in an arrested state of the mind is subject to mutation then the state of liberation must also be mutable. But that is not the case. In the arrested state of the mind when its latent impressions are going on increasing, the mind is mutating, but in the state of liberation the mind is resolved into its constituent cause. Therefore, there can be no further mutation therein. When Nirodha matures and reaches its limit and the latent impressions of fluctuations are exhausted, then the process of increase of Nirodha comes to a stop (*i.e.* a stop in the break-up of the arrested state by fluctuations) and the mind ceases to function. That is why the author of the Sūtra has later (IV.32) described Kaivalya or state of liberation as the state when the stages of succession of the mutation of the three Guṇas, or the three basic constituent principles, terminate. So long as the mind remains active, modifications of its constituents take place. When modification ceases the mind reverts to its constituent cause, *viz.* the unmanifest. With the end of arrested mind, the latent impressions thereof also disappear. Bhojarāja has given the following example—When gold is burnt with lead, the lead burns out along with the dross in the gold ; complete stoppage of the mind is like that.

Latent impression is not manifest cognition, but its subtle state of retention. It is not the case that with the suppression of a particular class of cognition, the latent impressions of that class also will disappear. For example, in childhood many forms of traits are not present, but the latent impressions thereof are not absent because they appear in youth. When there is attachment, anger is absent, but that does not mean that anger has disappeared. In fact, latent impressions have to be obliterated by latent impressions, *i.e.* impressions of fluctuations have to be suppressed by impressions of arrested state.

The characteristic of the arrested state of mind is that in every moment there is destruction of latent impressions of fluctuations and development of latent impressions of suspensions.

———

तस्य प्रशान्तवाहिता संस्कारात् ॥ १० ॥

भाष्यम्—निरोधसंस्कारान्निरोधसंस्काराभ्यासपाटवापेक्षा प्रशान्तवाहिता चित्तस्य भवति, तत्संस्कारमान्द्ये व्युत्थानधर्मिणा संस्कारेण निरोधधर्मसंस्कारोऽभिभूयत इति ॥ १० ॥

**Continuity** (1) **Of The Tranquil Mind (In An Arrested State) Is Ensured By Its Latent Impressions. 10.**

From the latent impressions of the arrested state of the mind, *i.e.* when proficiency is acquired in the art of keeping the mind in an arrested state, the mind attains a continuous undisturbed state. When the impression of the arrested state gets feeble, it is overcome by the latent impression of the manifest state, *i.e.* a state of fluctuation ensues.

(1) Praśānta-vāhitā [see I.13 (1)] means absence of emergence of cognition, when no modification is noticeable. Arrested state is the tranquil state of the mind. Through latent impressions of that state, tranquillity becomes continuous.

Tranquillity = Complete cessation of fluctuations.

———

सर्वार्थतैकाग्रतयोः क्षयोदयौ चित्तस्य समाधिपरिणामः ॥ ११ ॥

भाष्यम्—सर्वार्थता चित्तधर्मः, एकाग्रता चित्तधर्मः। सर्वार्थतायाः क्षयः तिरोभाव इत्यर्थः, एकाग्रताया उदय आविर्भाव इत्यर्थः, तयोर्धर्मित्वेनानुगतं चित्तम्। तदिदं चित्तमपायोपजननयोः स्वात्मभूतयोर्धर्मयोरनुगतं समाधीयते स चित्तस्य समाधिपरिणामः ॥ ११ ॥

**Diminution Of Attention To All And Sundry And Development Of One-Pointedness Is Called Samādhi-Pariṇāma Or Mutation Of The Concentrative Mind. 11.**

Attending to all objects (1) is a characteristic of the mind ; one-pointedness is also a characteristic of the mind. Diminution of the habit of attending to all objects means disappearance of that characteristic and development of one-pointedness means emergence of one-pointed state of the mind. It is the same mind that has both these characteristics. Mind gets engrossed under the influence of its own action, *viz.* the curtailment of its habit of serving all and the growth of its habit of attending to one. That is known as Samādhi-pariṇāma of the mind or mutation of the concentrative mind.

(1) Attending to all = Always receiving everything, *i.e.* restlessness. Mind being always engaged in taking in sound, touch, light, taste and smell and in thinking of the past and the future, is attending to all or being directed to all. To be naturally ready to take in everything is the habit of attending to all.

One-pointedness is likewise getting the attention fixed on one object—to be naturally preoccupied with one thing. Attenuation of the tendency of attending to all and the increase and development of the habit of attending to only one object, is the Samādhi-pariṇāma of the mind. The mind engaged in practising concentration is affected in that way.

Nirodha-pariṇāma or the mutation of the arrested state referred to before, relates to suppression and development of latent impressions only. Samādhi-pariṇāma is suppression and rise of both latent impressions and cognised modifications. The reduction of the latent impressions of attending to everything and the resultant cognised impressions, and the development of the latent impressions of one-pointedness, and cognised impressions arising therefrom, constitute the features of Samādhi-pariṇāma.

---

ततः पुनः शान्तोदितौ तुल्यप्रत्ययौ चित्तस्यैकाग्रतापरिणामः ॥ १२ ॥

भाष्यम्—समाहितचित्तस्य पूर्वप्रत्ययः शान्तः, उत्तरस्तत्सदृश उदितः। समाधिचित्तमुभयोरनुगतं पुनस्तथैव आ समाधिभ्रेषादिति। स खल्वयं धर्मिणश्चित्तस्यैकाग्रतापरिणामः ॥ १२ ॥

**There (In Samādhi) Again (In The State Of Concentration) The Past And The Present Modifications Being Similar It Is Ekāgratā-Pariṇāma Or Mutation Of The Stabilised State Of The Mind. 12.**

In a mind in the state of concentration the modification that appeared in the past is the same as that which rises subsequently, *viz.* manifest modification (1). A concentrated mind runs through both of them and until concentration is disturbed similar sequence of the same modification goes on. This is the mutation of the one-pointed state of the mind.

(1) In Samādhi, the past and the present modifications are the same. Such uniformity of flow is concentration. The appearance and disappearance of the same modification during Samādhi (concentration) is called mutation of one-pointedness. The word 'Tataḥ' in the Sūtra means 'in the state of concentration', *i.e.* in Samādhi.

One-pointedness relates to appearance and disappearance of the same knowledge or idea. Suppose a Yogin can concentrate for six hours; during that period the same notion appears and disappears in his mind. This flow of the same idea amounts to one-pointedness. Then the Yogin reaches the Samprajñāta stage. His mind is then habitually one-pointed and he would always be (not for a fixed period only) trying to keep his mind fixed on the same object. The mind would then abandon the habit of taking in all objects but rest only on one particular object. This is what is meant by Samāpatti or engrossment of the mind. That is called the Samādhi-pariṇāma (of the previous Sūtra).

When the Yogin, through knowledge acquired in Samprajñāta-yoga, gains discriminative knowledge and by practice of supreme renunciation can, for a time, arrest the mind entirely, and by practice again goes on increasing the arrested state, then the mind gets Nirodha-pariṇāma.

Mutation of one-pointedness or Ekāgratā-pariṇāma occurs in every concentration, mutation of concentration occurs in Samprajñāta-yoga and mutation of arrested mind happens in Asamprajñāta-yoga (*i.e.* alternatively arrested and manifested states).

Mutation of one-pointedness (Ekāgratā-pariṇama) relates to change of cognised modifications, mutation of concentration (Samādhi-pariṇāma) relates to changes of cognised as well as latent states of mind, and mutation of arrested state (Nirodha-pariṇāma) means change of latencies only. Thus it will be seen that one-pointedness takes place while there is any concentration. Samādhi-pariṇāma is possible only in habituated one-pointed state of the mind, while Nirodha-pariṇāma takes place only in a (habitually) arrested state of the mind which is called Nirodha-bhūmi.

The distinction between the three as given above should be carefully noted. The mutations mentioned above are with reference to the practice of Yoga to attain liberation. Arrested state of mind etc. also takes place in Yoga leading to a discarnate state (Videha-laya), but that does not lead to permanent cessation of the sequence of mutations.

———

एतेन भूतेन्द्रियेषु धर्मलक्षणावस्थापरिणामा व्याख्याताः ॥ १३ ॥

भाष्यम्—एतेन पूर्वोक्तेन चित्तपरिणामेन धर्मलक्षणावस्थारूपेण, भूतेन्द्रियेषु धर्मपरिणामो लक्षणपरिणामोऽवस्थापरिणामश्चोक्तो वेदितव्यः। तत्र व्युत्थान-निरोधयोर्धर्मयोरभिभवप्रादुर्भावौ धर्मिणि धर्मपरिणामः।

लक्षणपरिणामश्च निरोधस्त्रिलक्षणस्त्रिभिरध्वभिर्युक्तः, स खल्वनागतलक्षण-मध्वानं प्रथमं हित्वा धर्मत्वमनतिक्रान्तो वर्त्तमानं लक्षणं प्रतिपन्नो यत्रास्य स्वरूपेणाभिव्यक्तिः, एषोऽस्य द्वितीयोऽध्वा, न चातीतानागताभ्यां लक्षणाभ्यां वियुक्तः। तथा व्युत्थानं त्रिलक्षणं त्रिभिरध्वभिर्युक्तं, वर्त्तमानं लक्षणं हित्वा

धर्मत्वमनतिक्रान्तमतीतलक्षणं प्रतिपन्नम्, एषोऽस्य तृतीयोऽध्वा, न चानागतवर्त्तमानाभ्यां लक्षणाभ्यां वियुक्तम्। एवं पुनर्व्युत्थानमुपसम्पद्यमानमनागतं लक्षणं हित्वा धर्मत्वमनतिक्रान्तं वर्त्तमानं लक्षणं प्रतिपन्नं, यत्रास्य स्वरूपाभिव्यक्तौ सत्यां व्यापारः, एषोऽस्य द्वितीयोऽध्वा, न चातीतानागताभ्यां लक्षणाभ्यां वियुक्तमिति। एवं पुनर्निरोध एवं पुनर्व्युत्थानमिति।

तथाऽवस्थापरिणामः—तत्र निरोधक्षणेषु निरोधसंस्कारा बलवन्तो भवन्ति दुर्बला व्युत्थानसंस्कारा इति, एष धर्माणामवस्थापरिणामः। तत्र धर्मिणो धर्मैः परिणामः, धर्माणां लक्षणैः परिणामः, लक्षणानामप्यवस्थाभिः परिणाम इति। एवं धर्मलक्षणावस्थापरिणामैः शून्यं न क्षणमपि गुणवृत्तमवतिष्ठते। चलं च गुणवृत्तम्, गुणस्वाभाव्यन्तु प्रवृत्तिकारणमुक्तं गुणानामिति। एतेन भूतेन्द्रियेषु धर्मधर्मिभेदात् त्रिविधः परिणामो वेदितव्यः, परमार्थतस्त्वेक एव परिणामः। धर्मिस्वरूपमात्रो हि धर्मः, धर्मिविक्रियैवैषा धर्मद्वारा प्रपञ्च्यत इति। तत्र धर्मस्य धर्मिणि वर्त्तमानस्यैवाध्वस्वतीतानागतवर्त्तमानेषु भावान्यथात्वं भवति न द्रव्यान्यथात्वं, यथा सुवर्णभाजनस्य भित्त्वाऽन्यथाक्रियमाणस्य भावान्यथात्वं भवति न सुवर्णान्यथात्वमिति। अपर आह—धर्मानभ्यधिको धर्मी पूर्वतत्त्वानतिक्रमात्, पूर्वापरावस्थाभेदमनुपतितः कौटस्थ्येन विपरिवर्त्तेत यद्यन्वयी स्यादिति। अयमदोषः, कस्माद्, एकान्तानभ्युपगमात्। तदेतत् त्रैलोक्यं व्यक्तेरपैति, कस्मात्, नित्यत्वप्रतिषेधात्। अपेतमप्यस्ति विनाशप्रतिषेधात्। संसर्गाच्चास्य सौक्ष्म्यं सौक्ष्म्याच्चानुपलब्धिरिति।

लक्षणपरिणामो धर्मोऽध्वसु वर्त्तमानोऽतीतोऽतीतलक्षणयुक्तोऽनागतवर्त्तमानाभ्यां लक्षणाभ्यामवियुक्तः, तथानागतोऽनागतलक्षणयुक्तो वर्त्तमानातीताभ्यां लक्षणाभ्यामवियुक्तः। तथा वर्त्तमानो वर्त्तमानलक्षणयुक्तोऽतीतानागताभ्यां लक्षणाभ्यामवियुक्त इति। यथा पुरुष एकस्यां स्त्रियां रक्तो न शेषासु विरक्तो भवतीति।

अथ लक्षणपरिणामे सर्वस्य सर्वलक्षणयोगादध्वसङ्करः प्राप्नोतीति परैर्दोषश्चोद्यत इति, तस्य परिहारः—धर्माणां धर्मत्वमप्रसाध्यं, सति च धर्मत्वे लक्षणभेदोऽपि वाच्यः, न वर्त्तमानसमय एवास्य धर्मत्वम्, एवं हि न चित्तं रागधर्मकं स्यात् क्रोधकाले रागस्यासमुदाचारादिति। किञ्च, त्रयाणां लक्षणानां युगपदेकस्यां व्यक्तौ नास्ति सम्भवः क्रमेण तु स्वव्यञ्जकाञ्जनस्य भावो भवेदिति। उक्तं च 'रूपातिशया वृत्त्यतिशयाश्च परस्परेण विरुध्यन्ते सामान्यानि त्वतिशयैः

सह प्रवर्त्तन्ते' तस्मादसङ्करः। यथा रागस्यैव क्वचित् समुदाचार इति न तदानीमन्यत्राभावः, किन्तु केवलं सामान्येन समन्वागत इत्यस्ति तदा तत्र तस्य भावः, तथा लक्षणस्येति। न धर्मी त्र्यध्वा धर्मास्तु त्र्यध्वानः, ते लक्षिता अलक्षिताश्च तान्तामवस्थाम्प्राप्नुवन्तोऽन्यत्वेन प्रतिनिर्दिश्यन्ते अवस्थान्तरतो न द्रव्यान्तरतः, यथैका रेखा शतस्थाने शतं दशस्थाने दश एकं चैकस्थाने, यथा चैकत्वेऽपि स्त्री माता चोच्यते दुहिता च स्वसा चेति।

अवस्थापरिणामे कौटस्थ्यप्रसङ्गदोषः कैश्चिदुक्तः, कथम्, अध्वनो व्यापारेण व्यवहितत्वाद् यदा धर्मः स्वव्यापारं न करोति तदाऽनागतः, यदा करोति तदा वर्त्तमानः, यदा कृत्वा निवृत्तस्तदाऽतीत इत्येवं धर्मधर्मिणोर्लक्षणानामवस्थानां च कौटस्थ्यं प्राप्नोतीति परैर्दोष उच्यते। नासौ दोषः, कस्मात्, गुणिनित्यत्वेऽपि गुणानां विमर्दवैचित्र्यात्। यथा संस्थानमादिमद्धर्ममात्रं शब्दादीनां विनाश्य-विनाशिनाम्, एवं लिङ्गमादिमद्धर्ममात्रं सत्त्वादीनां गुणानां विनाश्यविनाशिनां, तस्मिन् विकारसंज्ञेति।

तत्रेदमुदाहरणं मृद्धर्मी पिण्डाकाराद् धर्माद् धर्मान्तरमुपसम्पद्यमानो धर्मतः परिणमते घटाकार इति। घटाकारोऽनागतं लक्षणं हित्वा वर्त्तमानलक्षणं प्रतिपद्यते, इति लक्षणतः परिणमते। घटो नवपुराणतां प्रतिक्षणमनुभवन्नवस्था-परिणामं प्रतिपद्यत इति। धर्मिणोऽपि धर्मान्तरमवस्था, धर्मस्यापि लक्षणान्तर-मवस्था इत्येक एव द्रव्यपरिणामो भेदेनोपदर्शित इति। एवं पदार्थान्तरेष्वपि योज्यमिति। एते धर्मलक्षणावस्थापरिणामा धर्मिस्वरूपमनतिक्रान्ताः। इत्येक एव परिणामः सर्वानमून् विशेषानभिप्लवते। अथ कोऽयं परिणामः?—अव-स्थितस्य द्रव्यस्य पूर्वधर्मनिवृत्तौ धर्मान्तरोत्पत्तिः परिणामः ॥ १३ ॥

**By These Are Explained The Three Changes, Viz. Of Essential Attributes Or Characteristics, Of Temporal Characters, And Of States Of The Bhūtas And The Indriyas (i.e. All The Knowable Phenomena). 13.**

The three changes mentioned before (1) are of essential characters or attributes (Dharma), temporal character (Lakṣaṇa), and state as old and new (Avasthā), of the mind. Likewise there are changes in the essential qualities or attributes, temporal characters and states, of objects of knowledge and organs (2). Of these changes, the suppression of fluctuating states and development of the arrested state of mind (Nirodha) are known as changes of attributes.

Temporal change is described in the following manner :—An arrested state of mind can be associated with three phases or periods of time as the past, present and the future. That phase of time which is yet to be, is known as the first period. When the arrested state of mind is not involved with the future period but is manifested in the present, retaining its essential character, that is known as its second period. At that time, however, it is not completely dissociated from its other two temporal characters of past and future.

Similarly a fluctuating mind has three temporal phases or characters. When one of its states merges into the past leaving the present without changing its essential character, it is in its third temporal phase as the past. Even then it is not dissociated from its unmanifest temporal features which it will have in the present and the future. The second period occurs when it is manifest with its usual character by its function or activity in the present. Still it is not dissociated from its temporal character of the past and future. Thus both arrested (Nirodha) and fluctuating states of mind have three temporal characters.

Change of state* : At the time of Nirodha, the latencies of arrest become powerful and the latencies of fluctuations become weak. This is known as the change of state of the characteristics or attributes. It is to be noted here that a change in the attributes involves a change in the thing qualified by these. The three temporal changes are, however, related to the attributes, and change of state (as old or new) is related to the temporal characters (3). The cycle of the

* Avasthā (lit. state) is a technical term used by the author of the Sūtra and has nothing to do with the meaning normally associated with it, *viz.* general physical condition of an object.

Guṇas cannot exist even for a moment without these mutations. The Guṇa-modifications, that is the products of the Guṇas, are ever changing since they are always mutating. The nature of the Guṇas (4) is said to be responsible for this tendency, *viz.* their transformation through action.

The three kinds of changes (5) that take place in the Bhūtas and the Indriyas (the objective world and the organs) and which rest on the distinction between an object and its attributes are known in the aforesaid manner. Fundamentally, however, there is only one kind of change when we consider that the object and its attributes are one and the same. Attributes are essentially the same as the object to which they belong and any changes in the object qualified by them are detailed by the description of the changes of attributes, of temporal character and of state as old and new. It is only the characteristic, present in an object, that changes into past, present and future ; the substance itself does not change. Thus when a gold vessel is molten to be made into something else, it is only the shape etc. that change but not the gold. Some say that an object or substance is nothing more than its attributes since the former never gives up its essential nature. If the substance persists through all its attributes, then because of its sameness in all conditions it would be changeless (6). Taking the above view, some object that this will mean that the substance or the object is eternal, but that is not so. The view-point of Sāṁkhya-yoga is correct, because it has nowhere been mentioned that an object is immutably eternal. On the other hand, it has been maintained that all things in this world, from Buddhi to all knowables, disappear from their manifest or present condition and vanish into the past ; thus it is not admitted that these are immutably eternal. Again, since these reappear, their complete annihilation is denied. When they merge into their cause, they stay in a subtle form which is not noticeable on account of its subtlety.

The temporal character of a thing exists in all the three

periods of time (though these may not be manifest all at once or simultaneously). That which is past, is not dissociated from the present and future temporal characters. Similarly the future temporal character is not independent of that of the present and the past, and the present is not independent of the past and the future.

Apropos of the above, some critics point out that if all the temporal characters are present in all the three periods then there would be an overlapping of the time-element without any clear-cut distinction (7). That objection can be refuted in this way. That the characteristics do exist requires no proof. Since the attributes are admitted, their difference due to the time-element must also be admitted. It is not only in the present period of time that all the attributes exhibit themselves. If it were so, the mind would not have the characteristic of attachment when it is in a state of anger, simply because the former is not manifest at the moment. Moreover, the three temporal characters (past, present and future) cannot be simultaneously present in the same individual. These may, however, appear in succession through functioning of their respective causes. And so it has been said : "The preponderance of the forms (the eight forms of piety, knowledge, etc. vide II. 15) and states of mind (pleasure, pain and stupor) are mutually subversive, the weaker of them co-exist (as subordinates) with the intense states." That is why there is no overlapping of periods. For example, attachment being highly manifested in respect of one object, does not necessarily cease to exist in respect of other objects, but only remains in an unmanifest form. The same is the case with respect to temporal characters. Objects do not have three phases but the characteristics have, *viz.* manifested as present and unmanifest as past or future. The characteristics are regarded as different as they get into different states—a distinction of states but not of the thing itself. Take, for instance, the digit 1 (one). When placed in the first column it means unity, in the second column it denotes ten and in the third it stands for hundred ; or, as the same woman is called mother, daughter or sister in reference to the relationships borne by her.

Regarding change of state (8) some hold that the thing with reference to which such changes take place must be permanent. The reason given is : when due to lack of proper time-element an attribute cannot function or fails to manifest itself it is considered as yet to be or belonging to the future. Again, when it can operate it is regarded as present. When it ceases to function after having operated it is considered as past. Thus since different attributes and the substance to which they belong, exist in one way or another, through all the periods of time, they must be permanent. In reply, it is said that although the substratum is permanent, the modifications cannot be regarded as permanent on account of the conflicting mutations that take place. Just as gross elements (having a cause) originate and perish, and are mutations of the relatively intransient subtle elements, *viz.* monads of sound, light, etc., so also Mahat or pure I-sense, is a perishing and originating evolute of the three Guṇas or ultimate constituent principles. It is for this reason that Mahat is termed a Vikāra or evolved form.

Here is an illustration of mutation from the empirical standpoint. The substance clay passes from a clod to the shape of a pot (its transformation into a pot is its change of characteristic). When we consider the shape of a pot at the present moment we are disregarding its future unmanifest form which will manifest in time. The pot undergoes change every moment from newness to oldness which is its change of state. Assumption of a different characteristic is a change of condition of an object, and a change of the time-element of a characteristic is also a change of condition. Thus change of conditions has been shown in three different categories. This rule is applicable to other objects also. These changes though three in number, do not transcend the original nature of the substratum, *i.e.* it does not become a different object altogether though transmuted. For this reason it is held that there is in reality only one kind of mutation which includes the other varieties, or in other words, change of characteristics which covers the other mutations. What then is this mutation? It is the manifestation of another characteristic on the disappearance of the previous characteristic of a substance which remains constant (9).

(1) The three mutations of a Yogin's mind mentioned in Sūtras III. 9, III.11 and III.12, are not the same as the changes of characteristics, changes relating to time and states (new or old) dealt with in this aphorism. By the word 'Etena' (by this) it is only meant that as there are changes in the state of the mind, so there are mutations in the Bhūtas and the Indriyas. The commentator has explained that in each one of the three conditions of the mind there can be mutations of characteristics, temporal characters and states.

(2) Change or mutation can be of three kinds—relating to the characteristics, relating to the temporal character, and relating to the state. That is how we understand and speak of the difference between objects. When one characteristic disappears and another rises, that is called change of characteristics. For example, when fluctuations cease and state of arrest appears we say that the mind has undergone a change of characteristics.

The three periods of time are related to temporal character. The difference that is signified by the variation in time-epochs is called temporal change. For example, we speak of state of flux having existed, and not present now; or state of arrest having existed before, it is also present now, and will be so in future. Temporal change is designated by the three periods—past, present and future.

Again, temporal change is also classified. There the distinction is not on the basis of characteristic or time. For example, one piece of diamond is first called new, then after some time it is called old. At both points of time it is 'present', but is distinguished as old and new. Here the change in characteristics has not been taken into account. In the mental sphere we can take the example of an arrested state of the mind. When the mind is in an arrested state, the latencies of suppression predominate and the latencies of fluctuation become weak. The distinction here is on the basis of strength and weakness of different latencies.

Of the changes mentioned above, only the change of characteristic is real and the other two are imaginary. As they have some usefulness in practice they have been accepted. The author of the Sūtra has introduced them as a prelude to past and future knowledge.

(3) Mutation of an object is perceived from a change of its characteristics. Change of characteristics is inferred from consideration of change of time. That is why the commentator has said that change of time takes place during the prevalence of the same characteristic. Again idea of change of temporal character is deduced from change of state. Without any change in temporal character, a difference is conceived from change of state. For example, in the arrested sate of the mind the latent impressions of suppression and fluctuation are both there, but as comparatively the latencies of arrest are stronger the distinction is imagined on the strength of latencies.

An object which is 'present' is not unconnected with its 'past' or 'future' existence, because what is 'present' to-day, was 'future' at one time, and will pass on to the 'past'. As a matter of fact, past and future states remain in an undistinguished form. The present characteristic of a thing is only manifested in its active or phenomenal state. Active nature (of an object) is its manifested state.

(4) Mutability is the nature of the Guṇas. Rajas means mutative state, which means changeability. The activity that is noticeable in all phenomena goes by the name of Rajas. There is no cause behind this activity ; it is one of the fundamental characters of all phenomena. When the three Guṇas are mentioned as primary causes of creation, the nature of the Guṇas is implied. It might be questioned in this connection that if by nature the Guṇas are changeable, then how can there be a cessation of the fluctuations of the mind ? The reply is that mutation, no doubt, follows from the nature of the Guṇas, but their conjoint action resulting in the formation of Buddhi etc., does not take place from the nature of the Guṇas alone. It depends on witnessing by Puruṣa. Witnessing on the part of Puruṣa is due to contact between Puruṣa and Prakṛti which itself is the outcome of nescience. When nescience ceases, the witnessing also comes to an end. Buddhi etc. also terminate at that time.

(5) Basically, the real nature of an object is an aggregate of its characteristics. In the following Sūtra, the author has described the nature of an object. A thing conforming to its past, present and future characteristics, has been called an object. In practice an object and its characteristics are regarded as different, but fundamentally looked at from the point of view of basic constituents where there is no past or future, a thing and its characteristics are regarded as the same ; in other

words, looked at from the viewpoints of the Guṇas, both are identical. In essence, there are only mutations. In practice, such of those mutations as are perceptible to our senses, are called 'present', and those which are not perceptible are called 'past' or 'future'. The underlying something on which the past, present and future characteristics are based, is the object or substratum. If putting aside the gross materialistic outlook, we regard every knowable object as only sentient, mutative and static principles, then there would be no past, present or future, but that would be the unmanifest condition. The real basis or substratum of everything is thus the unmanifest [III.15(2)]. In the manifest state there are variations in the three constituent principles. As there are innumerable variations, the characteristics would also be innumerable. That is why, the commentator says that the characteristics are the real nature of objects, and the mutations of objects are only made manifest by their characteristics, past, present or future. In reality, a thing has only mutations which are designated as characteristics, temporal character and states.

(6) A thing and its characteristics are essentially one and the same, but in practice they are regarded as different, because Tattva-dṛṣṭi or the reflective point of view and Vyavahāra-dṛṣṭi or the practical worldly point of view, are different. From the latter point of view, an object and its characteristics are regarded as different. If from the practical aspect these two are regarded as identical then the characteristics would appear to have no basis or to be really non-existent. It would be altogether illogical to call an existent thing as basically non-existent. From the point of view of Tattvas, the characteristics are ultimately reduced to the three Guṇas, *viz.* Sattva, Rajas and Tamas. At that stage there is no means of distinguishing an object from its characteristics. They are not non-eese, neither are they manifest ; so they exist in an unmanifest condition. Ultimately, also the object and its characteristics become one. Therefore, the Guṇas are neither phenomena nor noumena, they cannot be described by those terms.

From the practical point of view there must be past and future states. To call everything present would therefore be absurd from that point of view. A characteristic is only a practical indication, that is why it has to be expressed by the three temporal states, of which present is the one when it is known, and the past and the future are those when it is not known. The condition in which they basically exist is the substratum or the object.

In effect the whole creation also does exist in an unmanifest state. That is why the Sāṁkhya philosophy does not admit of total annihilation,

In the unmanifest state nothing can be realised on account of subtlety of the form. Subtlety means remaining unseparated from its associates or causes and thus in an unperceived state.

(7) In regard to time-element it can be objected that if the present is not separate from the past and the future, then the three are present simultaneousely and are overlapping. This objection is without any basis. Past and future are non-existent and therefore imaginary. To establish relationship in imagination with imaginary things is to form notions of the past and the future with reference to the present. That which is perceivable is regarded as manifest, and we call it the present. That which is unfit for direct perception or is subtle, we designate as past or future. Thus there is no chance of the manifest being assigned the three periods of time.

Herein the commentator has explained that even when a characteristic is not manifest, it exists. For example, when a mind is full of anger, it cannot be said that it has no feeling of attachment at the time. The characteristic of attachment may manifest itself the next moment.

(8) The commentator having explained the different states, proceeds to refute the objections that are raised. The critic says that since an object and its characteristics always exist, then an object, its characteristics, time-element and state are everlasting like immutable Awareness, *i.e.* what is called old is always there in a subtle form and what is called new is and will be there also. What remains always is everlastingly present ; therefore, what is called a state of change is, in fact, immutably everlasting.

In reply, it is pointed out that 'everlasting' does not necessarily imply everlasting in the same form. Only that which always remains in the same form is 'Kūṭastha' (or truly, *i.e.* immutably everlasting). The material cause of the everchanging world must be mutative. That is why, a naturally mutative entity called Pradhāna is mentioned as the material cause. Pradhāna though everlasting is mutative. Its mutations take the form of characteristics or manifestations as Buddhi etc. From the mutations, or appearance and disappearance of changes, the original cause is called changeably everlasting.

(9) The commentator concludes his observations by bringing out the distinctive features of mutation. The change in the form of a thing is its mutation. When we see that its previously noticed characteristic is not present, we say, it has changed.

Mutation of subjective matters is change of condition in relation to time. Mental fluctuations have no spatial existence. They exist only in time and their change is only emergence or subsidence, *i.e.* the appearance of some modifications at one time and of others at another time. Thus alteration of condition in reference to either space or time is change or mutation.

———

भाष्यम्—तत्र—

शान्तोदिताव्यपदेश्यधर्मानुपाती धर्मी ॥ १४ ॥

योग्यतावच्छिन्ना धर्मिणः शक्तिरेव धर्मः। स च फलप्रसवभेदानुमितसद्भाव एकस्याऽन्योऽन्यश्च परिदृष्टः। तत्र वर्तमानः स्वव्यापारमनुभवन् धर्मो धर्मान्तरेभ्यः शान्तेभ्यश्चाव्यपदेश्येभ्यश्च भिद्यते, यदा तु सामान्येन समन्वागतो भवति तदा धर्मिस्वरूपमात्रत्वात् कोऽसौ केन भिद्येत। तत्र त्रयः खलु धर्मिणो धर्माः शान्ता उदिता अव्यपदेश्याश्चेति, तत्र शान्ता ये कृत्वा व्यापारानुपरताः, सव्यापारा उदिताः, ते चानागतस्य लक्षणस्य समनन्तराः, वर्तमानस्यानन्तराः अतीताः। किमर्थमतीतस्यानन्तरा न भवन्ति वर्तमानाः, पूर्वपश्चिमताया अभावात्। यथाऽनागतवर्तमानयोः पूर्वपश्चिमता नैवमतीतस्य, तस्मान्नातीतस्यास्ति समनन्तरः, तदनागत एव समनन्तरो भवति वर्तमानस्येति।

अथाव्यपदेश्याः के? सर्वं सर्वात्मकमिति। यत्रोक्तं 'जलभूम्योः पारिणामिकं रसादिवैश्वरूप्यं स्थावरेषु दृष्टं तथा स्थावराणां जङ्गमेषु जङ्गमानां स्थावरेषु' इति, एवं जात्यनुच्छेदेन सर्वं सर्वात्मकमिति। देशकालाकारनिमित्तापबन्धान्न खलु समानकालमात्मनामभिव्यक्तिरिति। य एतेष्वभिव्यक्तानभिव्यक्तेषु धर्मेष्वनुपाती सामान्यविशेषात्मा सोऽन्वयी धर्मी।

यस्य तु धर्ममात्रमेवेदं निरन्वयं तस्य भोगाभावः, कस्मात्, अन्येन विज्ञानेन कृतस्य कर्मणोऽन्यत् कथं भोक्तृत्वेनाधिक्रियेत; तत् स्मृत्यभावश्च, नान्यदृष्टस्य स्मरणमन्यस्यास्तीति। वस्तुप्रत्यभिज्ञानाच्च स्थितोऽन्वयी धर्मी यो धर्मान्यथात्वमभ्युपगतः प्रत्यभिज्ञायते। तस्मान्नेदं धर्ममात्रं निरन्वयमिति ॥ १४ ॥

Of these—

**That Which Continues Its Existence All Through The Varying Characteristics, Namely The Quiscent, i.e. Past, The Uprisen, i.e. Present Or Unmanifest (But Remaining As Potent Force), i.e. Future, Is The Substratum (Or Object Characterised). 14.**

Characteristic is the inherent capability of an object particularised by its function (1). Its existence is inferred from the different results arising out of its actions. Moreover, an object is seen to possess various characteristics. Of these, that which has started functioning is called the present and it is different from those which are past or quiescent and future or unmanifest. But when a characteristic lies dormant in the substratum with its special trait being unmanifest for lack of suitable situation, how can it be realised at the time, to be separate from the substratum itself? The characteristics of a substratum are of three types, *viz.* quiescent or past, uprisen or present, and unmanifest or future. Of these, that which has ceased to function is said to be quiescent, that which is functioning is said to be uprisen or emergent, and it is immediately contiguous to and behind that which has not manifested itself. Similarly, the quiescent one is contiguous to and behind the present or the emergent one. It may be asked, why the present characteristics are not behind those of the past. The reason is that there is no relationship of 'before and after' between them as in the case of the future and the present. That is why there is nothing contiguous to and behind the past, and the future is before the present.

What is the unmanifest characteristic? Everything is essentially every other thing. It has been said in this connection: "Infinite variety of all forms of earth and water is seen in plants. Similarly, essentials of plants are seen in animals and of animals in plants etc." Thus on account of non-destructibility of matter everything else is said to contain the essence of everything. This, however, is subject to the limitations of space, time, form and cause ; so particular objects do not manifest themselves simultaneously. The characterised object is that constant which remains common to all these manifest and unmanifest characteristics and which is the substratum of both the general (past and future) and specific (present, *i.e.* manifest) forms (2).

Those who hold that the mind is only a series of changing states without a substratum, cannot account for its experiences (of happiness and sorrow) because how can the fruits of actions of one cogniser be possibly enjoyed by another cogniser ? Further, there would be no memory thereof, because no one can remember what has been seen by another. Since, however, objects (previously seen) are recalled and recognised as such and such, a substratum common to changing states (of mind and objects) must be assumed to exist. That is why this world cannot be regarded simply as a bundle of characteristics involving no substratum.

(1) Capability implies the property of being known by its action or otherwise. Fire has the property of burning. From the burn caused, its power to burn is known. Power to burn is called the characteristic of fire. This power is the cause of burning, and is particularised by the act of burning. Burning is the capability and the power to burn is the characteristic.

In fact, that attribute by which a thing is known is called its characteristic. It is of two types, *viz.* real and imaginary or merely semantic. These characteristics again are divided into two, *viz.* essential and ascribed, *e.g.* whiteness of the sun is essential, while presence of water in a desert is ascribed.

That which is only understood by the word, and cannot be understood without it, is linguistic characteristic, *e.g.* eternity. Non-existing things, mere abstractions etc. are instances of such characteristics.

Real characteristics are either external *i.e.* objective, or internal *i.e.* subjective. External ones are fundamentally of three kinds—knowability or sentience, mutativeness and inertia. Properties like sound, light, etc. are knowable, all manners of action are mutative ; and hardness, softness, etc. are static. Subjective characteristics are similarly three, *viz.* cognition, conation and retention, or feeling, willing and memory. These primary characteristics change but do not disappear altogether.

From these it would appear that what can be cognised in some form or other is called a characteristic. Of the cognisable properties that which is directly known is called the emergent or present, what was cognised before is quiescent or past, and which is considered fit to be known later is called unmanifest or future.

What is present is known directly, and what are past and future are conjectured as they are not manifest. The past and the future characteristics of an object may be innumerable. Since there is an intrinsic unity of all objects, all objects might change into anything else.

This is the outlook of the Sāṁkhya philosophy and its basic method of analysis. In its view causes are divisible into two—efficient and material. The changed condition of an object through a cause is the effect.

(2) Manifestation of a thing is dependent on space, time, shape and cause. Everything can be made of everything, but that does not mean that it can so happen without any cause. Examples of dependence on space are—a thing very close to the eye cannot be seen properly, but it can be seen a little farther away ; things are thought of as small or large on account of location at a distance or otherwise ; of dependence on time, the examples are—a child does not get old at once but gradually, two ideas do not occur at the same time but one after another ; of dependence on shape, instances are—a square die cannot give a round impression, a man is not born of a deer. Efficient cause is the real cause. Space, time, etc. are only practical variations of the efficient cause. Every cause, other than the material caus is the efficient cause. With appropriate efficient cause, unmanifest characteristics become manifest.

The commentator has explained here that the thing which we use as the aggregate of particular, *i.e.* visible or emergent characteristics, and conjecturable, *i.e.* general (not particular) or past and future characteristics, is the substratum.

When we see a characteristic we must understand that there is behind it a basic substratum which is an aggregate of all its characteristics. We cannot think of realities without recognising the existence of a substratum. It is not proper to say that an object is comprised only of its manifest features.

———

क्रमान्यत्वं परिणामान्यत्वे हेतुः ॥ १५ ॥

भाष्यम्—एकस्य धर्मिण एक एव परिणाम इति प्रसक्ते क्रमान्यत्वं परिणामान्यत्वे हेतुर्भवतीति, तद् यथा चूर्णमृत् पिण्डमृद् घटमृत् कपालमृत् कणमृदिति च क्रमः। यो यस्य धर्मस्य समनन्तरो धर्मः स तस्य क्रमः, पिण्डः प्रच्यवते घट उपजायत इति धर्मपरिणामक्रमः। लक्षणपरिणामक्रमः—घटस्यानागतभावाद्वर्त्तमानभावक्रमः, तथा पिण्डस्य वर्त्तमानभावादतीतभावक्रमः। नातीतस्यास्ति क्रमः, कस्मात्, पूर्वपरतायां सत्यां समनन्तरत्वं, सा तु नास्त्यतीतस्य, तस्माद्द्वयोरेव लक्षणयोः क्रमः। तथावस्थापरिणामक्रमोऽपि घटस्याभिनवस्य प्रान्ते पुराणता दृश्यते सा च क्षणपरम्परानुपातिना क्रमेणाभिव्यज्यमाना परां व्यक्तिमापद्यत इति, धर्मलक्षणाभ्यां च विशिष्टोऽयं तृतीयः परिणाम इति।

त एते क्रमाः, धर्मधर्मिभेदे सति प्रतिलब्धस्वरूपाः। धर्मोऽपि धर्मी भवत्यन्यधर्मस्वरूपापेक्षयेति। यदा तु परमार्थतो धर्मिण्यभेदोपचारस्तद्द्वारेण स एवाभिधीयते धर्मः, तदायमेकत्वेनैव क्रमः प्रत्यवभासते। चित्तस्य द्वये धर्माः, परिदृष्टाश्चापरिदृष्टाश्च, तत्र प्रत्ययात्मकाः परिदृष्टाः, वस्तुमात्रात्मका अपरिदृष्टाः। ते च सप्तैव भवन्ति अनुमानेन प्रापितवस्तुमात्रसद्भावाः, 'निरोध-धर्म-संस्काराः परिणामोऽथ जीवनम्। चेष्टा शक्तिश्च चित्तस्य धर्मा दर्शनवर्जिताः' इति ॥ १५ ॥

**Change Of Sequence (Of Characteristics) Is The Cause Of Mutative Differences. 15.**

Since one characteristic gives rise to only one mutation, difference in mutations must be due to change of sequence (1), for example, dust, clod, a pot, pot-shred or bits are sequences of earth. The characteristic which follows another characteristic, is its Krama or sequence. Clod disappears and pot appears—this is sequence of change of characteristic.

Sequence of changes of time : The appearance of a pot from its potential state represents temporal transition from the unmanifest to its present state, while the disappearance of the clod of earth (of which the pot is made) represents a temporal transition from the present state to the past. There is no further sequence (in this order) after past, and the past is not antecedent to any state, so there is nothing after it ; that is why only the present and the future have sequence.

Sequence of change of state is also similar ; for example, a new pot becomes old in course of time. The oldness is only the result of the sequence of change taking place every moment, which becomes eventually noticeable in the shape of oldness. [It is to be noticed that this oldness is not a state of decay but only a relative state of existence as distinguished from characteristic and temporal character—vide III.13 (2).] This is the third (idea of) change as distinguished from changes of characteristic and temporal character.

These sequences can only be perceived if there is a difference between the object and its characteristics etc. As compared to one characteristic, another characteristic might be its substratum (2). When in the ultimate analysis, the characteristics (Dharma) and the substratum (Dharmī) are perceived as identical, the substratum is then called Dharma, and the sequence of mutation exists alone. A mind has two kinds of characteristics, *viz.* patent and latent. Of these, the patent are those which are perceived (*e.g.* as cognition or feeling), while the latent are those which merely exist as subconscious. These subconscious characteristics are seven in number and their existence is established by inference. "Arrested state, latent impression of action, subliminal impression, change, life, effort, and power are the subconscious characteristics of the mind (3)."

(1) To a substratum a change occurs by the disappearance of one characteristic and the appearance of another. The difference of such changes is the result of their sequence, *i.e.* the changes differ according to the change of sequence. We do not perceive the actual succession of changes because these are momentary subtle mutations. We only see the end (result) of a mutation. The commentator has explained later that Kṣaṇa (time atom) means the minutest conception of time in which the smallest particle (of knowledge) in respect of a thing appears to change. Therefore real sequence is the momentary change of the minutest particle. Thus the successive vibrations of Tanmātras (subtle elements)

are the minute sequence of external mutations, while the mutation of the dimensionless Buddhi or pure I-sense is a minute sequence of internal change.

One change succeeding another is called its sequence. When a clod of earth becomes a pot, the character of pot is the sequence of the character of clod. This is the sequence of characteristic. Similar is the case of temporal character and states.

Present is the sequence of future, and past is the sequence of present. This is the sequence of temporal changes. When a new pot becomes old, without losing its temporal character of being existent and there is no change of characteristic, it is said to have undergone a change of state. Change of location is also a change of state. Sequence of change of characteristics has to be perceived by bearing in mind that a substratum distinct from its characteristics exists.

(2) It has been stated before that one characteristic can be the substratum of another characteristic. It has also been shown that in the ultimate analysis the characteristic and substratum merge together when they resolve in the unmanifest fundamental Pradhāna. After that it becomes futile to make a distinction between the substratum and the characteristic and it may only be said that action in the form of preponderance and subordination of the Guṇas exist in the potential state, but whose action it is, cannot be ascertained. The mutating force is the Rajas principle in equilibrium. Witnessing (by Puruṣa) of the uneven state of the three Guṇas, or mutation of Pradhāna as knowable, is the cause of the manifest Buddhi etc. When for lack of contact between Puruṣa and Prakṛti, there is no witnessing by Puruṣa, the sequence of unevenness of the Guṇas as manifestation (in the shape of Buddhi etc.) ceases. Then spiritual enlightenment also terminates due to absence of Buddhi, and the three Guṇas and their mutable nature are no longer witnessed by Puruṣa.

Witnessing the uneven state of mutation means seeing the preponderance of manifestation. In other words, preponderance of Sattva Guṇa is knowledge or cognition, preponderance of Rajas is effort or conation, and preponderance of Tamas is retention. Thus through overseeing of Prakṛti or Pradhāna, *i.e.* the three Guṇas by Puruṣa, the evolution of Buddhi etc. takes place.

(3) The commentator has incidentally spoken of the characteristics of the mind. The patent characteristics are cognition or knowledge and conation or tendency or effort ; the latent characteristic is retention. Of the characteristics making up conation some are seen and some are unseen. The commentator has divided the unseen characteristics into

seven classes as noted in the next paragraph. These unseen characteristics are of the nature of a thing, *i.e.* they are inferred as existing, but how they exist cannot be clearly comprehended. That which exists is an object or a reality.

Nirodha or arrested state = Complete stoppage of mental fluctuations.

Dharma = Impressions of virtuous and vicious actions with their three-fold consequences.

Saṁskāra here implies Vāsanā or subliminal impressions of the result of action and feelings retained in memory.

Pariṇāma or change = The imperceptible sequence of mutation of the mind.

Jīvana or life = The functions of the Prāṇas or the vital forces.

Cheṣṭā or effort = The unseen action of the mind which leads the senses to work.

Śakti or power = The subtle force behind manifest action and effort.

---

भाष्यम्—अतो योगिन उपात्तसर्वसाधनस्य बुभुत्सितार्थप्रतिपत्तये संयमस्य विषय उपक्षिप्यते—

परिणामत्रयसंयमादतीतानागतज्ञानम् ॥ १६ ॥

धर्मलक्षणावस्थापरिणामेषु संयमाद् योगिनां भवत्यतीतानागतज्ञानम् । धारणाध्यानसमाधित्रयमेकत्र संयम उक्तः, तेन परिणामत्रयं साक्षात्क्रियमाणमतीतानागतज्ञानं तेषु संपादयति ॥ १६ ॥

The objects of Saṁyama and their attainment by a Yogin are now being discussed.

**Knowledge Of The Past And The Future Can Be Derived Through Saṁyama On The Three Pariṇāmas (Changes). 16.**

When Saṁyama is practised on the changes of characteristic, temporal character and state, Yogins acquire knowledge relating to the past and the future. It has already been said that fixity, meditation and concentration on the same object, is Saṁyama. If the changes in the characteristic, temporal character and state of any object, can be realised through Saṁyama, knowledge of the past and the future of that object would be revealed (1).

(1) Nothing can remain hidden to the power of perception purified by concentration. Such power has to be applied to the sequence of changes for acquisition of knowledge of past, present and future.

We can know, through ordinary intelligence, the past and the present to some extent by applying the rules of cause and effect. All the details of a cause can be realised through Saṁyama and thus its effects can also be known. The effects, of which these in turn form the causes, can be traced by the same process. In this way knowledge about the past and the future is obtained.

The gross organs of sight or hearing are not the only channels of knowledge, as is proved by clairvoyance, telepathy, etc. That we can have knowledge of the future is amply proved by dreams that come true. When, therefore, mind has the capability of knowing the future, it cannot be denied that such power can be developed through practice.

———

शब्दार्थप्रत्ययानामितरेतराध्यासात्सङ्करस्तत्प्रविभागसंयमात्सर्वभूतरुतज्ञानम् ॥१७॥

भाष्यम्—तत्र वाग् वर्णेष्वेवार्थवती, श्रोत्रं च ध्वनिपरिणाममात्रविषयं, पदं पुनर्नादानुसंहारबुद्धिनिर्ग्राह्यम् इति। वर्णा एकसमयासंभवित्वात् परस्परनिरनुग्रहात्मानः, ते पदमसंस्पृश्यानुपस्थाप्याविर्भूतास्तिरोभूताश्चेति प्रत्येकमपदस्वरूपा उच्यन्ते। वर्णः पुनरेकैकः पदात्मा सर्वाभिधानशक्तिप्रचितः सहकारिवर्णान्तरप्रतियोगित्वाद् वैश्वरूप्यमिवापन्नः। पूर्वश्चोत्तरेणोत्तरश्च पूर्वेण विशेषेऽवस्थापित इत्येवं बहवो वर्णाः क्रमानुरोधिनोऽर्थसंकेतेनावच्छिन्ना इयन्त एते सर्वाभिधानशक्तिपरिवृत्ता गकारौकारविसर्जनीयाः सास्नादिमन्तमर्थं द्योतयन्तीति।

तदेतेषामर्थसंकेतेनावच्छिन्नामुपसंहृतध्वनिक्रमाणां य एको बुद्धिनिर्भासस्तत्पदं वाचकं वाच्यस्य संकेत्यते। तदेकं पदमेकबुद्धिविषयम् एकप्रयत्नाक्षिप्तम् अभागमक्रममवर्णं बौद्धमन्त्यवर्णप्रत्ययव्यापारोपस्थापितं परत्र प्रतिपिपादयिषया वर्णैरेवाभिधीयमानैः श्रूयमाणैश्च श्रोतृभिरनादिवाग्व्यवहारवासनानुविद्धया लोकबुद्ध्या सिद्धवत्संप्रतिपत्त्या प्रतीयते। तस्य संकेतबुद्धितः प्रविभाग एतावतामेवं जातीयकोऽनुसंहार एकस्यार्थस्य वाचक इति।

खंकेतस्तु पदपदार्थयोरितरेतराध्यासरूपः स्मृत्यात्मकः। योऽयं शब्दः सोऽयमर्थः, योऽर्थः स शब्द इत्येवमितरेतराविभागरूपः (मितरेतराध्यासरूपः) संकेतो भवति। इत्येवमेते शब्दार्थप्रत्यया इतरेतराध्यासात् संकीर्णाः, गौरिति शब्दो गौरित्यर्थो गौरिति ज्ञानम्। य एषां प्रविभागज्ञः स सर्ववित्।

सर्वपदेषु चास्ति वाक्यशक्तिः, वृक्ष इत्युक्ते अस्तीति गम्यते, न सत्तां पदार्थो व्यभिचरतीति। तथा न ह्यसाधना क्रियास्तीति, तथा च पचतीत्युक्ते सर्वकारकाणामाक्षेपो नियमार्थोऽनुवादः कर्त्तृकर्मकरणानां चैत्राग्नितण्डुलानामिति। दृष्टं च वाक्यार्थे पदरचनं, श्रोत्रियश्छन्दोऽधीते, जीवति प्राणान् धारयति। तत्र वाक्ये पदार्थाभिव्यक्तिः, ततः पदं प्रविभज्य व्याकरणीयं क्रियावाचकं कारकवाचकं वा। अन्यथा भवति, अश्वः, अजापय इत्येवमादिषु नामाख्यातसारूप्यादनिर्ज्ञातं कथं क्रियायां कारके वा व्याक्रियेतेति।

तेषां शब्दार्थप्रत्ययानां प्रविभागः, तद् यथा श्वेतते प्रासाद इति क्रियार्थः, श्वेतः प्रासाद इति कारकार्थः शब्दः। क्रियाकारकात्मा तदर्थः प्रत्ययश्च, कस्मात्, सोऽयमित्यभिसम्बन्धादेकाकार एव प्रत्ययः संकेते इति। यस्तु श्वेतोऽर्थः स शब्दप्रत्यययोरालंबनीभूतः, स हि स्वाभिरवस्थाभिर्विक्रियमाणो न शब्दसहगतो न बुद्धिसहगतः। एवं शब्द एवं प्रत्ययो नेतरेतरसहगत इति। अन्यथा शब्दोऽन्यथार्थोऽन्यथा प्रत्यय इति विभागः, एवं तत्प्रविभागसंयमाद्योगिनस्सर्वभूतरुतज्ञानं सम्पद्यत इति ॥ १७ ॥

**Word, Object Implied And The Idea Thereof Overlapping, Produce One Unified Impression. If Saṁyama Is Practised On Each Separately, Knowledge Of The Meaning Of The Sounds Produced By All Beings can Be Acquired (1). 17.**

With regard to these (word, implied object and its knowledge) (2), articulation relates only to the alphabets constituting the word (a). Hearing relates to the sound thereof (b). It is a mental process that seizes the sounds of the alphabets and binds them together relating to one idea (c). Sounds of alphabets being pronounced successively and not being present at the same time, do not form a word but simply appear and disappear. Individual letter-sounds (alphabets) lack the nature of a word (d). Each letter is the constituent part of a word and is pregnant with the possibility of expressing innumerable ideas on association with others taking innumerable forms (e). A preceding letter is connected with the subsequent one, and vice versa, in a particular relationship to imply a particular word. Thus groups of alphabets placed in sequence (f) are assigned by conventional usage meanings to indicate various objects. For example, in the word Gauḥ (=Cow), the G, Au, and Ḥ (गौः=ग्+ौ+ः) spoken conjointly indicate a species of animal with particular features.

Thus regulated by their import, the sounds of the alphabets pronounced one after another, are presented together to the intellect as one word, to indicate something for which the word, thus formed, is the conventional name. This word is in every case the object of a single mental process requiring a single effort, is undivided, has no sequence and is different from the individual alphabets. It is understood by the intellect by aggregating the latent impressions of the alphabets with those pronounced before or manifested by the exciting cause which is the human intellect (g). If a man were to convey information to another, he must express himself by these alphabetical sounds which, on being heard by another and being sanctioned by eternal usage, appear as something real (h). This sort of division of words (i) and assignment of different meanings grow out of convention and they come to be associated with particular things.

The convention here is the memory of the identity of the word and the thing identified (j). This word is the object, and the object is the word—this sort of identity in memory gives rise to the convention. Thus the word, the object and the conception of the object are connected with one another, *e.g.* the word 'cow', the object 'cow' and the conception of cow get identified with one another. He who knows the distinction among these three is all-knowing, *i.e.* he knows the meaning of all uttered words.

Every word has in itself the power of expressing a complete idea (k). When the word 'Vṛkṣa' (tree) is mentioned, it implies that the tree exists, inasmuch as an object signified by a word can never fail to exist. Similarly no action is possible without an actor. When the word 'Pachati' (one cooks) is mentioned it implies the existence of all the factors related to cooking. It is only for the purpose of specifying details that the agent, the object and the instrument of action, *e.g.* Chaitra (name of a person), rice and fire may be expressly mentioned. Words are also so constructed as to convey the meaning of a sentence. For example, the word 'Śrotriya' (reciter) implies one who recites Vedic hymns, the word 'Jīvati' (lives) means one has got the breath of life. As even a word by virtue of its meaning is capable of expressing a whole sentence, a word has to be analysed to see whether it is indicative of action or that which acts, *i.e.* it has to be joined to an appropriate word to fully explain it. For example, the words 'Bhavati', 'Aśvaḥ' or 'Ajāpaya' which have many meanings would remain ambiguous if used singly.

There is a distinction between words, the object and the conception (l). To illustrate this, take the following examples. 'Śvetate Prāsādaḥ' or 'The palace shines white' implies an action, while the words 'Śvetaḥ Prāsādaḥ' or 'a white mansion' signifies a state. A word in essence signifies both an action and a state and so does a concept. This happens because the process of whitening is identified with its result, *viz.* making white. As to the white object, it is the support for both the word and the idea. As it independently changes its state, it goes neither with the word nor with the idea. The word, its object and the idea are thus distinct. By practising Saṁyama on this distinction, a Yogin can acquire knowledge of the articulations of all creatures.

(l) Word—Uttered word.
Object—Object which that uttered word signifies.

Idea—The mental nature or the feeling of the speaker and the conception created in the listener on hearing the word.

Overlapping—Imposition of the significance of one on the other, *i.e.* considering one for the other. From this overlapping comes the unified impression, *i.e.* the word, its object and the idea conveyed by it, are considered as one. But in reality they are quite different. Take, for example, cow. The uttered word is in the organ of speech of the speaker, the creature implied is either at the pasture or in the cowshed and the idea created is in the mind of the listener. Dividing the process in this way, the Yogin learns to think of the three separately. When he meditates on the uttered word, only that fills his mind, or when he contemplates on the idea, only the idea will occupy his mind. When a proficient Yogin on hearing a word of unknown meaning applies Saṁyama to it, he can reach the vocal organ of the speaker. Thence his power of knowledge proceeds to the latter's mind producing the word and he comes to know the sense in which the word has been uttered.

(2) In this connection the commentator has described the principles of words and objects as accepted by the Sāṁkhya philosophers. They are very sound and logical. It is being explained here part by part.

(a) By the vocal organ only the alphabets (A, B, C) etc. are produced. An alphabet means the basic part of an utterable word. The words used by men are formed singly or by the combination of such alphabets. Besides, cries and similar sounds might also be experienced by combination of suitable alphabets. The ordinary alphabets cannot be used for uttering them. All creatures have their own alphabets for indicating their utterances. As all varieties of colours are produced by the combination of seven basic colours, so all types of words can be pronounced with the help of a few alphabets.

(b) The ear takes in sound only, it cannot comprehend meaning. It takes in the sound of the alphabets one after another as they are uttered successively.

(c) Word is a combination of alphabets. Except in the case of words which are expressed by one alphabet, the sounds of alphabets composing a word are appearing and disappearing, their unification for the purpose of conveying an idea is being made by the mind. The word is formed by the unifying process arising out of memory of impressions of alphabets appearing in succession. This is not applicable to words consisting of one alphabet only.

(d) Alphabets are the materials for words but they themselves are not words (except where it is a one-alphabet word). As the combination of alphabets can be innumerable, so the words are, as it were, innumerable.

(e) The alphabets individually or in combination can indicate all objects. It is by convention that a word is made to signify an object. That is how some arrangement of alphabets is used conventionally to convey a particular object.

(f) Although words are mostly formed by the use of serveral alphabets, the alphabets do not appear simultaneously at one moment but are uttered successively. As past and present things cannot be really combined, the combination is effected in the mind with the help of the sounds perceived. Thus a word is only a mentally aggregated phenomenon, so the agent for that is the mind. It is really the word thus formed mentally which signifies the meaning conventionally given to it.

(g) The uttered words have appearing and disappearing parts in the shape of alphabets, but the words formed mentally have no such parts. They are the objects of one mental conception. What is felt by the intellect is always present ; it never disappears. What is not perceived but remains unmanifest is a latent object. Thus a mental word is like a single perception. We also feel that we raise the idea of a word in one effort. Because it is a single present idea, it has no appearing and disappearing parts. Therefore it is indivisible and simultaneous. As an uttered word, which is a collection of alphabets, is divisible and sequential, the mentally formed word is unlike an alphabetically formed word. How is it formed mentally ? As the alphabets are heard one after the other, knowledge arises in respect of each, from the knowledge comes impression and from impression comes memory. After the impression of the last uttered alphabet, impressions of all the alphabets forming the word arise by force of memory in one process and give rise to a comprehensible ideation of the word.

(h) Although the mental word is without letters, yet in expressing it, the help of alphabets has to be taken which are based on the latent impressions of the knowledge formed at the time of hearing the sound. Human nature has the mould for the use of human words. In human beings proficiency in speaking is a speciality. A human child on account of appropriate latent impressions naturally learns the use of human words. This learning comes primarily through hearing. The child, as he learns the words, gets to know their conventional meanings also. This learning is done by traditional usage, *i.e.* it is learnt from older people, first only the words and then comes unification of words, objects and their ideas.

(i) The classification of words and their division according to meaning, are no doubt made by convention. 'That so many alphabets will form this word and it will indicate this object' is fixed by someone and followed by others. Although it is not known who has done this, it is certain that it has been fixed by somebody.

(j) The recollection of the overlapping of a word and its meaning, is convention. On account of this overlapping of word, object and memory or knowledge, they are inseparable. When the Yogin becomes conversant with their difference, or through concentration comes to know them individually, he can, through Nirvitarka knowledge, understand the subject referred to by all words.

(k) A sentence generally indicates a noun with a verb, or in other words, it implies a proposition. The capacity of the word implies its property of conveying a meaning. The word 'pot' taken by itself is a term but it implies 'the pot exists' when it is a proposition. Every term contains the essence of a proposition. When it is pronounced it implies the existence of something, *i.e.* a noun with a verb conveying an idea. When the word 'tree' is pronounced it implies that it exists, or existed or will exist, involving an implication of its states of existence.

There are words which have many meanings. When they are used by themselves, they are not comprehensible by ordinary knowledge but their meanings are revealed in Yogic knowledge.

(l) Here the difference between a word, its implied object and significance, is being illustrated by examples.

Having thus established the distinction among the three, the commentator is describing the benefits of practising Saṁyama.

---

संस्कारसाक्षात्करणात्पूर्वजातिज्ञानम् ॥ १८ ॥

भाष्यम्—द्वये खल्वमी संस्काराः स्मृतिक्लेशहेतवो वासनारूपाः, विपाकहेतवो धर्माधर्मरूपाः। ते पूर्वभवाभिसंस्कृताः परिणाम-चेष्टा-निरोध-शक्ति-जीवन-धर्मवदपरिदृष्टाश्चित्तधर्माः। तेषु संयमः संस्कारसाक्षात्क्रियायै समर्थः, न च देशकालनिमित्तानुभवैर्विना तेषामस्ति साक्षात्करणम्, तदित्थं संस्कारसाक्षात्करणात्पूर्वजातिज्ञानमुत्पद्यते योगिनः। परत्राप्येवमेव संस्कारसाक्षात्करणात्परजातिसंवेदनम्। अत्रेदमाख्यानं श्रूयते, भगवतो जैगीषव्यस्य संस्कारसाक्षात्करणाद्दशसु महासर्गेषु जन्मपरिणामक्रममनुपश्यतो विवेकजं ज्ञानं प्रादुरभवत्। अथ भगवानावट्यस्तनुधरस्तमुवाच, दशसु महासर्गेषु भव्यत्वादनभिभूतबुद्धिसत्त्वेन

त्वया नरकतिर्यग्गर्भसंभवं दुःखं संपश्यता देवमनुष्येषु पुनः पुनरुत्पद्यमानेन सुखदुःखयोः किमधिकमुपलब्धमिति। भगवन्तमावट्यं जैगीषव्य उवाच, दशसु महासर्गेषु भव्यत्वादनभिभूतबुद्धिसत्त्वेन मया नरकतिर्यग्भवं दुःखं संपश्यता देवमनुष्येषु पुनः पुनरुत्पद्यमानेन यत् किञ्चिदनुभूतं तत्सर्वं दुःखमेव प्रत्यवैमि। भगवानावट्य उवाच, यदिदमायुष्मतः प्रधानवशित्वमनुत्तमं च सन्तोषसुखं किमिदमपि दुःखपक्षे निक्षिप्तमिति। भगवान् जैगीषव्य उवाच, विषयसुखापेक्षयैवेदमनुत्तमं सन्तोषसुखमुक्तं, कैवल्यापेक्षया दुःखमेव। बुद्धिसत्त्वस्यायं धर्मस्त्रिगुणः, त्रिगुणश्च प्रत्ययो हेयपक्षे न्यस्त इति। दुःखस्वरूपस्तृष्णातन्तुः, तृष्णादुःखसन्तापापगमात्तु प्रसन्नमबाधं सर्वानुकूलं सुखमिदमुक्तमिति ॥ १८ ॥

**By The Realisation Of Latent Impressions, Knowledge Of Previous Birth Is Acquired** (1). **18.**

The latent impressions referred to in this Sūtra are of two kinds, *viz.* those appearing as Vāsanās causing memory and (indirectly) afflictions, and those responsible for fruition of right or wrong deeds (2) done in previous births. Like change, effort, arrested state, power, life and impressions of virtuous and vicious actions, they are unseen characteristics of Chitta. If Saṁyama is practised on impressions, they are realised, and since such realisation cannot arise without an idea of the place, time and cause of the incident concerned, the Yogin practising it comes to know of the previous birth. Knowledge of previous births of others can also be acquired in the same way. There is a story prevalent in this connection in the Śruti. Bhagavān Jaigīṣavya after having acquired knowledge of ten cycles of creation and the sequence of births therein through realisation of subliminal impressions, obtained discriminative knowledge. Then Bhagavān Āvaṭya, having assumed a corporeal form created at will, asked him : 'You have lived through ten cycles and because of enlightenment your intellect has not been clouded ; you have experienced sorrows of hell and animal life, and have repeatedly enjoyed pleasures as a Deva (celestial) and as a human being. Of these what have you enjoyed best ?' To this Bhagavān Jaigīṣavya replied : 'I have lived through ten cycles of creation and my mental essence has not been overpowered. I have experienced the sorrows of hell as well as of animal life. I have been born again and again as a Deva and as a man. But I consider all that I have been through, as pain.' Then Āvaṭya said : 'Oh long-lived one, tell me whether you count your mastery over the constituent principles and the unsurpassable pleasure of contentment amongst sorrows.' Jaigīṣavya replied : 'Pleasure of contentment has been ranked as superior to other enjoyments, but it is nothing but pain compared to the bliss of the state of liberation. This characteristic of contentment of mind is nothing but a composition of the three Guṇas, and everything connected with the Guṇas has been counted as that to be avoided. The state of desire is nothing but pain. When pain-producing desire is removed, contentment is said to become pleasant, unrestricted, and all-embracing (3).'

(1) Perception of latent impressions means memory or recollection of subliminal impressions. It is clear that if latent impressions are perceived it will bring forth knowledge of the previous life. Latent impressions have been gathered in previous lives. If, therefore, through concentration, the power of perception is directed exclusively to subliminal impressions, then their particulars will be revealed, *i.e.* where, in which life, and how they were gathered will be recollected.

(2) The subject of subliminal impressions has been dealt with in the comments on Sūtras II.12 and 15. Latent impressions are, like mutation etc., the result of an unseen characteristic of Chitta. For the purpose of perceiving latent impression, a particular personal latent impression has to be thought of. If that latent impression is forceful, the result of such thinking will be its vivification. Therefore, fixing the mind on any particular tendency or on any faculty of reception and getting engrossed thereon, will bring about a recollection of the cause of such latent impression in a previous birth and that is perception of the latent impression. In the case of a man, the particular latent impressions of the human species are the memory-producing Vāsanās. If the peculiarities

of the human form, its sense-organs, mind, etc. are thought upon and engrossed in, this will bring about a knowledge of their causes, *i.e.* it will be known why they have been cast into this particular mould and why they have adopted the virtuous or vicious ways in this life. Vāsanā has been explained before. Vāsanā is like a mould and actions of virtue and vice are like molten metal.

(3) The story of the conversation between Jaigīṣavya and Āvaṭya quoted above is not found in any extant literature. It might have been quoted from some obsolete Śruti.

Pleasant—unaffected by material pains.

Unrestricted—unbroken by any obstacle.

All-embracing—liked by everybody and favourably situated in all circumstances.

---

प्रत्ययस्य परचित्तज्ञानम् ॥ १६ ॥

भाष्यम्—प्रत्यये संयमात् प्रत्ययस्य साक्षात्करणात्ततः परचित्तज्ञानम् ॥ १६ ॥

**(By Practising Saṁyama) On Notions, Knowledge Of Other Minds Is Developed. 19.**

By practising Saṁyama on notions and thus realising them, knowledge of other minds can be acquired (1).

(1) Notions here refer to the notions prevailing in one's own mind as well as in other minds. Unless an idea in one's own mind can be isolated and perceived, how can the idea in another mind be realised ? First realising one's own idea, the mind has to be made vacant for the reception of the idea prevalent in another mind and then effort should be made to realise that. We come across many thought-readers, but they have not always acquired the power through Yoga ; many of them are born with that power. Keeping in view the person whose thought is to be read, the reader's mind has to be made vacant and when other thoughts rise therein they are the thoughts of the other person. Thought-readers cannot say how the thought is transferred, but they just feel that the thoughts are not their own. Some can read other people's thought without any effort when the other person is in the process of thinking of

something. Anything previously felt but since forgotten may also be sometimes known by a thought-reader.

---

न च तत्सालम्बनं तस्याविषयीभूतत्वात् ॥ २० ॥

भाष्यम्—रक्तं प्रत्ययं जानाति, अमुष्मिन्नालम्बने रक्तमिति न जानाति। परप्रत्ययस्य यदालम्बनं तद् योगिचित्तेन नालम्बनीकृतं, परप्रत्ययमात्रन्तु योगिचित्तस्य आलम्बनीभूतमिति ॥ २० ॥

**The Prop (Or Basis) Of The Notion Does Not Get Known Because That Is Not The Object Of The (Yogin's) Observation. 20.**

In the process of Saṁyama referred to in the previous Sūtra, the Yogin comes to know the nature of the notion (whether it is one of attachment or passion) but not what it is based on. It is so because only the nature of the modification in the other person's mind, and not the object on which it is based, comes in the Yogin's field of observation (1).

(1) Realisation of the feeling (of attachment, hate etc.) does not bring with it knowledge of the object which has generated that feeling, which is a mental state mostly independent of the object itself. The tiger is not present in the fright that develops on seeing it.

---

कायरूपसंयमात्तद्ग्राह्यशक्तिस्तम्भे चक्षुःप्रकाशाऽसम्प्रयोगेऽन्तर्द्धानम् ॥ २१ ॥

भाष्यम्—कायरूपे संयमाद्रूपस्य या ग्राह्या शक्तिस्तां प्रतिबध्नाति, ग्राह्यशक्तिस्तम्भे सति चक्षुःप्रकाशासम्प्रयोगेऽन्तर्द्धानमुत्पद्यते योगिनः। एतेन शब्दाद्यन्तर्द्धानमुक्तं वेदितव्यम् ॥ २१ ॥

**When Perceptibility Of The Body Is Suppressed By Practising Saṁyama On Its Visual Character, Disappearance Of The Body Is Effected Through Its Getting Beyond The Sphere Of Perception Of The Eye. 21.**

When Saṁyama is practised on the (visible) appearance of the body, the property of perceptibility possessed by it becomes ineffective. When that property is suppressed, the body ceases to be an object of observation by another person, and the Yogin can thus remain unseen by others. This implies that other faculties by which the body can be perceived, *e.g.* auditory perceptibility etc., can also be eliminated (1).

(1) Magicians follow this system. They exert their will-power on the spectators who see only such things as the former want them to see. This shows how extraordinary things can be brought about by will-power. It is no wonder, therefore, that Yogins can, if they so will, make their bodies totally imperceptible to others.

———

सोपक्रमं निरुपक्रमं च कर्म तत्संयमादपरान्तज्ञानमरिष्टेभ्यो वा ॥ २२ ॥

भाष्यम्—आयुर्विपाकं कर्म द्विविधं सोपक्रमं निरुपक्रमं च। तत्र यथा आर्द्रवस्त्रं वितानितं लघीयसा कालेन शुष्येत्तथा सोपक्रमं, यथा च तदेव सम्पिण्डितं चिरेण संशुष्येदेवं निरुपक्रमम्। यथा चाग्निः शुष्के कक्षे मुक्तो वातेन समन्ततो युक्तः क्षेपीयसा कालेन दहेत्तथा सोपक्रमं, यथा वा स एवाग्निस्तृणराशौ क्रमशोऽवयवेषु न्यस्तश्चिरेण दहेत्तथा निरुपक्रमम्। तदैकभविकमायुष्करं कर्म द्विविधं सोपक्रमं निरुपक्रमं च, तत्संयमाद् अपरान्तस्य प्रायणस्य ज्ञानम्। अरिष्टेभ्यो वेति। त्रिविधमरिष्टम् आध्यात्मिकमाधिभौतिकमाधिदैविकं चेति। तत्राध्यात्मिकं, घोषं स्वदेहे पिहितकर्णो न शृणोति, ज्योतिर्वा नेत्रेऽवष्टब्धे न पश्यति। तथाधिभौतिकं, यमपुरुषान् पश्यति, पितॄनतीतानकस्मात् पश्यति। आधिदैविकं, स्वर्गमकस्मात् सिद्धान् वा पश्यति, विपरीतं वा सर्वमिति। अनेन वा जानात्यपरान्तमुपस्थितमिति ॥ २२ ॥

**Karma Is Either Fast or Slow In Fructifying. By Practising Saṁyama On Karma Or On Portents, Fore-Knowledge Of Death Can Be Acquired. 22.**

Karma (action) which fructifies as span of life is of two kinds, some which fructify quickly (Sopakrama), and others which fructify slowly (Nirupakrama) (1). For example, when a wet cloth is spread out it dries quickly, whereas if kept in a lump it takes a longer time. Fast fructifying Karma is like fire which, fanned on all sides by wind, consumes dry grass quickly ; while slow fructifying Karma is like fire applied gradually in different places to a heap of grass, thus taking longer time to burn. Karma of one period of existence causing span of life is thus of two varieties. By practising Saṁyama on them knowledge of end of this life can be gathered. It can also be gained from portents.

Portents are of three kinds—personal, elemental and divine. The example of personal portents is not hearing any sound from within the body on closing the ears, or not seeing any effulgent light on the eyes being closed (pressed by fingers). The example of elemental portents is seeing the messengers of the god of death, or the wraiths of departed forefathers. The divine portents are seeing the heavens or the Siddhas (ethereals) suddenly, or seeing everything contrary to what has been seen before. Through such portents one comes to know that death is at hand.

(1) Reference has been made before to Karma with its three types of fruition. When Karmāśaya matures and brings forth birth, its result is the span of life and experience in the shape of enjoyment or suffering which continues throughout life. In this period, however, all the Karmas do not fructify all at once. They become ready to bear fruit according to their nature. That which has started action is said to be fructifying or Sopakrama and that which is inactive now but will produce result at some future time, is called slow in fruition or Nirupakrama. Take, for instance, the case of a man who on account of action in a previous birth will suffer severely at the age of forty which will end his

span of life in another three years. For forty years that Karma is said to remain slow in fruition.

On realisation of the three-fold latent impressions and the fast and slow fructifying Karmas amongst them, the particulars of their results become known. The Yogin can thereby know when his life will come to an end. The commentator has explained by illustration that Karmas which are restrained from manifestation by obstacles are slow in fruition and those which are not so restricted are fast in fruition. Portents also indicate approaching death.

———

मैत्र्यादिषु बलानि ॥ २३ ॥

भाष्यम्—मैत्रीकरुणामुदितेति तिस्रो भावनाः। तत्र भूतेषु सुखितेषु मैत्रीं भावयित्वा मैत्रीबलं लभते, दुःखितेषु करुणां भावयित्वा करुणाबलं लभते, पुण्यशीलेषु मुदितां भावयित्वा मुदिताबलं लभते। भावनातः समाधिर्यः स संयमः ततो बलान्यबन्ध्यवीर्याणि जायन्ते। पापशीलेषु उपेक्षा न तु भावना, ततश्च तस्यां नास्ति समाधिरिति, अतो न बलमुपेक्षातस्तत्र संयमाभावादिति ॥ २३ ॥

**Through Saṁyama On Friendliness (Amity) And Other Similar Virtues, Strength Is Obtained Therein. 23.**

Friendliness, compassion and goodwill are the three kinds of sentiments that are recommended. Of these, strength of friendliness is acquired through entertaining a feeling of friendliness towards a happy person. By cultivating a sentiment of compassion towards unhappy creatures, strength of compassion is developed. By a feeling of pleasure towards the virtuous, strength of goodwill is developed. The concentration resulting from contemplation on these feelings, is called Saṁyama, and it begets unfailing power. Indifference to sinners is not an object of contemplation ; that is why there cannot be any meditation on it. Therefore, it is not possible to practise Saṁyama on it and thus no power can be acquired through it (1).

(1) Through sentiment of friendliness, the Yogin completely destroys all feelings of envy and hatred, and on account of his will-power, other malicious persons consider him to be friendly, and unhappy people take him to be a source of comfort. A Yogin's mind gets completely free from harshness and malice and he becomes a favourite of the virtuous.

When these powers are acquired, the Yogin becomes capable of behaving in a friendly manner towards others and no desire of injuring others would ever darken his heart.

———

बलेषु हस्तिबलादीनि ॥ २४ ॥

भाष्यम्—हस्तिबले संयमाद् हस्तिबलो भवति, वैनतेयबले संयमाद् वैनतेयबलो भवति, वायुबले संयमाद् वायुबल इत्येवमादि ॥ २४ ॥

**By Practising Saṁyama On (Physical) Strength, The Strength Of Elephants Etc. Can Be Acquired. 24.**

If Saṁyama is practised on the strength of an elephant, power like that of an elephant is obtained. Similarly, the power of the king of birds (Garuḍa, son of Vinatā) can be acquired by Saṁyama on Garuḍa's strength, and the power of the wind by Saṁyama on the strength of Vāyu or wind, etc. (1).

(1) All physical culturists know that by consciously applying the will-power on particular muscles, their strength can be developed. Saṁyama on strength is only the highest form of the same process.

———

प्रवृत्त्यालोकन्यासात्सूक्ष्मव्यवहितविप्रकृष्टज्ञानम् ॥ २५ ॥

भाष्यम्—ज्योतिष्मती प्रवृत्तिरुक्ता मनसः, तस्या य आलोकस्तं योगी सूक्ष्मे वा व्यवहिते वा विप्रकृष्टे वा अर्थे विन्यस्य तमर्थमधिगच्छति ॥ २५ ॥

**By Applying The Effulgent Light Of The Higher Sense-Perception (Jyotiṣmatī) Knowledge Of Subtle Objects, Or Things Obstructed From View, Or Placed At A Great Distance, Can Be Acquired. 25.**

The light of the higher sense-perception of the mind has been mentioned before. With its help, *i.e.* through Sāttvika revelation, the Yogin can see things which are very subtle, or obstructed from view, or situated far away (1).

(1) The effulgent light of higher sense-perception has been explained in Sūtra I.36. On contemplation thereon a sense of all pervading revelation would be felt emanating from the heart. If that light is directed towards the object to be known, it will become known howsoever subtle it may be, or howsoever separated it may be. This is the highest attainment before which clairvoyance pales into insignificance. This knowledge is derived from contact of the objects with the all-pervading power of Buddhi and is not restricted like the knowledge coming by way of sense-channels.

———

भुवनज्ञानं सूर्ये संयमात् ॥ २६ ॥

भाष्यम्—तत्प्रस्तारः सप्तलोकाः। तत्रावीचेः प्रभृति मेरुपृष्ठं यावदित्येष भूर्लोकः, मेरुपृष्ठादारभ्य आध्रुवाद् ग्रहनक्षत्रताराविचित्रोऽन्तरिक्षलोकः। तत्परः स्वर्लोकः पञ्चविधः, माहेन्द्रस्तृतीयो लोकः, चतुर्थः प्राजापत्यो महर्लोकः। त्रिविधो ब्राह्मः, तद्यथा जनलोकस्तपोलोकः सत्यलोक इति। 'ब्राह्मस्त्रिभूमिको लोकः प्राजापत्यस्ततो महान्। माहेन्द्रश्च स्वरित्युक्तो दिवि तारा भुवि प्रजा ॥' इति संग्रहश्लोकः। तत्रावीचेरुपर्युपरि निविष्टाः षण्महानरकभूमयो घनसलिलानलानिलाकाशतमःप्रतिष्ठाः महाकालाम्बरीषरौरवमहारौरवकालसूत्रान्धतामिस्राः। यत्र स्वकर्मोपार्जितदुःखवेदनाः प्राणिनः कष्टमायुः दीर्घमाक्षिप्य जायन्ते। ततो महातलरसातलातलसुतलवितलतलातलपातालाख्यानि सप्तपातालानि। भूमिरियमष्टमी सप्तद्वीपा वसुमती, यस्याः सुमेरुर्मध्ये पर्वतराजः काञ्चनः, तस्य राजतवैदूर्यस्फटिकहेममणिमयानि शृङ्गाणि, तत्र वैदूर्यप्रभानुरागान्नीलोत्पलपत्रश्यामो

नभसो दक्षिणो भागः। श्वेतः पूर्वः, स्वच्छः पश्चिमः, कुरण्डकाभ उत्तरः। दक्षिणपार्श्वे चास्य जम्बुः, यतोऽयं जम्बुद्वीपः, तस्य सूर्यप्रचाराद् रात्रिन्दिवं लग्नमिव विवर्त्तते। तस्य नीलश्वेतश्रृङ्गवन्त उदीचीनास्त्रयः पर्वता द्विसहस्रायामाः, तदन्तरेषु त्रीणि वर्षाणि नव नव योजनसाहस्राणि रमणकं हिरण्मयमुत्तराः कुरव इति। निषधहेमकूटहिमशैला दक्षिणतो द्विसहस्रायामाः, तदन्तरेषु त्रीणि वर्षाणि नव नव योजनसाहस्राणि हरिवर्षं किम्पुरुषं भारतमिति।

सुमेरोः प्राचीना भद्राश्वा माल्यवत्सीमानः प्रतीचीनाः केतुमाला गन्धमादन-सीमानः, मध्ये वर्षमिलावृतम्। तदेतत् योजनशतसहस्रं सुमेरोर्दिशि दिशि तदर्धेन व्यूढम्। स खल्वयं शतसहस्रायामो जम्बुद्वीपस्ततो द्विगुणेन लवणो-दधिना वलयाकृतिना वेष्टितः। ततश्च द्विगुणा द्विगुणाः शाक-कुश-क्रौञ्च-शाल्मल-मगध-(गोमेध) पुष्कर-द्वीपाः। सप्तसमुद्राश्च सर्षपराशिकल्पाः सविचित्रशैलावतंसा इक्षुरससुरासर्पिर्दधिमण्डक्षीरस्वादूदकाः। सप्तसमुद्रवेष्टिता वलयाकृतयो लोका-लोकपर्वतपरीवाराः पञ्चाशद्योजनकोटिपरिसंख्याताः। तदेतत्सर्वं सुप्रतिष्ठित-संस्थानमण्डमध्ये व्यूढम्, अण्डं च प्रधानस्याणुरवयवो यथाकाशे खद्योतः। तत्र पाताले जलधौ पर्वतेष्वेतेषु देवनिकाया असुरगन्धर्व-किन्नर-किम्पुरुषयक्षराक्षस-भूतप्रेतपिशाचापस्मारकाप्सरोब्रह्मराक्षसकुष्माण्डविनायकाः प्रतिवसन्ति। सर्वेषु द्वीपेषु पुण्यात्मानो देवमनुष्याः।

सुमेरुस्त्रिदशानामुद्यानभूमिः, तत्र मिश्रवनं नन्दनं चैत्ररथं सुमानसमित्यु-द्यानानि, सुधर्मा देवसभा, सुदर्शनं पुरं, वैजयन्तः प्रासादः। ग्रहनक्षत्रतारकास्तु ध्रुवे निबद्धा वायुविक्षेपनियमेनोपलक्षितप्रचाराः सुमेरोरुपर्युपरि सन्निविष्टा विपरिवर्त्तन्ते। माहेन्द्रनिवासिनः षड्देवनिकायाः—त्रिदशा अग्निष्वात्ता याम्याः तुषिता अपरिनिर्मितवशवर्तिनः परिनिर्मितवशवर्तिनश्चेति। सर्वे संकल्पसिद्धा अणिमाद्यैश्वर्योपपन्नाः कल्पायुषो वृन्दारकाः कामभोगिन औपपादिकदेहा उत्त-मानुकूलाभिरप्सरोभिः कृतपरिवाराः। महति लोके प्राजापत्ये पञ्चविधो देव-निकायः—कुमुदाः ऋभवः प्रतर्दना अञ्जनाभाः प्रचिताभा इति, एते महाभूतवशिनो ध्यानाहाराः कल्पसहस्रायुषः। प्रथमे ब्रह्मणो जनलोके चतुर्विधो देवनिकायः—ब्रह्मपुरोहिता ब्रह्मकायिका ब्रह्ममहाकायिका (अजरा) अमरा इति, एते भूतेन्द्रियवशिनो द्विगुणद्विगुणोत्तरायुषः। द्वितीये तपसि लोके त्रिविधो देव-निकायः—आभास्वरा महाभास्वराः सत्यमहाभास्वरा इति। एते भूतेन्द्रियप्रकृति-वशिनो द्विगुणद्विगुणोत्तरायुषः, सर्वे ध्यानाहारा ऊर्ध्वरेतसः ऊर्ध्वमप्रतिहतज्ञाना

अधरभूमिष्वनावृतज्ञानविषयाः। तृतीये ब्रह्मणः सत्यलोके चत्वारो देवनिकायाः—अच्युताः शूद्धनिवासाः सत्याभाः संज्ञासंज्ञिनश्चेति। अकृतभवनन्यासाः स्वप्रतिष्ठा उपर्युपरिस्थिताः प्रधानवशिनो यावत्सर्गायुषः। तत्राच्युताः सवितर्कध्यानसुखाः, शुद्धनिवासाः सविचारध्यानसुखाः, सत्याभा आनन्दमात्रध्यानसुखाः, संज्ञासंज्ञिनश्चास्मितामात्रध्यानसुखाः, तेऽपि त्रैलोक्यमध्ये प्रतितिष्ठन्ति। त एते सप्त लोकाः सर्व एव ब्रह्मलोकाः। विदेहप्रकृतिलयास्तु मोक्षपदे वर्त्तन्ते, न लोकमध्ये न्यस्ता इति। एतद्योगिना साक्षात्कर्त्तव्यं सूर्यद्वारे संयमं कृत्वा ततोऽन्यत्रापि, एवन्तावदभ्यसेद् यावदिदं सर्वं दृष्टमिति ॥ २६ ॥

**(By Practising Saṁyama) On The Sun (The Point In The Body Known As The Solar Entrance) The Knowledge Of The Cosmic Regions Is Acquired** (1). **26.**

The cosmic regions are seven in number. Starting from Avīchi up to the summit of Meru is the Bhūḥloka (Loka = Region). The stellar region from the Meru to the pole-star (Dhruva), strewn with planets and stars, is called Antarīkṣa. Beyond that is the region known as Svaḥ-loka having five planes, of which the first one, Mahendra by name, is known as the third Loka. The fourth is the Mahaḥ-loka of Prajāpati. Then there are the three Brahmalokas, *viz.* Janaloka, Tapoloka and Satyaloka.

Then up to Avīchi, one placed above the other, are the six great hells wherein are the excesses of earth (Ghana), water (Salila), fire (Anala), air (Anila), void (Ākāśa) and darkness (Tamas) respectively and called the Mahākāla, Ambarīṣa, Raurava, Mahāraurava, Kālasūtra and Andhatāmiśra, in which creatures are born to suffer painful long lives as consequences of their accumulated sinful actions. Next come the seven nether worlds called Mahātala, Rasātala, Atala, Sutala, Vitala, Talātala, and Pātāla. The eighth is this earth called Vasumatī with its seven Dvīpas and the golden king of mountains called Sumeru in the middle. Its peaks on the four sides are of silver, emerald, crystal and gold

(2). On account of the sheen of the emerald, the southern region of the sky looks like the leaf of a blue lotus ; the eastern is white, the western bright and the northern yellow. On the right side is the Jambu (tree) whence it is called the Jambu-dvīpa. Its night and day go round with the motion of the sun, where the days and nights seem to be in contact. This has three northern mountain chains called Nīla, Śveta, and Śṛṅgavat covering an extent of nearly two thousand Yojanas. Surrounded by these mountains are three continents of nine thousand Yojanas each. They are known as Ramaṇaka, Hiraṇmaya and Uttarakuru. To the south are the three mountain chains called Niṣadha, Hemakūta and Himaśaila extending over two thousand Yojanas each, in the midst of which are situated the three continents of Harivarṣa, Kimpuruṣavarṣa and Bhāratavarṣa, each extending over nine thousand Yojanas. (1 Yojana = about 9 miles).

To the east of Sumeru is Bhadrāśva up to Mālyavat mountain and to the west is Ketumāla up to Gandhamādana mountain. In their midst is Ilāvṛtavarṣa. The diameter of Jambu-dvīpa is a hundred thousand Yojanas and stretches round Sumeru for fifty thousand Yojanas. These are surrounded by double their extent of salt-water ocean. After them are the Dvīpas called Śāka, Kuśa, Krauñcha, Śālmala, Magadha and Puṣkara, each twice the size of the one mentioned just before it, with beautiful mountains and surrounded by oceans, and spreading like a pile of mustard seeds. The seven oceans, except the first one of salt water, taste as sugarcane juice, wine, butter, curd, cream and milk (3). These are encompassed by seven seas, girdle-shaped and encircled by Lokāloka mountains, and are estimated to be five hundred millions of Yojanas. This configuration is well established inside the cosmic egg. The egg is a minute particle of Pradhāna like a firefly in the sky. In the nether worlds, in the seas and in the mountains live the Asuras, Gandharvas, Kinnaras, Kimpuruṣas, Yakṣas, Rākṣasas, Bhūtas, Pretas, Piśāchas, Apasmāras, Apsarās, Brahma-rākṣasas, Kuṣmāṇḍas, Vināyakas and such like divine beings, while in the Dvīpas live the virtuous Devas or heavenly beings and men (after their death).

Sumeru is the land of garden of the deities ; there are four gardens called Miśravana, Nandana, Chaitraratha and Sumānasa, the council of the deities called Sudharmā, the city called Sudarśanapura and the palace called Vaijayanta. The planets and stars, fastened by the pole-star and restrained by the movement of the wind, are going round the Sumeru at different points above it. In the Mahendraloka live six classes of deities, *viz.* Tridaśas, Agniṣvāttas, Yāmyas, Tuṣitas, Aparinirmita-vaśavartīs, and Parinirmita-vaśavartīs. They have all their desires fulfilled and are possessed of supernormal powers like power to reduce one's body, their spans of life extend over Kalpas ; they are held in reverence, are fond of pleasures, their bodies are not of parental origin, and they have families consisting of good-looking and docile Apsarās (nymphs). In the great Prājāpatya region there are five groups of deities—Kumudas, Ṛbhus, Pratardanas, Añjanābhas, and Prachitābhas. They have mastery over the gross elements, and meditation is their food. They live for a thousand Kalpas (eons). In Brahmā's first sphere called Janaloka, there are four classes of Devas—the Brahma-purohitas, the Brahma-kāyikas, the Brahma-mahākāyikas and the Amaras. They have power over the elements and the organs and have double the longevity of those mentioned before. In the second sphere called Tapoloka, there are three kinds of Devas, the Ābhāsvaras, the Mahābhāsvaras, and the Satya-mahābhāsvaras. They have mastery over the elements, the organs and the Tanmātras. Their longevity is twice that of the former, they live on meditation, have full control over their passions, have the capacity of knowing what is happening in regions above them, while knowledge of everything in regions below them is laid bare before them.

In the third sphere of Brahma, the Satyaloka, there are found four kinds of Devas—the Achyutas, the Śuddhanivāsas, the Satyābhas and the Saṁjñāsaṁjñīs. They have no material habitation, they live in themselves, each being one layer above the other, have control over the Pradhāna and live to the end of creation. Of these, the Achyutas enjoy the bliss of Savitarka meditation. The Śuddhanivāsas are occupied with the bliss of Savichāra meditation, the Satyābhas with Ānanda-mātra or blissful meditation and the Saṁjñāsaṁjñīs with Asmitā-mātra (pure I-sense) meditation. They also live within the three cosmic regions. All these seven regions come within Brahmaloka. But the discarnates and those whose bodies are resolved into primal matter and have reached the Mokṣa-like stage, do not reside in the phenomenal world.

Yogins should see all these by practising Saṁyama on the solar entrance (Sūryadvāra) or on any other region, until all these are seen thoroughly.

(1) The word 'sun' here implies the point in the body known as the solar entrance. Every commentator is agreed on this. From the words 'moon' and 'Dhruva' used in the two succeeding Sūtras one might think that 'sun' refers to the great luminary, but that is not so. In fact, 'moon' also refers to the point known as lunar entrance (Chandradvāra). 'Dhruva' has been fully explained by the commentator.

In determining the solar entrance, first Suṣumnā has to be fixed. Heart is the point of contact between the soul and the body. In other words, the most sentient part of the body is the heart. The chest is generally the centre of the 'I'-feeling ; therefore the part which is most sentient and which has the most subtle feeling is the heart. The current of subtle feeling flowing up from the heart towards the brain is the Suṣumnā. Suṣumnā is not to be looked for in the gross body, but is only to be located by meditation. According to the modern physiologists the Suṣumnā is located inside the spinal cord, but according to the ancients a particular nerve going up from the heart is called Suṣumnā. The Yogin wilfully suppressing the action of the body and thus any feelings therein, would last of all give up the sentient portion and become discarnate. This portion is called Suṣumnā. On account of some connection with the sun it is called the solar entrance. It is said in the Śāstras, "The lamp-like thing situated within the heart has innumerable rays, one of which goes up right through the solar region. After passing the Brahmaloka the departing soul gets to the highest point with the help of this ray." Thus one of the rays of the effulgent light mentioned before (I.36) is the Suṣumnā entrance or solar entrance.

On practising Saṁyama on this particular ray of effulgent light a knowledge of the whole universe is revealed. The regions of the universe are both gross and subtle and of them, Avīchi etc. are without illumination ; therefore, they cannot be seen with the gross material light. Ordinary sunlight cannot illumine them. It is only the developed power of sense-faculty, which does not wait for an illuminator but sees things by its own power of illumination, that can have knowledge of the universe. One reason for not taking the words 'solar entrance' to imply the sun, is that Saṁyama on the sun can reveal only the sun. How can it bring knowledge of other regions like Brahamaloka etc. ?

On account of similarity between the microcosm and the macrocosm, the identity of the Suṣumnā nerve and the regions of the universe has been spoken of. Every creature has its super-mundane soul, and all-pervading Buddhi is only limited by the action of the senses. As these limitations disappear the power of Buddhi goes on increasing and one goes up from higher to higher regions. Thus the elimination of the coverings on Buddhi is related to the attainment of different Lokas or regions. From the point of view of Buddhi there is no such thing as far or near. Thus Buddhi of each creature and the stellar regions are on the same plane, and the power of attaining them is gained when the Vṛttis or modifications of Buddhi are purified.

(2) Bhūḥ-loka is not this earth but the large ethereal region attached to this earth. Sumeru hill, the residence of the Devas, is also such a region ; it is not visible to the eye. The location of the different regions of the universe as described herein, was accepted by the ancient Yoga philosopher as being current at the time.

(3) The Dvīpas are inhabited by holy Devas and pious men after their death. The Dvīpas must therefore be subtle regions.

The nether worlds are located inside the Bhūḥ-loka (not this earth) and are also subtle regions. To one with a subtle vision the seven hells have the same appearance as the different parts of the gross earth. The creatures living in those regions are endowed with subtle organs of reception but as their powers are restrained they suffer misery, being unable to fulfil their wishes. In a nightmare the body cannot act on account of the organs being inactive, but the mind being active suffers like an ensnared beast ; so do creatures suffer in hell.

As in this world there are separate lower animals, so amongst the subtle-bodied creatures, the inhabitants of the seven hells form separate lower classes. The same gross region appears different according as the view-point is gross, subtle or mixed. What men see as earth, water or fire, those in hell see as hell and those in the nether regions look upon as their wonted abode. The Deva-lokas start form the top of Bhūḥ-loka. Top of Bhūḥ-loka does not mean top of the earth, but it is situated much above the aerial region of the earth.

Residents of the nether regions and the Devas who come into existence without parents, are regarded as separate species. As the denizens of hell are transformed human beings, so also are there human beings residing in heaven. They retain the memory of their human existence. That is why in the Upaniṣads two separate classes as Deva-gandharva and Manuṣya-gandharva have been mentioned.

Unless the constitution of the different regions of abode and the nature of the residents thereof, described in this Sūtra, are clearly understood the sanctity and greatness of the state of liberation would not be appreciated. Through piety the lower Deva regions are attained, while in accordance with the different Yogic states the higher Deva regions are reached.

The state of Kaivalya or liberation is beyond all Lokas and no one returns from there.

---

चन्द्रे ताराव्यूहज्ञानम् ।। २७ ।।

भाष्यम्—चन्द्रे संयमं कृत्वा ताराव्यूहं विजानीयात् ।। २७ ।।

**(By Practising Saṁyama) On The Moon (The Lunar Entrance) Knowledge Of The Arrangements Of Stars Is Acquired. 27.**

By Saṁyama on the lunar entrance (of the body) the disposition of the stellar system would be known (1).

(1) As sun in the last Sūtra refers to the solar entrance so moon here refers to the lunar entrance (*i.e.* not the satellite). But they are not exactly of the same nature. While those who travel with the ray going through the solar region, reach Brahmaloka, departing souls reaching the lunar region, have to return to the earth. As the sun is self-

luminous, so is the knowledge of the solar entrance. The light of the moon is reflected light. The power of perception required to know a luminous object is of the kind required to know the (luminous) stellar systems. By development of the knowledge attainable through the senses, *i.e.* by proficiency in knowledge of gross objects, arrangement of stellar regions can be known.

Since the soul leaving the body by means of one of the sense-energies, *e.g.* eye etc., reaches the lunar region, this passage is called the moon (or lunar entrance).

---

ध्रुवे तद्गतिज्ञानम् ॥ २८ ॥

भाष्यम्—ततो ध्रुवे संयमं कृत्वा ताराणां गतिं जानीयाद्, ऊर्ध्वविमानेषु कृतसंयमस्तानि विजानीयात् ॥ २८ ॥

**(By Practising Saṁyama) On The Pole-Star, Motion Of The Stars Is known. 28.**

After that, by practising Saṁyama on the fixed pole-star the movement of the stars is to be known. By Saṁyama on the high aerial vehicle (void) of celestial bodies, their motions are to be known (1).

(1) After the stars are known, their movements can be known by external means. Pole-star mentioned here is therefore the ordinary pole-star. The commentator has included it amongst the higher stellar regions. Fixing the gaze on the pole-star, if one can get steadfastly engrossed in the sky, the movement of the stars will be known. In fact, the movement of the stars is known with reference to one's own stillness.

---

नाभिचक्रे कायव्यूहज्ञानम् ॥ २९ ॥

भाष्यम्—नाभिचक्रे संयमं कृत्वा कायव्यूहं विजानीयात्। वातपित्त-

श्लेष्माणस्त्रयो दोषाः सन्ति। धातवः सप्त त्वग्लोहितमांसस्नाय्वस्थिमज्जाशुक्राणि, पूर्वं पूर्वमेषां वाह्यमित्येष विन्यासः ॥ २९ ॥

**(By Practising Saṁyama) On The Navel Plexus, Knowledge Of The Composition Of The Body Is Derived. 29.**

The composition of the body and the arrangement of the organs are to be known by practising Saṁyama on the plexus of the navel. The humours are three in number, *viz.* wind, bile and phlegm (1). The seven corporeal elements are skin, blood, flesh, sinew, bone, marrow and semen, amongst which each element is exterior to the one mentioned next.

(1) As by taking the solar entrance as the principal item, and applying Saṁyama to other appropriate objects, knowledge is gained of the cosmic region, so by taking the plexus or nerve-organs round the navel as the central point, knowledge can be gained of the body as a whole.

In the Āyurvedic system of medicine, disturbance or imbalance of wind, bile, and phlegm is regarded as the root of all ailments. Suśruta says that this division follows the three Guṇas or constituent principles, *viz.* Sattva, Rajas and Tamas. Thus wind is disturbance of the sentient functions, bile of the mutative functions and phlegm of the retentive functions. In fact, a review of their symptoms supports this view.

As the whole world has benefited from Sāṁkhya philosophy obtaining therefrom the highest code of conduct like Ahiṁsā, truth, etc. and the doctrines of Yoga, so has mankind gained the first principles of medical science from it.

---

कण्ठकूपे क्षुत्पिपासानिवृत्तिः ॥ ३० ॥

भाष्यम्—जिह्वाया अधस्तात्तन्तुः, ततोऽधस्तात्कण्ठः, ततोऽधस्तात्कूपः, तत्र संयमात्क्षुत्पिपासे न बाधेते ॥ ३० ॥

**(By Practising Saṁyama) On The Trachea, Hunger And Thirst Can Be Subdued. 30.**

Below the tongue are the vocal cords and the larynx, and below that is the trachea. One practising Saṁyama on the trachea is not affected by hunger and thirst (1).

(1) When by Saṁyama on the trachea a calm and placid feeling is gained, the feelings of hunger and thirst are also conquered. The feelings of hunger and thirst arise in the alimentary canal no doubt, but sometimes nervous action can be better controlled from a distance.

———

कूर्मनाड्यां स्थैर्यम् ॥ ३१ ॥

भाष्यम्—कूपादध उरसि कूर्माकारा नाड़ी, तस्यां कृतसंयमः स्थिरपदं लभते, यथा सर्पो गोधा वेति ॥ ३१ ॥

**Calmness Is Attained By Saṁyama On The Bronchial Tube. 31.**

Within the chest, below the trachea is a tortoise-shaped tubular structure, by Saṁyama on which one attains freedom from restlessness, like a snake or an iguana (1).

(1) Below the trachea are the bronchial tubes. It can be easily felt that if the breathing mechanism is calmed, calmness of the whole body follows. As a snake or an iguana can stay inert like a piece of stone, so also can Yogins. If the body does not move, the mind can also be made calm along with it. The calmness referred to in the Sūtra refers to calmness of the mind, because the powers referred to herein are of the nature of knowledge.

———

मूर्द्धज्योतिषि सिद्धदर्शनम् ॥ ३२ ॥

भाष्यम्—शिरःकपालेऽन्तश्छिद्रं प्रभास्वरं ज्योतिः, तत्र संयमात् सिद्धानां द्यावापृथिव्योरन्तरालचारिणां दर्शनम् ॥ ३२ ॥

**(By Practising Saṁyama) On The Coronal Light, Siddhas Can Be Seen. 32.**

In the skull there is a small hole through which emanates effulgent light. By practising Saṁyama on that light Siddhas who frequent the space between the earth and the sky, can be seen (1).

(1) The light is to be thought of as within the head specially at the back. Siddhas are a kind of Devas or aerial beings.

———

प्रातिभाद्वा सर्वम् ॥ ३३ ॥

भाष्यम्—प्रातिभन्नाम तारकं, तद्विवेकजस्य ज्ञानस्य पूर्वरूपं यथोदये प्रभा भास्करस्य। तेन वा सर्वमेव जानाति योगी प्रातिभस्य ज्ञानस्योत्पत्ताविति ॥ ३३ ॥

**From Knowledge Known As Prātibha (Intuition), Everything Becomes Known. 33.**

Prātibha, *i.e.* Tāraka knowledge is the state of knowledge before attainment of discriminative knowledge, like the light of dawn preceding the sunrise. By that also, *i.e.* when Prātibha knowledge is attained, the Yogin comes to know everything (1).

(1) Discriminative knowledge has been discussed in Sūtras III.52-54. The enlightenment preceding it illumines everything like the light of dawn.

———

हृदये चित्तसंवित् ॥ ३४ ॥

भाष्यम्—यदिदमस्मिन्ब्रह्मपुरे दहरम्पुण्डरीकं वेश्म तत्र विज्ञानं, तस्मिन्संयमाच्चित्तसंवित् ॥ ३४ ॥

**(By Practising Saṁyama) On The Heart, Knowledge Of The Mind Is Acquired. 34.**

The citadel of Brahma (the heart), shaped like a lotus with a small aperture in it, is the seat of knowledge. By Saṁyama on this, perception of Chitta arises (1).

(1) The word 'Saṁvit' used in the Sūtra implies knowledge of Chitta. By practising Saṁyama on the heart, fluctuations of Chitta, which are but mutations of Buddhi, are correctly apprehended. In the comments on Sūtras I.28 and III.26, the heart and meditation therein have been dealt with. The brain is no doubt the mechanism of knowledge, but for arriving at the I-sense, meditation on the heart is the easier method. And if from the heart, one watches the action of the mind, one can realise its different fluctuations. The fluctuations are not spatial like light, sound, etc. Realisation of fluctuations of the mind is, in fact, realisation of the flow of activity that exists in the knowledge of light, sound, etc. The main root of knowledge is the pure I-sense. That is realised through meditation on the heart, and is only a step towards the knowledge about Puruṣa, mentioned hereafter.

———

सत्त्वपुरुषयोरत्यन्तासङ्कीर्णयोः प्रत्ययाविशेषो भोगः परार्थत्वात्स्वार्थसंयमात् पुरुषज्ञानम् ॥ ३५ ॥

भाष्यम्—बुद्धिसत्त्वं प्रख्याशीलं समानसत्त्वोपनिबन्धने रजस्तमसी वशीकृत्य सत्त्वपुरुषान्यताप्रत्ययेन परिणतं, तस्माच्च सत्त्वात् परिणामिनोऽत्यन्तविधर्मा शुद्धोऽन्यश्चितिमात्ररूपः पुरुषः। तयोरत्यन्तासङ्कीर्णयोः प्रत्ययाविशेषो भोगः पुरुषस्य, दर्शितविषयत्वात्। स भोगप्रत्ययः सत्त्वस्य परार्थत्वाद् दृश्यः। यस्तु तस्माद्विशिष्टश्चितिमात्ररूपोऽन्यः पौरुषेयः प्रत्ययस्तत्र संयमात्पुरुषविषया प्रज्ञा

जायते। न च पुरुषप्रत्ययेन बुद्धिसत्त्वात्मना पुरुषो दृश्यते, पुरुष एव प्रत्ययं स्वात्मावलम्बनं पश्यति, तथाह्युक्तं 'विज्ञातारमरे केन विजानीयाद्' इति ॥ ३५ ॥

**Experience (Of Pleasure Or Pain) Arises From A Conception Which Does Not Distinguish Between The Two Extremely Different Entities, Viz. Buddhisattva And Puruṣa. Such Experience Exists For Another (i.e. Puruṣa). That Is Why Through Saṁyama On Puruṣa (Who Oversees All Experience And Also Their Complete Cessation), A Knowledge Regarding Puruṣa Is Acquired. 35.**

Buddhisattva is sentient. Inseparably associated with it are Rajas and Tamas Guṇas. By subduing or counteracting the force of the other two, Buddhisattva proceeds to realise the distinction between Buddhi and Puruṣa (1).

Puruṣa is altogether different in nature from Buddhi. He is pure, distinct and absolute Consciousness. Conception of the two distinct entities (Buddhisattva and Puruṣa) as the same, is experience (Bhoga) and it is ascribed to Puruṣa, because in reality what is seen or experienced is presented to Puruṣa by Buddhi. The conception of experience is of Buddhi and as it is serving another it is regarded as the knowable of the Seer. If a conception is formed of that (*i.e.* of Puruṣa), which is distinct from experience and nothing but absolute Consciousness, and Saṁyama is practised on that, then is knowledge regarding Puruṣa acquired. Puruṣa is not, however, realised by this intellectual conception of Him. Moreover, Puruṣa is the Knower of the conception formed of Him. It has therefore been said in the Upaniṣad : "What will the Knower be known by."

(1) It has been explained before that Viveka-khyāti or discriminative enlightenment is a characteristic of Buddhi, *i.e.* it is a kind of mental modification. That is the final Sāttvika form of Buddhi. When the Rājasika and Tāmasika dross of Buddhi is overcome, then only this discriminative knowledge arises. Puruṣa, however, is different even from this

highly sentient Buddhi in a state of discriminative knowledge, because after all Buddhi is mutable etc. (See II.20).

To consider such Buddhi and Puruṣa as identical, *i.e.* to have the conception of both at one and the same time, is known as Bhoga or experience (of pleasure and pain). As knowledge, experience is a form of fluctuation of Buddhi. And because it is a fluctuation of Buddhi it is an object of knowledge. And being a knowable, it behaves as an object made known by the Seer. A knowable serves as an object of another, while Puruṣa owns the knowable object. This has been explained in Sūtra II.20. The owner is one who has property of his own, *i.e.* a proprietor. According to context that proprietor is either the self-established Puruṣa or Buddhi associated with the conception of Puruṣa. Here Buddhi, having the knowledge about Puruṣa, is referred to as the object on which Saṁyama has to be practised. In this connection the commentator has stated that when Buddhi, which is only the conventional receiver and is the pure I-sense, assumes the look of Puruṣa, it is the object of Saṁyama. In other words, what is thought of as Puruṣa in ordinary use, is not the real Puruṣa but has only the appearance of Puruṣa and it is nothing but Buddhi simulating the absolute Knower. By Saṁyama on this form of knowledge of Puruṣa, a knowledge regarding the real Puruṣa is acquired. On this, the question might be asked—is Puruṣa the object of the knowledge of Buddhi ? No, that is not so ; that is why the commentator has said—a knowledge relating to Puruṣa is acquired, *i.e.* Buddhi does not reveal Puruṣa who is self-expressive. Buddhi or pure I-sense, therefore, thinks 'I am self-expressive'. That is Puruṣa-like Buddhi. Such knowledge as derived from the Śāstras, or from inference, however, is not pure knowledge of Puruṣa. After the true nature and function of the mind has been grasped through Samādhi, the knowledge of Puruṣa as distinct from the mind dawns and that is the pure knowledge of Puruṣa. On one side of that knowledge is the absolutely conscious Puruṣa, devoid of any objectivity and on the other side is the sense of experience which is working on behalf of another (*i.e.* Puruṣa). The one in the middle, that is the pure I-sense, therefore, is the object of Saṁyama. Thus the knowledge that is derived from this Saṁyama is the highest knowledge relating to Puruṣa. Thereafter on the cessation of Buddhi, the Self becomes self-established and reaches the state of liberation, or the state of being-in-Itself.

Puruṣa cannot be objectively realised by Buddhi. Then what is this knowledge of Puruṣa ? In reply the commentator states that Buddhi (being divested of all other knowables) which is shaped after Puruṣa, when witnessed by Him, is knowledge of Puruṣa. Buddhi shaped after

Puruṣa has been explained before. 'I am the Seer (knower)'—this form of knowledge is Buddhi shaped after Puruṣa. Puruṣa by Himself cannot be the object of Saṁyama but the pseudo-Puruṣa or pure I-sense, the 'I' regarding itself as the Seer, is the subject of Saṁyama.

———

ततः प्रातिभश्रावणवेदनाऽऽदर्शाऽऽस्वादवार्त्ता जायन्ते ॥ ३६ ॥

भाष्यम्—प्रातिभात्सूक्ष्मव्यवहितविप्रकृष्टातीतानागतज्ञानं श्रावणाद्दिव्यशब्द-श्रवणं वेदनाद्दिव्यस्पर्शाधिगम आदर्शाद्दिव्यरूपसंविद् आस्वादाद्दिव्यरससंविद् वार्त्तातो दिव्यगन्धविज्ञानम् । इत्येतानि नित्यं जायन्ते ॥ ३६ ॥

**Thence (From The Knowledge Of Puruṣa) Arise Prātibha (Prescience), Śrāvaṇa (Supernormal Power Of Hearing), Vedana (Supernormal Power Of Touch), Ādarśa (Supernormal Power Of Sight), Āsvāda (Supernormal Power Of Taste) And Vārtā (Supernormal Power Of Smell). 36.**

From Prātibha, a prescience is acquired of the knowledge of the subtle, the obstructed, the remote, the past and the future. From Śrāvaṇa, divine sounds become audible; from Vedana, the divine sense of touch is felt; from Ādarśa, comes the divine sense of light; from Āsvāda, comes the cognition of divine taste, and from smell, the cognition of heavenly odours. These always (inevitably) arise (with the knowledge of Puruṣa) (1).

(1) When the knowledge of Puruṣa is acquired, these faculties are developed involuntarily, *i.e.* without the application of Saṁyama. The author has thus far described the supernormal powers in the shape of knowledge. Supernormal powers in respect of action and potentiality thereof are now being dealt with.

———

ते समाधावुपसर्गा व्युत्थाने सिद्धयः ॥ ३७ ॥

भाष्यम्—ते प्रातिभादयः समाहितचित्तस्योत्पद्यमाना उपसर्गास्तद्दर्शन-प्रत्यनीकत्वाद् व्युत्थितचित्तस्योत्पद्यमानाः सिद्धयः ॥ ३७ ॥

**They (These Powers) Are Impediments To Samādhi, But Are Acquisitions In A Normal Fluctuating State Of The Mind. 37.**

When powers like prescience etc. mentioned before are acquired, they prove to be hindrances to the attainment of Samādhi because they stand in the way of realisation of the ultimate truth by an engrossed mind. When the mind is fluctuating they are acquisitions (1).

(1) In Samādhi there is only one object as the prop of a concentrated mind, hence the attainment of powers mentioned before causes disturbance to such a mind. When aided by the knowledge of the various Tattvas (principles), and by the practice of renunciation the mind becomes one-pointed, and is completely closed (to permeation of knowledge) then only can the state of the Self being-in-Itself be reached. Attainment of powers is inimical to that (vide I.30).

———

बन्धकारणशैथिल्यात् प्रचारसंवेदनाच्च चित्तस्य परशरीरावेशः ॥ ३८ ॥

भाष्यम्—लोलीभूतस्य मनसोऽप्रतिष्ठस्य शरीरे कर्माशयवशाद्बन्धः प्रतिष्ठेत्यर्थः ; तस्य कर्मणो बन्धकारणस्य शैथिल्यं समाधिबलाद् भवति। प्रचारसंवेदनं च चित्तस्य समाधिजमेव, कर्मबन्धक्षयात् स्वचित्तस्य प्रचारसंवेदनाच्च योगी चित्तं स्वशरीरान्निष्कृष्य शरीरान्तरेषु निक्षिपति। निक्षिप्तं चित्तं चेन्द्रियाण्यनुपतन्ति यथा मधुकरराजानं मक्षिका उत्पतन्तमनूत्पतन्ति निविशमानमनु निविशन्ते तथेन्द्रियाणि परशरीरावेशे चित्तमनुविधीयन्त इति ॥ ३८ ॥

**When The Cause Of Bondage Gets Weakened And The Movements Of The Mind Are Known, The Mind Can Get Into Another Body. 38.**

Being restless by nature, the mind gets tied up with the body on account of latent impressions of previous actions (1). Through the power of concentration the ties created by previous actions become loosened, and the movements of the mind are known. When the bonds of previous actions become weak and the movements of the mind over the nerves are known, the Yogin can withdraw the mind from his own body and project it into another person's body. As when a queen-bee flies all bees follow it, and when it settles down others do the same, so do the sense-energies (Indriyas) follow the mind as it enters another body.

(1) Influenced by the notion 'I am the body', the mind flits from object to object every moment. The impression 'I am not the body', does not last long in a distracted mind. That is what causes attachment to the body. Moreover, the body is the result of latent impressions of previous actions. As long as activity goes on, the mind containing the latent impressions of actions will continue to be associated with the body. When through concentration the knowledge 'I am not the body' gets established and the actions of the body stop, the mind becomes free from the body. Through subtle insight gained by concentration, the movement of the mind along the nerves comes to be known. Thus a Yogin's mind can also enter into another body and influence it.

---

उदानजयाज्जलपङ्ककण्टकादिष्वसङ्ग उत्क्रान्तिश्च ॥ ३९ ॥

भाष्यम्—समस्तेन्द्रियवृत्तिः प्राणादिलक्षणा जीवनम्। तस्य क्रिया पञ्चतयी, प्राणो मुखनासिकागतिराहृदयवृत्तिः, समं नयनात् समानश्चानाभिवृत्तिः, अपनयनादपान आपादतलवृत्तिः, उन्नयनादुदान आशिरोवृत्तिः, व्यापी व्यान इति। तेषाम्प्रधानः प्राणः। उदानजयाज्जलपङ्ककण्टकादिष्वसङ्ग उत्क्रान्तिश्च प्रायणकाले भवति, तां वशित्वेन प्रतिपद्यते ॥ ३९ ॥

**By Conquering The Vital Force Called Udāna The Chance Of Immersion In Water Or Mud, Or Entanglement In The Thorns, Is Avoided And Exit From The Body At Will Is Assured. 39.**

Action of the senses characterised by the vital forces, is life. Its action is fivefold. Movement of Prāṇa is limited to the mouth and the nose, and its action extends up to the heart. Samāna distributes (the nourishment from food) to all parts equally and its sphere of action is up to the navel. Apāna is so called because it carries the wastes away and it acts down to the soles of the feet. Udāna is the vital force with upward direction and it goes right up to the head. The vital force Vyāna is spread all over the body. Of these forces, the chief is the Prāṇa. Mastery over the vital force Udāna eliminates the possibility of immersion in water or mud and assures exit (through Archi and similar passages) at the time of death. It also makes the exit from the body (*i.e.* death) occur at will (1).

(1) The vital force called Udāna supports the nerve wherein feeling of the bodily humours resides. All feelings are carried by the sense channels upward to the brain. By practising Saṁyama on this upward flow and meditating on the presence of the sentient Sattva Guṇa in all the humours of the body, the body is felt to be light. If Chitta is fixed on Udāna in the Suṣumnā nerve it will facilitate the voluntary exit through Archi and similar other passages.

———

समानजयाज्ज्वलनम् ॥ ४० ॥

भाष्यम्—जितसमानस्तेजस उपध्मानं कृत्वा ज्वलति ॥ ४० ॥

**By Conquering The Vital Force Called Samāna, Effulgence Is Acquired. 40.**

The Yogin who has overcome Samāna can generate radiance in the body and become effulgent (1).

(1) By the vital force called Samāna, all parts of the body are properly nourished, *i.e.* the energy supplied by food is evenly distributed. By conquering that vital force a Yogin gets an aura around his body.

———

श्रोत्राकाशयोस्सम्बन्धसंयमाद्दिव्यं श्रोत्रम् ॥ ४१ ॥

भाष्यम्—सर्वश्रोत्राणामाकाशं प्रतिष्ठा सर्वशब्दानां च, यथोक्तं 'तुल्यदेशश्रवणानामेकदेशश्रुतित्वं सर्वेषाम्भवति' इति। तच्चैतदाकाशस्य लिङ्गमनावरणं चोक्तम्। तथाऽमूर्त्तस्यानावरणादर्शनाद्विभुत्वमपि प्रख्यातमाकाशस्य। शब्दग्रहणानुमितं श्रोत्रं बधिराबधिरयोरेकः शब्दं गृह्णात्यपरो न गृह्णातीति, तस्मात् श्रोत्रमेव शब्दविषयम्। श्रोत्राकाशयोः सम्बन्धे कृतसंयमस्य योगिनो दिव्यं श्रोत्रं प्रवर्त्तते ॥ ४१ ॥

**By Saṁyama On The Relationship Between Ākāśa And The Power Of Hearing, Divine Sense Of Hearing Is Gained. 41.**

All powers of hearing and all sounds abide in Ākāśa. It has thus been said : "Since the sense of hearing of all beings has a bearing on the identical sound element, it is related to that single element (1)." It is that conditioned hearing which is the Liṅga or indicator of Ākāśa, and absence of obstruction (void) is also mentioned as its Liṅga or indicator. Moreover, it is found that a formless thing or a thing intangible is not obstructed by anything (as it can stay anywhere) ; thus the all-pervasiveness of Ākāśa is established. From the perception of sound, existence of the organ of hearing can be inferred. One who is deaf does not perceive sound, while one who is not so perceives it. Sound is thus the object of the organ of hearing only. The Yogin who practises Saṁyama on the relationship between the organ of hearing and Ākāśa, develops subtle sense of hearing.

(1) Ākāśa has the property of sound. The property of sound is the most unobstructible because it can penetrate other things more easily

than heat, light, etc. It can be argued that the vibration of solid, liquid or gaseous things causes sound, therefore, sound is their property. In one sense it is true, but the vibration only manifests itself taking them as support. If a search were made to find out where the energy of vibration resides, it will be seen that externally it resides basically in the sources of heat, electricity, etc., and internally in the mind. All kinds of external sound vibrations are principally produced by heat etc. ; by volition too the organ of speech is made to vibrate to produce sound. Although in speech the sound is produced by the vibrating tissues of the throat, it is really a sort of transference of muscular energy.

What is that power which manifests itself as sound, heat or light ? In reply it must be admitted that it is itself without (*i.e.* beyond) any sound, heat or light. That which is free from these attributes, is called void or vacancy or Ākāśa. By a vague concept it is called emptiness or void, but that has no real existence. But the energy that manifests itself as sound, light, etc., does exist. If a thing has to be conceived as existing but without any property of sound, light, etc., it has to be imagined as Ākāśa or void. The most correct conception of such a void can be in terms of sound. When a sound is heard it generates a knowledge of something external but that knowledge is devoid of any form. Thus an external entity full of sound but without any substance is Ākāśa. Moreover, all vibrations indicate a void as there can be no vibration where there is no vacancy. Solid, liquid and gaseous things can emit sound by vibration on account of this vacancy. This vacancy or voidness can be relative, just as compared to a solid a gaseous substance is more void. Absolute void is an inconceivable thing but comparative void is a reality.

Ear, the gross organ of hearing, must have void in it as it can receive vibrations. The sense-organ relating to void is the organ of hearing. All sense-organs are formed of similar affinity with appropriate elements. In other words, the ossicles etc., the solid parts of the organ of hearing, being susceptible to vibrations of the relatively vacant air, the ear is considered to be akin to void.

The kinship of I-sense with void is the relationship between the ear and Ākāśa. And by Saṁyama thereon, there is a development of I-sense on Sāttvika lines and growth of void towards non-obstructiveness. This is known as divine or subtle sense of hearing.

The meaning of the quotation from Pañchaśikha is that all organs of hearing, being made of identical sound element, are all attuned to Ākāśa. This is the material side of the sense of hearing. From the point of view of energy all senses are modifications of I-sense.

———

कायाकाशयोस्सम्बन्धसंयमाल्लघुतूलसमापत्तेश्चाकाशगमनम् ॥ ४२ ॥

भाष्यम्—यत्र कायस्तत्राकाशं तस्यावकाशदानात्कायस्य, तेन सम्बन्धः प्राप्तिः (सम्बन्धावाप्तिरिति पाठान्तरम्)। तत्र कृतसंयमो जित्वा तत्सम्बन्धं लघुषु तूलादिष्वापरमाणुभ्यः समापत्तिं लब्ध्वा जितसम्बन्धो लघुः, लघुत्वाच्च जले पादाभ्यां विहरति, ततस्तूर्णनाभितन्तुमात्रे विहृत्य रश्मिषु विहरति ततो यथेष्टमाकाशगतिरस्य भवतीति ॥ ४२ ॥

**By Practising Saṁyama On The Relationship Between The Body And Ākāśa And By Concentrating On The Lightness Of Cotton Wool, Passage Through The Sky Can Be Secured. 42.**

Wherever there is body, there is Ākāśa, because void provides room for the body. That is why the relationship between Ākāśa and the body is one of the former pervading the latter. By Saṁyama on that relationship, *i.e.* by realising it, the Yogin becomes light and can move through the sky. Or by meditation on cotton wool or other light things down to atoms, Yogin becomes light. By becoming light he can walk on water and then on cobwebs and on rays of light. Thereafter he can move to the sky at will (1).

(1) If Saṁyama is practised on the relationship between the body and Ākāśa, *i.e.* on the existence of the body in the midst of void, the power to move unobstructed at will is acquired.

Ākāśa has the property of sound. Sound is nothing but a flow of activity without any form. To think that the body is nothing but a collection of activities and is vacant like Ākāśa, is to think of the relationship between the body and Ākāśa. This is done by contemplating an unstruck sound (Anāhata-nāda) pervading the body. That is why it has been said in another Śāstra that by contemplation on a particular unstruck sound, movement to the sky is accomplished.

Again, if one gets engrossed in the lightness of cotton wool or other similar light things, the particles of the body lose their heaviness and become light. In fact, the material constituents of the body like flesh and blood are really modifications of I-sense. Heaviness is a modification of I-sense and if by power of Samādhi the opposite idea is conceived, the materials of the body change to lightness. From lightness of body and from mastery over the relationship between the body and Ākāśa the power of unobstructed movement is acquired, resulting in the ability to move to the sky.

In spiritist literature there are records of mediums having gone up the air during seances. A famous medium (D. D. Home) used to go up in the air like this. During Prāṇāyāma, as the body is to be thought of as light as air, it sometimes actually becomes light. Mention is made of this in Haṭha-yoga literature. Mental contemplation is at the root of all these.

There is a deep truth underlying the statement that body becomes light by contemplation. Weight means force towards the centre of the earth. That force varies according to the nature of material objects. What is a body or any material object ? It is nothing but a collection of minute particles, say the ancients. Modern science holds a similar view—the minute particles or atoms are made up of even smaller particles like electrons, protons and neutrons. Electrons move round a nucleus consisting of protons and neutrons millions of times in a second and between these two subtle entities there is a lot of gap (as between the sun and the planets). Our ego acting on the materials constituting the body shapes them into the form of a body and makes it feel heavy. By concentrating on the relationship between the body and Ākāśa, it is possible to transform that ego. The Sūtra can be explained in this way.

———

वहिरकल्पिता वृत्तिर्महाविदेहा ततः प्रकाशावरणक्षयः ॥ ४३ ॥

भाष्यम्—शरीराद्वहिर्मनसो वृत्तिलाभो विदेहा नाम धारणा। सा यदि शरीरप्रतिष्ठस्य मनसो वहिर्वृत्तिमात्रेण भवति सा कल्पितेत्युच्यते, या तु शरीर-निरपेक्षा वहिर्भूतस्यैव मनसो वहिर्वृत्तिः सा खल्वकल्पिता। तत्र कल्पितया साधयत्यकल्पितां महाविदेहामिति, यया परशरीराण्याविशन्ति योगिनः। ततश्च धारणातः प्रकाशात्मनो बुद्धिसत्त्वस्य यदावरणं क्लेशकर्मविपाकत्रयं रजस्तमोमूलं तस्य च क्षयो भवति ॥ ४३ ॥

**When The Unimagined Conception Can Be Held Outside, i.e. Unconnected With The Body, It Is Called Mahāvideha Or The Great Discarnate. By Saṁyama On That The Veil Over Illumination (Of Buddhisattva) Is Removed. 43.**

The fluctuation or notion of the mind when conceived as outside the body, is called discarnate fixity or Videha Dhāraṇā (1). If that Dhāraṇā or fixity is caused by an external conception of the mind held within the body, it is called Kalpita (imagined). If, however, the fixity of a mind, independent of the body, relates to a conception outside the body it is known as Akalpita (unimagined or actual). Amongst these the fluctuations relating to Mahāvideha fixity have to be practised with the help of the imagined fixity. By such unimagined fixity a Yogin's mind can enter another body. By such fixity the veil over sentient Buddhi, in the shape of Kleśa (affliction), Karma(action) and threefold Vipāka (fruition) originating from Rajas and Tamas, is removed.

(1) When through practice of Dhāraṇā on any external object (all-pervading Ākāśa is the most suitable) one deeply contemplates 'I am there', and thereby makes the mind stay there, that is, when one really feels that one is there (and not within the body), one attains discarnate fixity. When the mind is felt to be both inside the body and outside, it is called imagined fixity. When the mind, being freed of the body, gains fixity outside, it is called Mahāvideha fixity. Thereby is attained the removal of the veil referred to in the commentary. The feeling 'I am the body' is the grossest of the veils over knowledge which is thinned or destroyed by this Saṁyama.

———

स्थूलस्वरूपसूक्ष्मान्वयार्थवत्त्वसंयमाद्भूतजयः ॥ ४४ ॥

भाष्यम्—तत्र पार्थिवाद्याः शब्दादयो विशेषाः सहाकारादिभिर्धर्मैः स्थूल-शब्देन परिभाषिताः, एतद्भूतानां प्रथमं रूपम्। द्वितीयं रूपं स्वसामान्यं,

मूर्त्तिर्भूमिः, स्नेहो जलं, वह्निरुष्णता, वायुः प्रणामी, सर्वतोगतिराकाश इति, एतत् स्वरूपशब्देनोच्यते, अस्य सामान्यस्य शब्दादयो विशेषाः। तथा चोक्तम् 'एकजातिसमन्वितानामेषां धर्ममात्रव्यावृत्ति'रिति। सामान्यविशेषसमुदायोऽत्र द्रव्यम्, द्विष्ठो हि समूहः। प्रत्यस्तमितभेदावयवानुगतः—शरीरं वृक्षो यूथं वनमिति। शब्देनोपात्तभेदावयवानुगतः समूहः—उभये देवमनुष्याः, समूहस्य देवा एको भागो मनुष्या द्वितीयो भागः, ताभ्यामेवाभिधीयते समूहः। स च भेदाभेदविवक्षितः, आम्राणां वनं ब्राह्मणानां सङ्घः, आम्रवणं ब्राह्मणसङ्घ इति। स पुनर्द्विविधो युतसिद्धावयवोऽयुतसिद्धावयवश्च, युतसिद्धावयवः समूहो वनं सङ्घ इति, अयुतसिद्धावयवः सङ्घातः शरीरं वृक्षः परमाणुरिति। 'अयुतसिद्धावयवभेदानुगतः समूहो द्रव्यमिति' पतञ्जलिः, एतत्स्वरूपमित्युक्तम्।

अथ किमेषां सूक्ष्मरूपं, तन्मात्रं भूतकारणम्। तस्यैकोऽवयवः परमाणुः सामान्यविशेषात्माऽयुतसिद्धावयवभेदानुगतः समुदाय इति, एवं सर्वतन्मात्राणि, एतत्तृतीयम्। अथ भूतानां चतुर्थं रूपं ख्यातिक्रियास्थितिशीला गुणाः कार्यस्वभावानुपातिनोऽन्वयशब्देनोक्ताः। अथैषां पञ्चमं रूपमर्थवत्त्वं, भोगापवर्गार्थता गुणेष्वन्वयिनी गुणास्तन्मात्रभूतभौतिकेष्विति सर्वमर्थवत्। तेष्विदानीं भूतेषु पञ्चसु पञ्चरूपेषु संयमात्तस्य तस्य रूपस्य स्वरूपदर्शनं जयश्च प्रादुर्भवति, तत्र पञ्चभूतस्वरूपाणि जित्वा भूतजयी भवति, तज्जयाद्वत्सानुसारिण्य इव गावोऽस्य सङ्कल्पानुविधायिन्यो भूतप्रकृतयो भवन्ति ॥ ४४ ॥

**By Saṁyama On The Grossness, The Essential Character, The Subtlety, The Inherence And The Objectiveness Which Are The Five Forms Of The Bhūtas Or Elements, Mastery Over Bhūtas Is Obtained. 44.**

Of these five forms, the distinctive properties of each, *e.g.* sound, earth, etc. and the properties like shape etc. are technically called grossness. This is the first form of the Bhūtas (1). The second is its generic form, each peculiar to itself. For example, the feature of earth is its natural hardness, of water liquidity, of fire heat, of wind mobility, of Ākāśa all-pervasiveness. This second form is called essential attribute. This generic form has sound etc. as its particulars. It has been said in this connection : "These (elements) belonging as they do to the same class are yet distinguished from one another by specific properties." Here (according to Sāṁkhya philosophy) a substance is an aggregate of generic and specific attributes. That aggregate is of two kinds— (i) in which conception of the distinction of individual parts has disappeared, *e.g.* a body, a tree, a herd, a forest; and (ii) in which the different parts are indicated by terms which show the distinction, *e.g.* 'Devas-and-men', one part being Devas, and the other part men. The two together form one group. In the conception of aggregate the distinction of individual parts may or may not be mentioned, for instance, we may say 'a grove of mango trees', 'a gathering of Brahmins', or 'a mango-grove', 'a Brahmin-gathering'. Again the collection is two-fold—(i) that of which the parts exist when separated (Yuta-siddhāvayava) and (ii) that of which the parts are not separable (Aytua-siddhāvayava). 'A forest', or 'an assemblage', is a group where the parts are separate from each other. A body or a tree or an atom etc. is a whole of which the parts are not separable. Patañjali says that an object is a collection, the different component parts of which do not exist separately. This has been called the essential attribute or Swarūpa of the Bhūtas.

Now, what is the subtle form of the Bhūtas? The answer is 'It is Tanmātra—the source of the Bhūtas' (2). It has one single (*i.e.* ultimate) part which is an atom. It is a composite substance (Ayuta-siddhāvayava) consisting of both generic and specific qualities. All Tanmātras are like this; this is the third form of the Bhūtas.

The fourth form of the Bhūtas relates to its properties of manifestation (knowability), activity and retentiveness. These three being akin to the modifications of the three Guṇas, have been described by the word inherence, *i.e.* as their inherent qualities.

The fifth form of the Bhūtas is objectivity. Experience and release therefrom are inherent in the Guṇas and the Guṇas are inherent in the Tanmātras, the Bhūtas and material objects. For this reason everything is objective. By practising Saṁyama on the Tattva formed last, *i.e.* on the five Bhūtas (3) having the five forms, the proper aspects of the five forms can be realised and subjugated. By subjugating the five forms, the Yogin gains mastery over the Bhūtas. As a result thereof, the Bhūtas and the Tanmātras follow the will of the Yogin as a cow follows its calf.

(1) Gross form—that which is first perceived by senses. With a shape, endowed with special qualities, existing in a material form is the gross form of an object, *e.g.* a pot or a cloth etc.

Essential character—more particularised than gross form. The different forms of Bhūtas by contact with which is derived knowledge of sound, touch, etc. constitute their essential character. The sense of smell arises out of contact with minute particles, so hardness is the substantive nature of earth element, the special property of which is smell. The special peculiar feature is the essential character as distinguished from gross nature.

The sense of taste is felt on contact with a liquid substance ; therefore the essential character of the Ap-bhūta is liquidity. Light generally exists in some form of heat. The source of Tejas or light and colours is the sun which is hot. Therefore the essential character of the light (Tejas) Bhūta is heat. The hot and cold feelings arise out of contact of the skin with air. Air is mobile and not static. Thus the essential character of the Vāyu-bhūta, with its special property of touch, is mobility.

Perception of sound is associated with knowledge of unobstructiveness. Thus the substantive nature of Ākāśa which has the special property of sound is non-obstructiveness. In particular forms of sound etc. these features are common. Sāṁkhya philosophers have said in this connection that objects of the same class are differentiated by their separate characteristics or by their particular shapes. In other words, the gross material objects made of the common five Bhūtas, are differentiated as pot, cloth etc. by their specific characteristics.

Thereafter the commentator explains the distinctive feature of substances through examples. The peculiar nature of Bhūtas which follows its particular form is known as its essential character.

That which we term collectively as 'whole' is basically as follows. Body, tree, etc. represent one kind of 'whole' which may have different parts but the emphasis is not on the latter. Another kind of 'whole', *e.g.* 'both Deva-and-men', draws attention to the distinction in the form of Devas (heavenly beings) and men. When the 'whole' is expressed by words then it may be spoken of in two ways like 'a collection of Brahmins' and 'a Brahmin-collection'. In the first the distinctive parts are explicit, while in the second they are not. Body, tree, etc. are 'whole's where the parts are not separable, while 'forest', 'an assemblage', etc. are 'whole's of which the parts are separable. In the first the parts are intimately connected with each other, while in the second the parts are conventionally associated for convenience of expression. Thus a 'whole' in which the parts are inseparable is called a substance.

(2) The subtle form of Bhūtas is Tanmātra. Tanmātra has been explained previously in II.19. Tanmātra has no consituent parts, because it is an atom (not to be confused with the atom in physical sciences). Being the minutest particle or the limit of diminutiveness, its further division in parts is inconceivable. The minutest form in which properties like sound etc. become perceivable in Samādhi is Tanmātra. That is why it is said to consist of one part only, *i.e.* it has no parts. The knowledge of that minute particle is not spatial but takes place in time, because spatial existence is noticeable only if it has a physical dimension. Sequence of knowledge of such minute particles is a knowledge of their mutation. An atom is in itself general and affords material for particulars (*i.e.* Bhūtas). That is why it is both general and particular. It is also particular because it is a special modified form of I-sense. An atom has therefore been defined as something whose different parts are not knowable and, therefore, indescribable.

The fourth form of Bhūtas is their manifestation (knowability), activity and retentiveness. I-sense gives rise to Tanmātra. I-sense again is sentient, active and retentive. All these three qualities are present in Bhūtas ; so they are called the constituent qualities of Bhūtas. In other words, all things made of Bhūtas like body etc. are Sāttvika, Rājasika and Tāmasika. That is how all Bhūtas become knowable, active and retentive.

The fifth form of Bhūtas is its objectiveness in asmuch as it can be the object of experiences and of salvation (by renunciation). By its property of being an object of experience, it causes happiness or misery and creates the body that experiences both, while by renouncing both one attains salvation.

(3) By practising Saṁyama on the Bhūta principle formed last (*i.e.* after Tanmātra) in which all the five forms are present (which are

not present in the Tanmātras), these have to be gradually realised and conquered and thus mastery over them is acquired. With the acquisition of such mastery comes the knowledge of all their particulars and the ability to change them at will. With the realisation of the essential character, the basis underlying the properties like hardness etc. becomes known and the power to change them at will is acquired.

With mastery over the subtle form, *viz.* Tanmātras, the essential nature of properties like sound etc. comes to be known and those properties can be changed at will.

Realisation of the inherent form leads to mastery over all organs, made of Bhūtas, through which pleasure and pain are experienced. On realisation of the objectiveness the power to renounce Bhūtas for a spiritual goal, is acquired. By attaining a state beyond the touch of pleasure, pain or stupor caused by Bhūtas, a Yogin can become completely indifferent to external objects. This is how Bhūtas and their causes (Tanmātras) are realised. The cause of an object is its Prakṛti. Puruṣa-like Buddhi as mentioned in III.35 may also be termed Prakṛti, which is not the same as the primal principle (Tattva) because it still forms part of Buddhi.

———

ततोऽणिमादिप्रादुर्भावः कायसम्पत्तद्धर्मानभिघातश्च ॥ ४५ ॥

भाष्यम्—तत्राणिमा भवत्यणुः, लघिमा लघुर्भवति, महिमा महान् भवति, प्राप्तिरङ्गुल्यग्रेणापि स्पृशति चन्द्रमसम्, प्राकाम्यमिच्छानभिघातो भूमावुन्मज्जति निमज्जति यथोदके, वशित्वम् भूतभौतिकेषु वशी भवति अवश्यश्चान्येषाम्, ईशितृत्वं तेषां प्रभवाप्ययव्यूहानामीष्टे। यत्रकामावसायित्वं सत्यसङ्कल्पता यथा सङ्कल्पस्तथा भूतप्रकृतीनामवस्थानं, न च शक्तोऽपि पदार्थविपर्यासं करोति, कस्माद्, अन्यस्य यत्रकामावसायिनः पूर्वसिद्धस्य तथाभूतेषु सङ्कल्पादिति। एतान्यष्टावैश्वर्याणि। कायसम्पद् वक्ष्यमाणा। तद्धर्मानभिघातश्च पृथ्वी मूर्त्या न निरुणद्धि योगिनः शरीरादिक्रियां, शिलामप्यनुप्रविशतीति, नापः स्निग्धाः क्लेदयन्ति, नाग्निरुष्णो दहति, न वायुः प्रणामी वहति, अनावरणात्मकेऽप्याकाशे भवत्यावृतकायः, सिद्धानामप्यदृश्यो भवति ॥ ४५ ॥

**Thence Develop The Power Of Minification And Other Bodily Acquisitions. There Is Also No Resistance By Its Characteristics. 45.**

Of these—

Minification (Aṇimā) is that by which one can reduce one's size to that of an atom. Lightness (Laghimā) is that by which one can decrease one's weight. Largeness (Mahimā) is that by which one can increase one's size or stature. Attaining (Prāpti) is that by which one can touch the moon by fingertips. Irresistible will (Prākāmya) is that by which one can go through solid earth or cannot be immersed in water. Control (Vaśitva) is that by which one can have control over the Bhūtas and which they are made of, *i.e.* Tanmātras, and cannot be swayed by others. Mastery (Īśitṛtva) is that by which one can control appearance, disappearance and aggregation of Bhūtas and objects made thereof. Resolution (Yatrakāmāvasāitva) is that by which one can determine at will the Bhūtas and their nature and their stayings as desired.

Yogins with such powers do not utilise them for disturbing the disposition of the world because they do not or cannot go against the will of a previously perfected One who has brought about the existing disposition of things. These are the eight attainments. The supernormal powers of the body will be mentioned later.

Example of non-obstruction to the characteristics of the body is the inability of the earth, through its hardness, to arrest the functioning of the organs of the Yogin's body. His body can go even through a stone, the fluidity of water cannot make the body wet, fire cannot burn him, the blowing wind does not move him and even in Ākāśa which by nature does not obstruct anything he can hide himself, so that he can disappear from view, even of Siddhas (1).

(1) Attaining implies distant things coming near, *e.g.* touching the moon at will. Mastery implies power to regulate the formation, retention

or destruction of objects at will. Resolution implies that Bhūtas and their constituents can be made to stay as desired.

In spite of the acquisition of such powers Yogins do not or cannot alter the disposition of things. The reason for this is that Hiraṇyagarbha, the previously perfected One, as creator of the universe had acquired such powers before and the disposition of the universe is still under His control. In other words, the resolution of the previous Siddha that the world should continue as it is, in which its inhabitants can work and enjoy or suffer according to their deserts, being still in force, the later Siddhas cannot bring about a change in the disposition of things in this world. They can, however, exercise their powers in respect of things which are outside the influence of Īśvara.

By the term 'previously perfected One' used by the commentator, the creator, protector and destroyer of the universe—the Saguṇa Īśvara—is referred to. In the Sāṁkhya philosophy it has been said : "He is all-knowing and all-powerful." So the views of Sāṁkhya and Yoga philosophies are the same.

———

रूपलावण्यबलवज्रसंहननत्वानि कायसम्पत् ।। ४६ ।।

भाष्यम्—दर्शनीयः कान्तिमान् अतिशयबलो वज्रसंहननश्चेति ।। ४६ ।।

**Perfection Of Body Consists In Beauty, Grace, Strength And Adamantine Hardness. 46.**

To be presentable, lovely, full of strength and hard as adamant, is to have a perfect body.

———

ग्रहणस्वरूपास्मितान्वयार्थवत्त्वसंयमादिन्द्रियजयः ।। ४७ ।।

भाष्यम्—सामान्यविशेषात्मा शब्दादिर्ग्राह्यः, तेष्विन्द्रियाणां वृत्तिर्ग्रहणं, न च तत्सामान्यमात्रग्रहणाकारं, कथमनालोचितः स विषयविशेष इन्द्रियेण मनसानुव्यवसीयेतेति । स्वरूपं पुनः प्रकाशात्मनो बुद्धिसत्त्वस्य सामान्यविशेषयो-रयुतसिद्धावयवभेदानुगतः समूहो द्रव्यमिन्द्रियम् । तेषां तृतीयं रूपमस्मिता-

लक्षणोऽहंकारः, तस्य सामान्यस्येन्द्रियाणि विशेषाः। चतुर्थं रूपं व्यवसायात्मकाः प्रकाशक्रियास्थितिशीला गुणा येषामिन्द्रियाणि साहंकाराणि परिणामाः। पञ्चमं रूपं गुणेषु यदनुगतं पुरुषार्थवत्त्वमिति। पञ्चस्वेतेषु इन्द्रियरूपेषु यथाक्रमं संयमः, तत्र तत्र जयं कृत्वा पञ्चरूपजयादिन्द्रियजयः प्रादुर्भवति योगिनः ॥ ४७ ॥

**By Saṁyama On The Receptivity, Essential Character, I-sense, Inherent Quality And Objectiveness Of The Five Organs, Mastery Over Them Can Be Acquired. 47.**

Sounds etc. in their general and particular aspects are knowables. Reception is the action of the senses on the knowables (1). The senses are not receivers of the general aspect alone. Because in that case how can an object which has not been dealt with by the senses (*i.e.* particulars which have not been dealt with or have only been superficially perceived by the senses) be reflected upon by the mind ?

Essential Character—An organ is an object with inseparable parts consisting of the general and particular qualities of the sentient principle of Buddhi (thus that kind of 'whole' is the essential nature of an organ).

The third form is the principle of individuality characterised by I-sense. The senses are the specialised forms of that generic appearance.

The fourth form of the organs is their receptive qualities of sentience, mutation and retention. The organs together with Ahaṁkāra or individuality are the mutations of the primal cause, *viz.* the three Guṇas. Their being objects of the Self, a quality ever present in the Guṇas, is the fifth form of the organs.

By practising Saṁyama successively on these five aspects of the organs and mastering them one by one, the Yogin develops the power of subjugating the organs.

(1) The first form of the senses (here the organs of perception) is their receptivity, *i.e.* the channel through which the objects are

received. Sound etc. excite the sense-organs and thus activate the I-sense relating to it, and this causes a knowledge of sound etc. That active state of the sense is its receptivity. Objects like sound etc. (object referred to here is the mental state due to the exciting cause which produces the sense of sound etc.) are both general and particular. [See in this connection notes at I.7(3).] Thus perception of sound etc. in their general or particular aspects, is reception. As there is reflective thought of particulars so they are also received by the senses, *i.e.* on account of the primary reception of the particulars, there can be representation thereof.

The parts of the senses which produce knowledge are the particular formations of the sentient Buddhi. The distinctive features of such formations constitute the essential character of each of the organs, *e.g.* eyes for one kind, ear for another, etc.

The third form of the senses is the I-sense which is really the material cause of the senses. Cognition is the active state of the I-sense within a particular organ of perception. That activity of the I-sense, common to different senses, is the third form of the senses.

Their fourth form is sentience, mutation and retentivity, *i.e.* perception, movement and retention related to reception. As explained earlier in respect of Bhūtas, this is the inherent quality of the senses (see III.44). The three Guṇas are the material cause of I-sense also.

Being instruments for experience of pleasure and pain, and for attainment of salvation, the senses serve as objects of Self. This objectiveness is the fifth form of the organs.

For the same reasons the organs of action and the Prāṇas have five such forms.

When the various forms of the senses are mastered, complete control over the senses and their causes is attained. Mastery over the five forms means ability to create at will organs of one's choice, of both superior and inferior types.

———

ततो मनोजवित्वं विकरणभावः प्रधानजयश्च ॥ ४८ ॥

भाष्यम्—कायस्यानुत्तमो गतिलाभो मनोजवित्वं, विदेहानामिन्द्रियाणामभिप्रेतदेशकालविषयापेक्षो वृत्तिलाभो विकरणभावः, सर्वप्रकृतिविकारवशित्वं

प्रधानजय इति। एतास्तिस्रः सिद्धयो मधुप्रतीका उच्यन्ते, एताश्च करणपञ्चक-रूपजयादधिगम्यन्ते ॥ ४८ ॥

**Thence Come Powers Of Rapid Movement As Of The Mind, Action Of Organs Independent Of The Body And Mastery Over Pradhāna, The Primordial Cause. 48.**

Speed as of the mind means that the body acquires the best possible speed of movement. Action of organs, independent of the body, means their action (without the necessity of the presence of the body), at any desired place, or time, or on any object. Mastery over the primordial cause means subjugation of the constituent causes and their modifications. These three attainments are called Madhu-pratīka. These arise from the subjugation of the five forms of organs (1).

(1) The other associated result of the mastery over the senses is fleetness of the body as of the mind, derived from the ability to make up instantaneously an organ at any place by converting the power of the all-pervading mind. It also enables the organs to function independently of the body. Power over the primordial cause is the ultimate limit of the power of action.

---

सत्त्वपुरुषान्यताख्यातिमात्रस्य सर्वभावाधिष्ठातृत्वं सर्वज्ञातृत्वं च ॥ ४९ ॥

भाष्यम्—निर्धूतरजस्तमोमलस्य बुद्धिसत्त्वस्य परे वैशारद्ये परस्यां वशीकार-संज्ञायां वर्त्तमानस्य सत्त्वपुरुषान्यताख्यातिमात्ररूपप्रतिष्ठस्य सर्वभावाधिष्ठातृत्वं, सर्वात्मानो गुणा व्यवसायव्यवसेयात्मकाः स्वामिनं क्षेत्रज्ञं प्रत्यशेषदृश्यात्मत्वेनोप-तिष्ठन्त इत्यर्थः। सर्वज्ञातृत्वं सर्वात्मनां गुणानां शान्तोदिताव्यपदेश्यधर्मत्वेन व्यवस्थितानामक्रमोपारूढं विवेकजं ज्ञानमित्यर्थः। इत्येषा विशोका नाम सिद्धिः, यां प्राप्य योगी सर्वज्ञः क्षीणक्लेशबन्धनो वशी विहरति ॥ ४९ ॥

### To One Established In The Discernment Between Buddhi And Puruṣa Come Supremacy Over All Beings And Omniscience. 49.

When Buddhi-sattva, freed from the taint of Rajas and Tamas, attains perfection and becomes transparently clear, in that extreme Vaśīkāra-saṁjñā state, the Yogin's mind established in the knowledge of the distinction between Buddhi-sattva and Puruṣa, acquires power over all phases of existence (1), *i.e.* all objective and subjective forms of the Guṇas appear before his mind's eye in an infinite variety. Omniscience means simultaneous knowledge of mutations of all-pervading Guṇas in their past, present and future states of existence and it is called Vivekaja-jñāna. This attainment is called Viśokā and on acquiring this, the Yogin becomes all-knowing and free from all afflictions.

(1) Having spoken first of attainments in knowledge and then of attainments in respect of action, the commentator states how either kind of attainment can be fully developed.

The Yogin whose mind is full of discriminative knowledge, becomes omniscient and omnipotent. Omniscience implies simultaneous knowledge of all past, present and future characteristics of all things. Supremacy over all beings implies contact with all phases of things, they being knowable all at the same time. As the Seer coming into contact with Buddhi as an object, brings it under his control, so by establishing contact with the basic constituent he brings everything under him. It is said in the Śruti in this connection : "When Puruṣa is realised, omniscience is acquired."

———

तद्वैराग्यादपि दोषवीजक्षये कैवल्यम् ॥ ५० ॥

भाष्यम्—यदास्यैवं भवति क्लेशकर्मक्षये सत्त्वस्यायं विवेकप्रत्ययो धर्मः, सत्त्वं च हेयपक्षे न्यस्तं पुरुषश्चापरिणामी शुद्धोऽन्यः सत्त्वादिति। एवमस्य ततो विरज्यमानस्य यानि क्लेशवीजानि दग्धशालिवीजकल्पान्यप्रसवसमर्थानि तानि

सह मनसा प्रत्यस्तं गच्छन्ति। तेषु प्रलीनेषु पुरुषः पुनरिदं तापत्रयं न भुङ्क्ते। तदैतेषां गुणानां मनसि कर्मक्लेशविपाकस्वरूपेणाभिव्यक्तानां चरितार्थानां प्रति-प्रसवे पुरुषस्यात्यन्तिको गुणवियोगः कैवल्यं, तदा स्वरूपप्रतिष्ठा चितिशक्तिरेव पुरुष इति ॥ ५० ।'

### By Renunciation Of That (Viśokā Attainment) Even, Comes Liberation On Account Of The Destruction Of The Seeds Of Evil. 50.

On the attenuation of afflictions and actions arising out of them, the Yogin realises that discriminative knowledge is but a characteristic of Buddhi, and that Buddhi-sattva is one among the objects to be discarded and that Puruṣa is immutable, pure and different from Sattva Guṇa. On the attainment of such enlightenment the Yogin begins to lose his desire for Buddhi-sattva, and the seeds of affliction, rendered unproductive like roasted seeds, die out with his mind. When they (the seeds of affliction) totally disappear Puruṣa does not suffer from the threefold sorrow. Then the Guṇas, whose mutations exist in the mind as Kleśas and resultant actions, having fulfilled their purpose, recede to the unmanifest state and thus bring about their complete separation from Puruṣa. This is liberation. In that state Puruṣa is nothing but metemperic Consciousness established in Itself (1).

(1) It has been explained before that when afflictive actions are completely attenuated by the acquisition of discriminative enlightenment, they become unproductive as roasted seeds. Then dawns the idea that discrimination being a characteristic of Buddhi is to be forsaken along with Buddhi itself; the Yogin attains such enlightenment in the form of supreme renunciation and feels the desire to forsake everything. Thence are abandoned discrimination, the attainments acquired by discriminative knowledge and Buddhi where they dwell. Then Buddhi merges into the unmanifest and consequently contact between the Guṇas and Puruṣa is completely severed. That is the state of liberation of Puruṣa.

When the powers of omnipotence and omniscience are acquired the Yogin becomes like almighty Īśvara. That is the highest state of Buddhi.

Puruṣa with such adjuncts, *i.e.* such adjuncts and their Seer combined, is called Mahān Ātmā or the Great Self. The adjuncts by themselves are also called Mahat-tattva. In this state Yogins live in some tangible sphere, as manifested adjuncts can only exist in a manifested world.

The state immediately higher than this is that of liberation. In it the mind ceases to be operative and hence all knowledge like omniscience etc. disappear. It is beyond the manifested world and has been described in the Upaniṣads as unseen, unusable, unperceivable and unmanifest (quiescent) state. To abide in the state beyond supernormal powers and omniscience, in which the Self remains alone is liberation.

———

स्थान्युपनिमन्त्रणे सङ्गस्मयाकरणं पुनरनिष्टप्रसङ्गात् ॥ ५१ ॥

भाष्यम्—चत्वारः खल्वमी योगिनः—प्रथमकल्पिकः, मधुभूमिकः, प्रज्ञाज्योतिः, अतिक्रान्तभावनीयश्चेति। तत्राभ्यासी प्रवृत्तमात्रज्योतिः प्रथमः। ऋतम्भरप्रज्ञो द्वितीयः। भूतेन्द्रियजयी तृतीयः सर्वेषु भावितेषु भावनीयेषु कृतरक्षाबन्धः कृतकर्त्तव्यसाधनादिमान्। चतुर्थो यस्त्वतिक्रान्तभावनीयस्तस्य चित्तप्रतिसर्ग एकोऽर्थः, सप्तविधास्य प्रान्तभूमिप्रज्ञा। तत्र मधुमतीं भूमिं साक्षात्कुर्वतो ब्राह्मणस्य स्थानिनो देवाः सत्त्वशुद्धिमनुपश्यन्तः स्थानैरुपनिमन्त्रयन्ते, भोरिह आस्यतामिह रम्यतां, कमनीयोऽयं भोगः, कमनीयेयं कन्या, रसायनमिदं जरामृत्युं बाधते, वैहायसमिदं यानम्, अमी कल्पद्रुमाः, पुण्या मन्दाकिनी, सिद्धा महर्षयः, उत्तमा अनुकूला अप्सरसः, दिव्ये श्रोत्रचक्षुषी, वज्रोपमः कायः, स्वगुणैः सर्वमिदमुपार्जितमायुष्मता, प्रतिपद्यतामिदमक्षयमजरममरस्थानं देवानां प्रियमिति।

एवमभिधीयमानः सङ्गदोषान् भावयेत्। घोरेषु संसाराङ्गारेषु पच्यमानेन मया जननमरणान्धकारे विपरिवर्त्तमानेन कथञ्चिदासादितः क्लेशतिमिरविनाशो योगप्रदीपः, तस्य चैते तृष्णायोनयो विषयवायवः प्रतिपक्षाः, स खल्वहं लब्धालोकः कथमनया विषयमृगतृष्णाया वञ्चितस्तस्यैव पुनः प्रदीप्तस्य संसाराग्नेरात्मानमिन्धनीकुर्य्यामिति। स्वस्ति वः स्वप्नोपमेभ्यः कृपणजनप्रार्थनीयेभ्यो विषयेभ्य इत्येवन्निश्चितमतिः समाधिं भावयेत्। सङ्गमकृत्वा स्मयमपि न कुर्य्यादेवमहं देवानामपि प्रार्थनीय इति। स्मयादयं सुस्थितंमन्यतया मृत्युना केशेषु गृहीतमिवात्मानं न भावयिष्यति, तथा चास्य छिद्रान्तरप्रेक्षी नित्यं यत्नोपचर्यः प्रमादो लब्धविवरः क्लेशानुत्तम्भयिष्यति, ततः पुनरनिष्टप्रसङ्गः। एवमस्य

सङ्गस्मयावकुर्वतो भावितोऽर्थो दृढीभविष्यति, भावनीयश्चार्थोऽभिमुखीभविष्यतीति ॥ ५१ ॥

**When Invited By The Celestial Beings That Invitation Should Not Be Accepted Nor Should It Cause Vanity Because It Involves Possibility Of Undesirable Consequences. 51.**

Yogins are of four classes—(1) Prathama-kalpika, (2) Madhu-bhūmika, (3) Prajñā-jyoti and (4) Atikrānta-bhāvanīya. Of these the first are those who are engaged in devotional practices and in whom the supernormal powers of perception are just dawning. The second are those who have got Ṛtambhara wisdom. The third are those who have mastered the Bhūtas and the organs, who retain all those powers which are acquired and are devoutly engaged in the quest of further attainments. The fourth are those who have gone beyond acquisition of attainments and whose only remaining objective is elimination of the action of the mind. Theirs is the sevenfold ultimate insight.

The celestial beings residing in high regions noticing the purity of the intellect of those who have attained unalloyed truth Madhumatī (Madhu-bhūmika stage), try to invite them by tempting them with enjoyments available in their regions in the following manner : 'Oh Great Soul, come and sit here and enjoy yourself. It is lovely here. Here is a lovely lady. This elixir prevents death and decay. Here is a vehicle which can take you to the skies. The tree which fulfils all wishes is here. This is the holy river Mandākinī and here are the perfected Siddhas and the great seers. Beautiful and obedient nymphs, supernormal eyes and ears, body of adamantine strength, are all here. You have earned all these by your virtues. Come, take all these. All this is everlasting, indestructible, undying and loved by the deities.'

Accosted in this way, he should ponder thus on the danger of coming in contact with them : 'Baked in the fierce flames of births, and tossed between life and death, I have somehow obtained the light of Yoga which destroys the darkness of afflictions, but this thirstful atmosphere of attachment is antagonistic to that light. Having got that light why should I again be deluded by this mirage of pleasure and make myself a fuel of that burning fire of the cycle of births? Oh, ye pitiable, dreamy seekers of pleasures, may you be happy.' With this firm conviction in his mind, the Yogin should practise concentration. Not having formed any attachment, let him not also feel a sense of gratification that he is coveted by the celestial beings. Through self-gratification a false sense of security arises and man forgets that death has got him by the hair. In that way delusion would creep into the mind, as it is ever watchful for a chance, and strengthen the afflictions and make recurrence of mischief possible.

By avoiding contact with others and the feeling of pride in the above manner, the Yogin becomes firm in his contemplation which would lead him eventually to the object contemplated upon.

---

क्षणतत्क्रमयोः संयमाद्विवेकजं ज्ञानम् ॥ ५२ ॥

भाष्यम्—यथापकर्षपर्यन्तं द्रव्यं परमाणुरेवं परमापकर्षपर्यन्तः कालः क्षणः। यावता वा समयेन चलितः परमाणुः पूर्वदेशं जह्यादुत्तरदेशमुपसम्पद्येत स कालः क्षणः, तत्प्रवाहाविच्छेदस्तु क्रमः। क्षणतत्क्रमयोर्नास्ति वस्तुसमाहार इति बुद्धिसमाहारो मुहूर्त्ताहोरात्रादयः। स खल्वयं कालो वस्तुशून्यो बुद्धिनिर्माणः शब्दज्ञानानुपाती लौकिकानां व्युत्थितदर्शनानां वस्तुस्वरूप इवावभासते। क्षणस्तु वस्तुपतितः क्रमावलम्बी, क्रमश्च क्षणानन्तर्यात्मा, तं कालविदः काल इत्याचक्षते योगिनः। न च द्वौ क्षणौ सह भवतः, क्रमश्च न द्वयोः सहभुवोरसम्भवात्, पूर्वस्मादुत्तरभाविनो यदानन्तर्यं क्षणस्य स क्रमः।

तस्माद् वर्त्तमान एवैकः क्षणो न पूर्वोत्तरक्षणाः सन्तीति, तस्मान्नास्ति तत्समाहारः। ये तु भूतभाविनः क्षणास्ते परिणामान्विता व्याख्येयाः। तेनैकेन क्षणेन कृत्स्नो लोकः परिणाममनुभवति, तत्क्षणोपारूढ़ाः खल्वमी धर्माः। तयोः क्षणतत्क्रमयोः संयमात्तयोः साक्षात्करणम्। ततश्च विवेकजं ज्ञानं प्रादुर्भवति ॥५२॥

**Differentiating Knowledge Of The Self And The Non-Self Comes From Practising Saṁyama On Moment And Its Sequence. 52.**

As the minimal object is an atom (or minutest particle) (1), so minimal time is a moment. In other words, the time taken by an atom in motion in leaving one point in space and reaching the adjacent point, is a moment. The continuous flow of these is Krama or sequence. In such sequence there is no real aggregate of moments. Muhūrta (a measure of time covering 48 minutes), day, night, etc. are all aggregates formed by mental conception. Time (2) is not a substantive reality but only a mental concept, which comes into the mind as a verbal knowledge, but to an ordinary person it might appear as something real. Moment, however, is relative to objects and rests upon sequence because sequence is succession of moments, which is called by Yogins with knowledge of time as time (3). Two moments are never present at the same time. There can be no succession of two co-existing moments, which is impossible. When a later moment succeeds an earlier one without interruption it is called a sequence.

For that reason (what we call) the present is but a single moment, and an earlier or a later moment does not exist. Thus there is no combination of the past, present and future. Those which are past and future are to be explained as inherent in the mutations, *i.e.* past and future are only a general—quiescent and unmanifest—conception of mutability with the result that we consider the absent mutations as occurrences in either past or future moments. In that one present moment the whole universe is experiencing a change as all those characteristics—past, present and future—exist in that one present moment. By practising Saṁyama on moment and its sequence, knowledge is acquired of their characteristics, and from that flows knowledge of discernment.

(1) It has been said before that Tanmātras or the atoms of sound etc. are their subtlest form. Any further discrimination will altogether eliminate the atom from the field of perception, *i.e.* by becoming subtler and subtler it reaches a point where its varieties disappear and it remains only as a particle or atom of cognition of that property. Thus parts of an atom are not comprehensible. As an atom is the minutest part of space or of the property of a thing, so is a moment the minutest particle of time. A moment is an atom of time ; the period in which the minutest mutation is cognised by a Yogin is a moment. The commentator, by way of illustration, has said that the time in which the movement of an atom becomes noticeable is a moment. Since part of an atom is not conceivable, when an atom leaves the whole of the space occupied by it and moves on to occupy the next space, then its mutation in the form of motion becomes noticeable ; the time taken is called the moment. As in the cognition of an atom there is an indistinct conception of space, so an indistinct conception of space exists in its mutations also.

Whether an atom moves fast or slow, when a concept of its change of place arises, that would be a moment. Until an atom moves out of its occupied place, its mutation would not be noticeable. Thus when it moves fast the moments would appear to be contiguous, while when it moves slowly the moments would appear at intervals with break. The time period in a moment will, however, in both cases reveal a single mutation. Knowledge of Tanmātra consists of a series of perceptions each lasting for a moment. The succession of moments, *i.e.* their flow without a break, is called its sequence.

It must be remembered that even this description of an atom is a semantic concept like the definition of a point in geometry.

(2) Here the commentator has said the last word on time. We say that everything exists or will exist in time, but it is not correct to say that there is such a thing as time, because it will give rise to the question : 'Wherein does time exist ?' That which is absent is either past or future. Absent means non-existent. Therefore, past or future is non-

existent. But we are apt to say that the threefold time (past, present and future) exists. That is only a semantic concept of a non-existent thing. To treat an unreal thing as real with the help of words is called Vikalpa or vague notion of an unreality. Time is such a thing. Two moments do not exist at the same time. Therefore, flow of moments collected together in thought, *i.e.* built up in imagination, is called time. When we say 'Time exists', it implies 'Time exists in time', which is really a contradiction in terms. When we say 'Ram exists' we mean that Ram is present, but what does the expression 'Time exists' imply? That would convey nothing but a semantic concept, because time has no basic substratum.

Where there is nothing we call it void or empty space, but as without a thing there can be no conception of 'where', therefore, 'where' without a thing, *i.e.* void, is nothing. Similarly, unreal time expressed in words is a semantic concept only implying the idea of container. Without the help of words, time cannot be conceived. Ordinarily, however, time is taken as a real object. To Yogins engaged in meditation beyond the confusion of words and objects denoted by them, there is no such thing as time.

(3) Yogins do not call time an entity but only a succession of moments. Moments to them are periods wherein mutations of real objects are perceived.

A thing or an object is what exists. Moment is not a thing but the container of a thing which exists. Past or future cannot therefore be the containers of things as the latter do not exist.

Past and future moments are containers of non-existent things, *i.e.* they are unreal, whereas the present is the container of a thing which exists, that is the difference. The question might be asked in this connection: 'As the past and future things are said to exist, why their containers, *viz.* the past and the future, be regarded as containers of unreal things?' In reply it can be said that when we use the term 'exists' we imply that it is present, and therefore it is contained in the present moment. Thus only the present is the container of things, *i.e.* a real container, in which everything is undergoing mutation. What we cannot see with our limited power of perception, we call past or future. What is past or future? It is only not being cognised as present. To a person whose power of cognition is not restricted there is nothing past or future, everything is present. Therefore only the present is a reality or the real container of things. By practising Saṁyama on (that present) moment, *i.e.* on the characteristic of an object mutating in that moment and on its sequence, *i.e.* on the flow of mutations that takes place every moment, discriminative knowledge is acquired. When the minutest mutations in things and the flow thereof are known, the subtlest power of discrimination is attained. What has been spoken of in the next aphorism is discriminative knowledge, and is the same as omniscience referred to in Sūtra 49 ante.*

———

भाष्यम्—तस्य विषयविशेष उपक्षिप्यते—

जातिलक्षणदेशैरन्यतानवच्छेदात्तुल्ययोस्ततः प्रतिपत्तिः ॥ ५३ ॥

तुल्ययोः देशलक्षणसारूप्ये जातिभेदोऽन्यताया हेतुः, गौरियं वड़वेयमिति। तुल्यदेशजातीयत्वे लक्षणमन्यत्वकरं, कालाक्षी गौः स्वस्तिमती गौरिति। द्वयोरामलकयोर्जातिलक्षणसारूप्याद्देशभेदोऽन्यत्वकरः—इदं पूर्वमिदमुत्तरमिति। यदा तु पूर्वमामलकमन्यव्यग्रस्य ज्ञातुरुत्तरदेश उपावर्त्यते तदा तुल्यदेशत्वे पूर्वमेतदुत्तरमेतदिति प्रविभागानुपपत्तिः असन्दिग्धेन च तत्त्वज्ञानेन भवितव्यम्, इत्यत इदमुक्तं ततः प्रतिपत्तिः विवेकजज्ञानादिति। कथं, पूर्वामलकसहक्षणो देश उत्तरामलकसहक्षणादेशाद्‌ भिन्नः। ते चामलके स्वदेशक्षणानुभवभिन्ने अन्यदेशक्षणानुभवस्तु तयोरन्यत्वे हेतुरिति। एतेन दृष्टान्तेन परमाणोस्तुल्यजातिलक्षणदेशस्य पूर्वपरमाणुदेशसहक्षणसाक्षात्करणादुत्तरस्य परमाणोस्तद्देशानुपपत्तावुत्तरस्य तद्देशानुभवो भिन्नः सहक्षणभेदात् तयोरीश्वरस्य योगिनोऽन्यत्वप्रत्ययो भवतीति। अपरे तु वर्णयन्ति येऽन्त्या विशेषास्तेऽन्यताप्रत्ययं कुर्वन्तीति। तत्रापि देशलक्षणभेदो मूर्त्ति-व्यवधि-जातिभेदश्चान्यत्वहेतुः। क्षणभेदस्तु योगिबुद्धिगम्य एवेति, अत उक्तं, 'मूर्त्तिव्यवधिजातिभेदाभावान्नास्ति मूलपृथक्त्वम्' इति वार्षगण्यः ॥ ५३ ॥

The particular aspects of things which are the object of this knowledge of discernment are being mentioned—

*It should be noted that the knowledge of discernment resulting in omniscience, mentioned in this and subsequent Sūtras, is an attainment and though of the highest order, is secondary to the discriminative knowledge of Sūtra 26, Book II, which directly leads to and is indispensable for obtaining liberation.

**When Species, Temporal Character And Position Of Two Different Things Being Indiscernible They Look Alike, They Can Be Differentiated Thereby (By This Knowledge)** (1). **53.**

Two similar things having common position and temporal character may differ by virtue of their species, *e.g.* a cow and a mare. Position and species being the same, distinguishing marks might denote difference, *e.g.* a black-eyed cow and an auspicious cow. Between the two myrobalans which are the same in species and look, their position distinguishes them—one being put first and the other behind it. To an ordinary observer if the position is reversed while he is not looking, he cannot detect the difference, but the power (to differentiate) comes through certain and correct knowledge. That is why it has been said in the Sūtra that from knowledge of discernment comes proficiency in perceiving differences. How ? The space correlated to the moment of time of the anterior myrobalan is different from the space correlated to the moment of time of the posterior one. Therefore, the two fruits are separate in the sequential notion of the movements in time correlated to their distinct positions in space. The sequential notion of space correlated to another moment of time is the means of their distinction. From this (gross) illustration it is understood that although the species, time and position of two atoms might be the same, yet by discovering the correlation of every atomic position in space to a different moment of time, the sequential notion of such a position in space can be known to be different by an advanced Yogin. Others (Vaiśeṣikas) say that it is the ultimate particulars which cause the notion of the distinction. In their opinion also, difference in position and time as well as difference in perceivability, in location (2) and in species, are responsible for distinctness. That change in moment is the ultimate difference and that is known only to Yogins. That is why it has been said by Vārṣagaṇya : "Since there is no diversity in characteristics, shape and species in the primal cause there is no distinction or perceptible heterogeneity therein."

(1) Ordinarily many things look alike, and we cannot notice their difference. Take two newly minted coins, placed one after the other. If they are changed in position we cannot say which is which, but if they are put under the microscope, we shall be able to discover some difference which will enable us to say which is the first and which is the second. Knowledge of discernment is like that. Subtlest difference is noticed by it. The change that takes place in a moment is the subtlest change ; there is nothing subtler than that. This knowledge is the knowledge of that change.

Knowledge of difference arises in three ways—through distinction in species, through distinction in temporal characters and through distinction in position. If there are two things in which such distinctions are not noticeable, then ordinarily their difference would not be known, but through discerning knowledge that is known.

Take two balls of gold, one made earlier and the other later. Change their places and no man with ordinary knowledge can say which was made first and which later, because there is no distinction in their species, temporal character or position. Both are of the same species, have the same temporal character and are equally placed. Through this discerning knowledge their difference would, however, be known, because the one made earlier has undergone a longer sequence of mutations. By perceiving it the Yogin can determine which is the first and which is the second. The commentator has explained this with illustration. Momentary change correlated to point of space, implies the change which a thing has undergone in a particular place as long as it was there.

A Yogin does not, of course, want to know the difference between the myrobalans or the balls of gold, but by realising the subtle difference between atoms he acquires knowledge of the Tattvas or of the past and the future. This is what has been stated in the next aphorism.

(2) According to other schools of thought, the ultimate particulars or the distinguishing characteristics give rise to a knowledge of distinction. This view also points to the three kinds of differentiating causes because its protagonists also maintain that the final differentiating particulars are difference in position, difference in characteristics, difference in shape and difference in species. 'Mūrti', according to commentators on Vyāsa's commentary, is collocation or figure, but it would be more appropriate to

say that it relates to the special features or characteristics as sound etc. Vyavadhi = shape. The peculiar colour of a brick which is discernible to the eye and which cannot be completely expressed in words, is its Mūrti or special characteristic, and its shape as comprehensible by the senses, is its Vyavadhi.

The distinction in characteristic, shape, etc. is comprehensible by ordinary intelligence but distinction from the consideration of moments (atoms of time) is only perceived by the intellect of a Yogin. There is no further distinction beyond the moment which is the ultimate distinction. That is why Vārṣagaṇya has said : "In the primal cause there is no such difference (or perceptible heterogeneity), because there is no distinction at that stage," *i.e.* in the unmanifest state, or the ultimate state of the three Guṇas or constituent principles, there is no diversity. In the unmanifest state when the Guṇas are in equilibrium, all distinctions disappear. Or in other words, the change that takes place every moment is the minutest distinction. The perception of that momentary change is the subtlest form of cognition. Things subtler than these cannot be perceived, they are thus unmanifest. Since an unmanifest thing cannot be perceived, there is no chance of perceiving any difference therein. Therefore in the unmanifest state, which is at the root of things, no difference is imaginable.

———

तारकं सर्वविषयं सर्वथाविषयमक्रमं चेति विवेकजं ज्ञानम् ॥ ५४ ॥

भाष्यम्—तारकमिति स्वप्रतिभोत्थमनौपदेशिकमित्यर्थः, सर्वविषयं नास्य किञ्चिदविषयीभूतमित्यर्थः। सर्वथाविषयमतीतानागतप्रत्युत्पन्नं सर्वं पर्यायैः सर्वथा जानातीत्यर्थः, अक्रममिति एकक्षणोपारूढं सर्वं सर्वथा गृह्णातीत्यर्थः। एतद्विवेकजं ज्ञानं परिपूर्णमस्यैवांशो योगप्रदीपः, मधुमतीं भूमिमुपादाय यावदस्य परिसमाप्तिरिति ॥ ५४ ॥

**Knowledge Of Discernment Is Tāraka Or Intuitional, Is Comprehensive Of All Things And Of All Times And Has No Sequence. 54.**

Tāraka means that the knowledge comes from one's inborn faculty and does not depend on instruction from others. 'All-comprehensive' implies that nothing is outside its scope. 'Of all times' means that all things past, present and future with all their respective features, are within its scope. 'Has no sequence' means that all things appear as presented to the intellect at the same moment. This discerning knowledge is complete. Yoga-pradīpa or the lamp of Yoga (1) is a part thereof and it extends from Madhumatī or Ṛtambharā Prajñā to the seven kinds of ultimate knowledge.

(1) Lamp of Yoga means Yoga full of light of knowledge, which is Samprajñāta-yoga or secondary discriminative knowledge. Discriminative enlightenment is also Samprajñāta-yoga but it is the highest or supreme discriminative knowledge (Parama-prasaṁkhyāna). In this connection commentaries on I.2 should be seen. Through discriminative knowledge afflictions become like roasted seeds, while discriminative enlightenment brings about a complete cessation of the activities of the mind. Discriminative knowledge is fulfilment of knowledge. The light of Yoga is of its first part. Ṛtambharā Prajñā is the secondary discriminative knowledge. After attainment of Madhumatī stage, and until the mind is dissolved, the mind remains full of that knowledge.

———

भाष्यम्—प्राप्तविवेकजज्ञानस्याप्राप्तविवेकजज्ञानस्य वा—

सत्त्वपुरुषयोः शुद्धिसाम्ये कैवल्यमिति ॥ ५५ ॥

यदा निर्धूतरजस्तमोमलं बुद्धिसत्त्वं पुरुषस्यान्यताप्रत्ययमात्राधिकारं दग्धक्लेशवीजं भवति तदा पुरुषस्य शुद्धिसारूप्यमिवापन्नं भवति। तदा पुरुषस्योपचरितभोगाभावः शुद्धिः। एतस्यामवस्थायां कैवल्यं भवतीश्वरस्यानीश्वरस्य वा विवेकजज्ञानभागिन इतरस्य वा। न हि दग्धक्लेशवीजस्य ज्ञाने पुनरपेक्षा काचिदस्ति, सत्त्वशुद्धिद्वारेणैतत्समाधिजमैश्वर्यञ्च ज्ञानञ्चोपक्रान्तम्। परमार्थतस्तु ज्ञानाददर्शनं निवर्त्तते। तस्मिन्निवृत्ते न सन्त्युत्तरे क्लेशाः। क्लेशाभावात्कर्मविपाकाभावः, चरिताधिकाराश्चैतस्यामवस्थायां गुणा न पुरुषस्य पुनर्दृश्यत्वेनो-

पतिष्ठन्ते, तत्पुरुषस्य कैवल्यं, तदा पुरुषः स्वरूपमात्रज्योतिरमलः केवली भवति ॥ ५५ ॥

इति श्रीपातञ्जले सांख्यप्रवचने वैयासिके विभूतिपादस्तृतीयः ।

Irrespective of whether this secondary discriminative discernment is acquired or not—

**When Equality Is Established Between Buddhi-Sattva And Puruṣa In Their Purity, Liberation Takes Place (1). 55.**

When Buddhi-sattva being freed of all Rajas and Tamas impurities, is occupied with only discriminative discernment of Puruṣa and thus comes to acquire the state where seeds of affliction become roasted, then it becomes like Puruṣa on account of its purity. The absence of any imputation of experience of pleasure or pain is purity of Puruṣa. In this condition, whether omnipotent or not, whether endowed with secondary discriminative knowledge or not, one becomes liberated. When the seed of affliction is burnt out, nothing else is needed for the fulfilment of the ultimate spiritual knowledge. It has been stated before that various powers and knowledge are attainable through concentration. Speaking from the point of view of spiritual advancement one can say (2) that through discriminative discernment, the process of misapprehension is stopped, and after that, afflictions do not arise in future. There would then be no fruition of actions for want of afflictions. In that state, the Guṇas having fulfilled their objective, no longer present themselves for being witnessed by Puruṣa. That is known as the state of liberation of Puruṣa. Then Puruṣa shining in His own light becomes free from dross and all contacts.

(Here concludes the chapter on Supernormal Powers being the third part of the comments of Vyāsa known as Sāṁkhya-pravachana on the Yoga-philosophy of Patañjali.)

(1) Discriminative enlightenment leads to liberation but not so the intuitional discriminative knowledge known as Tāraka ; the latter stands in the way of attaining liberation. Thus, without practising the attainment of knowledge of discernment, liberation is attainable. Such knowledge implies both attainment of intuitive knowledge referred to in Sūtra III.54 ante, and discriminative enligtenment dealt with in IV. 26.

When Buddhi-sattva becomes pure as Puruṣa and the two appear alike, it leads to achievement of Kaivalya or liberation. This purity and likeness do not by themselves constitute Kaivalya, but are the cause of its attainment. Buddhi's likeness through purity implies likeness to the purity of Puruṣa. When Chitta is established in the unalloyed knowledge 'I am Puruṣa' then Buddhi or pure I-sense resembles Puruṣa. As Puruṣa is pure and free from all contacts, Buddhi appears to be like that. This is the purity of Buddhi-sattva and its resemblance to Puruṣa. In that state Buddhi-sattva is also completely free from the dross of Rajas and Tamas. That is its purest state. Puruṣa is naturally pure and self-existent, so His purity and alikeness are only imputed and not real. As the sun freed from cloud is called pure, so is the purity of Puruṣa. Impurity of Puruṣa means association with experience. When experience is not ascribed to Puruṣa, He is said to be pure. Puruṣa is said to be unlike Himself when He is identified with the modifications of Buddhi, *i.e.* the fluctuating state of Chitta. When the fluctuations cease, Puruṣa is said to be self-existent. Puruṣa is said to be like Himself when He is in Himself without reference to anything else.

When Buddhi becomes like Puruṣa, it ceases functioning. Therefore in ordinary parlance it has to be said that Puruṣa who was appearing as Buddhi now looks like Himself. That is Kaivalya or liberation. In the state of Kaivalya Puruṣa remains in Himself and the functioning of Buddhi ceases. Therefore on attainment of Kaivalya no change of state takes place in Puruṣa, only Buddhi ceases to function.

(2) Highest spiritual goal is complete cessation of misery. In practices for attainment of spiritual progress, discerning (Tāraka) knowledge and attainment of supernormal powers are not necessary, because complete annihilation of sorrow cannot be effected through supernormal knowledge or powers. Nescience or wrong knowledge is the root cause of afflictions and can be destroyed by discriminative enlightenment only. Then Chitta ceases to function and miseries disappear once and for all. That is the highest spiritual attainment.

———

BOOK IV

# ON THE SELF-IN-ITSELF OR LIBERATION

जन्मौषधिमन्त्रतपःसमाधिजाः सिद्धयः ॥ १ ॥

भाष्यम्—देहान्तरिता जन्मना सिद्धिः, ओषधिभिः—असुरभवनेषु रसायनेनेत्येवमादि, मन्त्रैः—आकाशगमनाणिमादिलाभः, तपसा—संकल्पसिद्धिः कामरूपी यत्र तत्र कामग इत्येवमादि । समाधिजाः सिद्धयो व्याख्याताः ॥ १ ॥

**Supernormal Powers Come With Birth Or Are Attained Through Herbs, Incantations, Austerities Or Concentration. 1.**

Supernormal powers arising at the time of changing the bodily frame show themselves with birth. By herbs, as for example with chemicals in an Asura's (demon's) abode, medicinal powers are acquired. By Mantras or incantations, powers like flying or reducing one's size are attained. By practising Tapas or austerities, power of fulfilment of wishes, *e.g.* going to any wished-for place etc., is acquired. The powers attainable through concentration have been explained before (1).

(1) Some of the supernormal powers mentioned before have been known to have been acquired without Yogic concentration. With some, the powers manifest themselves with birth, *i.e.* with the process of being embodied in a particular way. For example, powers of clairvoyance or of thought-reading have been found to be produced by particular dispositions. These have nothing to do with Yoga. Similarly, as a consequence of being incarnated in a celestial body as a result of virtuous deeds, the supernormal powers associated with such forms also appear.

Herbs also induce supernormal powers. Some in a state of stupor through the application of anaesthetics like chloroform etc. acquire the power of going out of the body. It has also been reported that by the application of hemlock all over the body similar power is acquired. Witches were supposed to practise this method. The commentator has mentioned about the abode of demons but nobody knows where it is, but it is certain that supernormal powers on a small scale can be acquired by the application of drugs. Through competence acquired in a previous birth by constant repetition of Mantras and by consequent well-developed will, insignificant powers like mesmerism etc. may appear in the present life.

Similarly, by practising severe austerities, superior powers can be acquired. On account of intensive will-power developed thereby, changes might take place in the body which would conduce to fructifying the virtuous latent impressions of an antecedent life. This is how supernormal powers can be attained without Yoga. The powers manifested from birth etc. are the result of Karmāśaya or latencies made fruitful or effective through causes like birth, medicine, incantations etc.

———

भाष्यम्—तत्र कायेन्द्रियाणामन्यजातीयपरिणतानाम्—

जात्यन्तरपरिणामः प्रकृत्यापूरात् ॥ २ ॥

पूर्वपरिणामापाय उत्तरपरिणामोपजनस्तेषामपूर्वावयवानुप्रवेशाद् भवति। कायेन्द्रियप्रकृतयश्च स्वं स्वं विकारमनुगृह्णन्त्यापूरेण धर्मादिनिमित्तमपेक्षमाणा इति ॥ २ ॥

Of these, the mutation of body and organs into those of one born in a different species—

**Takes Place Through The Filling In Of Their Innate Nature. 2.**

The destruction of their former state and the appearance of a new one, take place through impenetration of the new constituents. By impenetration of the innate nature of the body and the organs each one of them assumes the form, according to its own type of mutation (1). In this process of impenetration, respective dispositions (of body and the organs) depend upon causes such as pious or impious acts (for their manifestation).

(1) The mind and the organs found in men are of the human mould. Similarly, there are organs which are appropriate to the nature of Devas (in heaven), demons (in hell), animals, etc. In all creatures the nature or mould of all the modifications possible in each of the organs, is inherently present. When there is mutation from one species into another, the mould which is brought into play by the most appropriate cause, impenetrates the new form and shapes the organs accordingly. How that impenetration takes place has been explained in the next Sūtra.

———

निमित्तमप्रयोजकं प्रकृतीनां वरणभेदस्तु ततः क्षेत्रिकवत् ।। ३ ।।

भाष्यम्—न हि धर्मादिनिमित्तं प्रयोजकं प्रकृतीनां भवति, न कार्येण कारणं प्रवर्त्यते इति, कथन्तर्हि, वरणभेदस्तु ततः क्षेत्रिकवद्, यथा क्षेत्रिकः केदारादपाम्पूरणात् केदारान्तरं पिप्लावयिषुः समं निम्नं निम्नतरं वा नापः पाणिनापकर्षति, आवरणं तु आसां भिनत्ति, तस्मिन्भिन्ने स्वयमेवापः केदारान्तरमाप्लावयन्ति, तथा धर्मः प्रकृतीनामावरणमधर्मं भिनत्ति, तस्मिन्भिन्ने स्वयमेव प्रकृतयः स्वं स्वं विकारमाप्लावयन्ति। यथा वा स एव क्षेत्रिकस्तस्मिन्नेव केदारे न प्रभवत्यौदकान् भौमान् वा रसान् धान्यमूलान्यनुप्रवेशयितुं किन्तर्हि मुद्गगवेधुकश्यामाकादीन्ततोऽपकर्षति, अपकृष्टेषु तेषु स्वयमेव रसा धान्यमूलान्यनुप्रविशन्ति, तथा धर्मो निवृत्तिमात्रे कारणमधर्मस्य, शुद्ध्यशुद्ध्योरत्यन्तविरोधात्। न तु प्रकृतिप्रवृत्तौ धर्मो हेतुर्भवतीति। अत्र नन्दीश्वरादय उदाहार्याः। विपर्ययेणाप्यधर्मो धर्मं बाधते, ततश्चाशुद्धिपरिणाम इति, तत्रापि नहुषाजगरादय उदाहार्याः ।। ३ ।।

**Causes Do Not Put The Nature Into Motion, Only The Removal Of Obstacles Takes Place Through Them. This Is Like A Farmer Breaking Down The Barrier To Let The Water Flow (The Hindrances Being Removed By The Causes, The Nature Impenetrates By Itself). 3.**

Causes like virtuous acts etc. do not bring nature into play. Effect never guides the cause. Then how does this happen ? 'Like a farmer breaking down a barrier.' A farmer wanting to fill a plot of land with water does not push the mass of water with his hands, but only effects a breach in the ridge separating it from a plot of land of the same or higher level containing water, when water flows automatically into the other plot ; similarly when a particular trait, *e.g.* piety, pierces the veil of the opposite trait, *i.e.* impiety, enveloping the organs, the innate nature of the body and the organs automatically fills up their appropriate mutations. Or as a farmer cannot make the sap go into the roots of the corn, but only removes the weeds when the sap automatically goes into the roots, so virtue suppresses or overcomes impiety, as virtue and impiety are very much opposed to each other. Virtue is thus not the (direct) cause of bringing about the modification of nature (1). In this respect the case of Nandīśvara has been cited as an example. Thus in an opposite instance impiety overcomes piety and the mutation is due to impiety. Transformation of Nahuṣa into a python is an illustration of this.

(1) As a piece of stone can be said to hold in it innumerable forms, so each of the organs can be said to hold capabilities of innumerable dispositions. As by removing the unwanted excess, a piece of stone can be made to show up any image without any addition, so is the case with the organs. As removing the superfluity is the cause of emergence of the image, so the different dispositions of the organs may be revealed by the removal of the obstacles. Nature reveals itself by its characteristics. When the characteristic hostile to the nature which is to appear is destroyed, that innate nature will impenetrate into the organ and shape it accordingly. For example, clairaudience is the nature or characteristic of the divine sense of hearing, whose nature is hearing from a distance. That cannot be acquired by cultivating the human sense of hearing. When however the human sense of hearing is shut out by following the prescribed form of Saṁyama, divine hearing will manifest itself. Divine hearing is not manufactured thereby, because the cause thereof, *viz.* Saṁyama upon the relationship between the organ of hearing and the Ākāśa, is not its constituent cause. The term 'Dharma' used in the commentary refers to the appropriate cause of manifestation of a parti-

cular capacity inherent in nature, while 'Adharma' means antagonistic causes.

Power of hearing is the cause, and hearing is its effect. Effect does not guide the cause, *i.e.* under the influence of the effect the cause is not guided in producing a result Therefore only practising hearing, no other form of hearing can be developed. Hearing is not the material cause of the power of hearing.

The power of hearing exists and it can be of different types according to the variations of the three Guṇas. If the characteristic of one such variation is suppressed, another will appear in it through impenetration. The human nature is opposed to divine nature. Therefore through the cause, in the shape of suppression of human nature, divine nature manifests itself. To illustrate this point, the author of the Sūtra has cited the case of the farmer letting in water, while the commentator has mentioned the example of removal of weeds. Cause does not guide nature but only defeats the contrary properities, which helps nature to impenetrate and manifest itself.

In the story of Nandīśvara referred to above, he having by his piety and pious acts overcome impiety, his divine nature manifested itself in his present life which changed him into a Deva. Similarly, it is stated in the Purāṇas that King Nahuṣa having suppressed piety through impiety was transformed into a huge python in his life-time.

———

भाष्यम्—यदा तु योगी बहून् कायान् निर्मिमीते तदा किमेकमनस्कास्ते भवन्त्यथानेकमनस्का इति—

निर्माणचित्तान्यस्मितामात्रात् ॥ ४ ॥

अस्मितामात्रं चित्तकारणमुपादाय निर्माणचित्तानि करोति, ततः सचित्तानि भवन्ति ॥ ४ ॥

When the Yogin constructs many bodies, have they only one mind or many minds? (In reply to such a question it is being said—)

**All Created Minds Are Constructed From Pure I-sense. 4.**

Taking pure I-sense (1), which is the cause of the mind, the Yogin makes the minds, from which the constructed bodies are provided with minds.

(1) When the mind of a Yogin becomes barren and unproductive as a burnt seed through acquisition of discriminative knowledge, its natural activities cease for want of latent impressions. Such Yogins, however, give instructions on spiritual knowledge and piety for the benefit of all creatures. As to how that can be possible it is said that this is done by them with self-created minds, *i.e.* by their pure I-sense, in other words, by their the then I-sense free from fluctuations and latencies thereof. These created minds can be terminated at will, that is why they do not collect latencies of nescience and thus do not give rise to bondage.

If, however, the Yogin arrests the action of the mind with a view to perpetual stoppage, no mind is created any more. But if the Yogin arrests the function of the mind for a limited period, then the mind starts functioning again after that period and he can bring a constructed mind into existence.

This suggests how Īśvara with His created mind can, at the end of each cycle of creation, favour those who are qualified for liberation [vide I.24 (4)]. Just as an archer who wants to shoot an arrow over a short distance makes only a small effort, so a Yogin by exercising the required amount of power arrests the working of the mind for a limited period. Yogins can thus shut out the working of their minds either for a limited period, or for ever, when it would not rise again.

———

प्रवृत्तिभेदे प्रयोजकं चित्तमेकमनेकेषाम् ।। ५ ।।

भाष्यम्—बहूनां चित्तानां कथमेकचित्ताभिप्रायपुरःसरा प्रवृत्तिरिति सर्व-चित्तानां प्रयोजकं चित्तमेकं निर्मिमीते ततः प्रवृत्तिभेदः ।। ५ ।।

**One (Principal) Mind Directs The Many Created Minds In The Varietty Of Their Activities. 5.**

How is it that the activities of many minds are regulated by the will of one mind ? The Yogin creates one mind as the director of the many created minds, and this accounts for the difference in their activities (1).

(1) Yogins can construct many created minds at the same time. The question might then arise—how can many minds be directed in the same way ? In reply it has been said that one efficient basic mind might be the director of many minds just as one internal organ (mind) is the director of different Prāṇas and organs. Of course, it is not possible to observe the working of all the minds simultaneously, but the observation appears to be simultaneous just as a whirling lighted stick seems to be a wheel of light, or as hundred lotus leaves are simultaneously pierced. When knowledge of discrimination (Tāraka Jñāna—see III.54) which has no sequence, is acquired, all things are observed simultaneously. In other words, the directing and the many directed minds, as well as their objects, act as though they were simultaneous. In spite of the fact that the activities of the different minds are different, their simultaneous actions are rendered possible in the above manner and there is no overlapping.

To understand how one mind acts on another mind (encased in another body), it has to be borne in mind that the mind is by nature all-pervading (IV.10) and is related to all states ; that is why there is nothing far or near, spatially speaking, with reference to the mind. As the mind of the magician, which functions like the dominant mind, acts on the minds of the spectators and produces mass-hypnotism, so does the dominant created mind of a Yogin act on other secondary created minds.

The ability to produce constructed minds might be acquired through complete control of the organs and the elements or by other means without gaining discriminative knowledge, but the minds so created will have the afflictive latencies. It is thus seen that there are superior and inferior categories of constructed minds. Supernormal powers appearing with birth or gained through herbs or drugs, are of a lower order and in some cases might be counted as a disease. Powers acquired through austerities or incantations performed with the specific object of acquiring supernormal powers, though a little superior to others, produce latencies. But the actions of such devotees will no doubt be more Sāttvika in nature than those of the others.

The constructed mind full of knowledge of discernment and without any afflictive latency, is endowed with the highest efficiency, and only the best form of action in the shape of imparting instructions on virtue and piety is possible with it; different kinds of work like those done by persons who have not acquired discriminative knowledge are not possible with such a mind. Persons who have ceased experiencing pleasure and pain and have reached a state of liberation do not, obviously, assume a created mind for the purpose of enjoyment or for destroying the effects of their past actions.

It should be noted that here mention has been made of one pure I-sense creating different minds directing their respective bodies. The root of mutative ego is pure I-sense which is always unitary. As the different functional limbs of the body are guided by the same mind which appears to be moving about therein (like the whirling light appearing as an unbroken wheel of fire), so many bodies with subordinate minds work under the guidance of a master mind. But the creation of many Jīvas, *i.e.* individuals, is not possible. Therefore, a successful Yogin creating many minds will have but one ego and he will thus be called one Jīva. That different creatures have different egos is a well-established fact. Therefore, there is no room for supposing that one Jīva becomes many or many Jīvas merge into one.

---

तत्र ध्यानजमनाशयम् ॥ ६ ॥

भाष्यम्—पञ्चविधं निर्माणचित्तं जन्मौषधिमन्त्रतपःसमाधिजाः सिद्धय इति। तत्र यदेव ध्यानजं चित्तं तदेवानाशयं तस्यैव नास्त्याशयो रागादिप्रवृत्तिर्नातः पुण्यपापाभिसम्बन्धः, क्षीणक्लेशत्वाद् योगिन इति। इतरेषां तु विद्यते कर्माशयः ॥ ६ ॥

**Of These (Minds With Supernormal Powers) Those Obtained Through Meditation Are Without Any Subliminal Imprints. 6.**

Constructed minds or minds which have attained supernormal powers (1) are of five varieties, *viz.* those obtained with birth, or acquired through drugs, incantations, austerities and concentration. Of these, the mind obtained through meditation is free from afflictive latencies of attachment etc. That is why it has no connection with (worldly) virtue or vice, as afflictions of Yogins are fully attenuated. Others, *i.e.*

those who have acquired supernormal powers in other ways, have the latent impressions of their previous actions still left in their minds.

(1) The constructed minds referred to here, stand for minds which have acquired supernormal powers through incantation etc. The words 'through meditation' used in the Sūtra refer to minds acquired through Yogic concentration. No latent impression of Yoga or concentration can exist in a present mind because the very fact of being born indicates that Samādhi had not been attained in a previous birth. Therefore, a mind perfected through Yoga cannot be produced by impenetration of nature, based on past latent impressions but it appears through the impenetration of a nature not experienced before. Other attainments are derived from impressions of previous actions, but Samādhi cannot be had as a result of any action in a previous birth because if anyone attains Samādhi in his lifetime he will not be born again. When Samādhi is attained, liberation is secured in that birth and there is no further birth with a gross body. Thus acquisition of powers through Yogic concentration is not the outcome of previous latent impressions. In powers acquired through other means, *i.e.* by virtue of birth etc., the person having them exercises those powers involuntarily, whereas in powers acquired through Yogic concentration the case is different as each exercise of power is completely voluntary. In this case the power is employed for the purpose of destroying afflictions such as desires, hatred, etc. and is thus destructive of latent impressions. This attainment, therefore, is not the result of previous impressions, nor does it accumulate impressions. This latter function has been referred to by the commentator.

———

भाष्यम्—यतः—

कर्माशुक्लाकृष्णं योगिनस्त्रिविधमितरेषाम् ॥ ७ ॥

चतुष्पात्खल्वियं कर्मजातिः—कृष्णा शुक्लकृष्णा शुक्ला अशुक्लाकृष्णा चेति। तत्र कृष्णा दुरात्मनां, शुक्लकृष्णा वहिःसाधनसाध्या तत्र परपीड़ानुग्रहद्वारेण कर्माशयप्रचयः, शुक्ला तपःस्वाध्यायध्यानवतां, सा हि केवले मनस्यायतत्वादवहिः-साधनाधीना न परान् पीड़यित्वा भवति, अशुक्लाकृष्णा सन्न्यासिनां क्षीणक्लेशानां

चरमदेहानामिति। तत्राशुक्लं योगिन एव फलसन्न्यासाद्, अकृष्णं चानुपादानात्। इतरेषान्तु भूतानां पूर्वमेव त्रिविधमिति ॥ ७ ॥

Consequently (that is, in view of the fact that a Yogin's mind is free from impressions whereas minds of others are full of them)—

**The Actions Of Yogins Are Neither White Nor Black, Whereas The Actions Of Others Are Of Three Kinds. 7.**

Karma is of four kinds—black, black-and-white, white and neither white nor black. Of these the action of villains is black, while black-and-white Karma is brought about by external means and gathers latencies, as it hurts or benefits others. White Karma is of those who are engaged in austerities, religious study and meditation, which being mental are free from external action and thus not likely to injure or benefit others. The last variety, *viz.* neither white nor black Karma is the last phase in the bodily existence of Yogins who have reduced their afflictions. The action of such Yogins is not white (1) on account of their spirit of renunciation, and not black as they refrain from all prohibited actions. In respect of others, the actions are of the other three varieties.

(1) The actions of villains are black. The actions of ordinary men are black-and-white, because they do good as well as evil. It is difficult to conduct a household without either. Even in the harmless occupation of tilling the soil, lives of insects have to be taken or cattle have to be tortured. In trying to save one's wealth others have to be denied. In these and in many other ways domestic life entails pain to others. At the same time good work can also be done. That is why the action of ordinary men is regarded as black-and-white. The actions of those who are engaged in austerities and meditation alone, or in activities independent of external means, are purely white, because causing pain to others is not inevitable in such cases.

The type of work Yogins do brings about a cessation of the fluctuations of the mind, and consequently, of piety and impiety of the mind.

In other words, the latencies of piety or impiety and coresponding conduct having ceased, actions of the Yogins are neither white nor black. As a matter of fact they not only do not do any evil, but the good deeds they perform are done without any hope of reward and in a spirit of renunciation in order to shut out the spirit of enjoyment. The austerities and religious studies etc. of Yogins are for attenuating afflictions, while their renunciation is not for enjoying the fruits of their labour but for developing a spirit of detachment from pleasure and pain and thus stopping the fluctuations of the mind. On the attainment of discriminative enlightenment, actions of the body cease to be the cause of bondage and being directed towards arrest of the fluctuations of the mind, are neither white nor black.

———

ततस्तद्विपाकानुगुणानामेवाभिव्यक्तिर्वासनानाम् ॥ ८ ॥

भाष्यम्—तत इति त्रिविधात् कर्मणः। तद्विपाकानुगुणानामेवेति यज्जातीयस्य कर्मणो यो विपाकस्तस्यानुगुणा या वासनाः कर्मविपाकमनुशेरते तासामेवाभिव्यक्तिः। न हि दैवं कर्म विपच्यमानं नारकतिर्यङ्मनुष्यवासनाभिव्यक्तिनिमित्तं भवति, किन्तु दैवानुगुणा एवास्य वासना व्यज्यन्ते। नारकतिर्यङ्मनुष्येषु चैवं समानश्चर्चः ॥ ८ ॥

**Thence (From The Other Three Varieties Of Karma) Are Manifested The Subconscious Impressions Appropriate To Their Consequences. 8.**

The word 'thence' refers to the other three varieties of Karma. Tadvipākānuguṇa = the after-effects of an action give rise to subconscious impressions which follow the pattern of feeling produced by the experience arising out of such action. These remain collected in the mind and become manifest in due course. Action of a divine being does not result in bringing out the subconscious impressions of actions performed in previous births in hell or in animal or in human forms, but only brings out the appropriate divine impressions. Such rule applies also to the subconscious impressions of actions performed in hell or in animal or human forms(1).

(1) Latent impressions of actions which produce results are called Karmāśaya ; while the latent impression of feelings arising out of the threefold consequences of action, *e.g.* birth, life-span, and experience of pleasure and pain, is called Vāsanā or subliminal imprint. The comments in Sūtra II.12 should be seen in this connection. Take, for instance, a human being who is born as such as a result of his previous actions ; he goes over his allotted span, enjoying various pains and pleasures. The impressions acquired in the course of his existence as a human being, *i.e.* of the human body and its organs, of its span of life, and of its pleasures and pains go to form the human Vāsanā. The latent impressions of actions performed in that birth are Karmāśaya. Suppose, he acts like a beast in the lifetime as a result of which he is next born a beast. He, however, retains his human Vāsanā. In this way innumerable Vāsanās accumulate in the mind, including some Vāsanās acquired in previous animal births. The animal-like actions in this human life will impel the manifestation of those animal Vāsanās. That is why it has been said that Karmāśaya or latent impression of action manifests the appropriate Vāsanā. The nature of that Vāsanā regulates the birth and enjoyment of pleasure and pain therein. For example, a dog enjoys licking, a man enjoys similar pleasure differently. If on account of good work done in human life, pleasure is vouchsafed in a dog-life that pleasure will be enjoyed in a dog's way. The outcome of Vāsanā is memory. Memory here refers to the memory of births, longevity and experience of pleasure and pain. Memory of birth means memory of the body and of the nature of its organs in a particular species. Memory of longevity refers to the memory of the duration of existence in a particular form. The last named refers to the memory of experience of pleasure and pain in a particular life. Memory is a sort of knowledge or modification of the mind. For each modification there is an associated feeling. Therefore, each memory of experience of pleasure and pain is shaped by a corresponding latent impression of previous experience which is the Vāsanā or subconscious impression of that feeling. Same is the case with longevity-Vāsanā and Vāsanā of particular births.

जातिदेशकालव्यवहितानामप्यानन्तर्यं स्मृतिसंस्कारयोरेकरूपत्वात् ॥ ९ ॥

भाष्यम्—वृषदंशविपाकोदयः स्वव्यञ्जकाञ्जनाभिव्यक्तः स यदि जातिशतेन वा दूरदेशतया वा कल्पशतेन वा व्यवहितः पुनश्च स्वव्यञ्जकाञ्जन एवोदियाद् द्रागित्येव पूर्वानुभूतवृषदंशविपाकाभिसंस्कृता वासना उपादाय व्यज्येत। कस्मात्, यतो व्यवहितानामप्यासां सदृशं कर्माभिव्यञ्जकं निमित्तीभूतमित्यानन्तर्यमेव, कुतश्च, स्मृतिसंस्कारयोरेकरूपत्वात्, यथानुभवास्तथा संस्काराः, ते च कर्मवासनानुरूपाः। यथा च वासनास्तथा स्मृतिः, इति जातिदेशकालव्यवहितेभ्यः संस्कारेभ्यः स्मृतिः स्मृतेश्च पुनः संस्कारा इत्येते स्मृतिसंस्काराः कर्माशयवृत्तिलाभवशात् व्यज्यन्ते। अतश्च व्यवहितानामपि निमित्तनैमित्तिकभावानुच्छेदादानन्तर्यमेव सिद्धमिति ॥ ९ ॥

**On Account Of Similarity Between Memory And Corresponding Latent Impressions, The Subconscious Impressions Of Feelings Appear Simultaneously Even When They Are Separated By Birth, Space And Time (1). 9.**

The fruition of actions involving birth as a cat, when put in motion by the causes of their manifestation, will take place simultaneously even though they might have taken place after an interval of a hundred births, at a great distance or many eons before, because, although separated from each other, all actions of the same nature involving birth as a cat will be set in motion. Their simultaneous appearance happens on account of affinity between memory and latent impressions. As the feelings are, so are the latent impressions. These again correspond to the subconscious impressions of Karma-vāsanā. And as the subconscious impression of the feeling produced by an action is, so is its memory. Thus from latent impressions, though separated by births, space and time, memory arises and from such memory again arise latent impressions. That is how memory and impressions manifest themselves, being brought into play by Karmāśaya or latent impressions of actions. Thus even though separated by births, there is sequential non-interruption because there is no break in the relation of cause and effect.

(1) As the impression of a feeling experienced long ago at a far off place, emerges in the mind at once when there is an exciting cause, so does Vāsanā. Even though much time might have elapsed since the collection of a latent impression, its recollection does not take time at all but rises immediately. Effort to recollect might take time but when the memory comes, it comes at once. The intervening impressions do not cause any intervention in the memory. This has been explained by the commentator with the help of an illustration. For example, in the case of intervention of births in different species one is born as a man and then, on account of evil deeds done, he is born as an animal a hundred times, and then he is born again as a man. In spite of the intervention of a hundred animal births, the human Vāsanā will come up to the surface when he is born a man. The same rule applies in the case of intervention of space and time. The reason for this is the affinity between latency and memory. As the latency is, so is the memory. Memory is the re-cognition of the latent impression. As memory is only cognitive transformation of latent impression, there cannot be any gap between the two.

The manifestation of Vāsanā is caused by Karmāśaya. From that arises clear memory. Karmāśaya is the unfailing cause of memory. Thus from latency arises memory, and from memory latency is formed, and so the cycle goes on.

———

तासामनादित्वं चाशिषो नित्यत्वात् ॥ १० ॥

भाष्यम्—तासां वासनानामाशिषो नित्यत्वादनादित्वम्। येयमात्माशीर्मा न भूवं भूयासमिति सर्वस्य दृश्यते सा न स्वाभाविकी, कस्मात्, जातमात्रस्य जन्तोरननुभूतमरणधर्मकस्य द्वेषदुःखानुस्मृतिनिमित्तो मरणत्रासः कथं भवेत्? न च स्वाभाविकं वस्तु निमित्तमुपादत्ते तस्मादनादिवासनानुविद्धमिदं चित्तं निमित्तवशात् काश्चिदेव वासनाः प्रतिलभ्य पुरुषस्य भोगायोपावर्त्तत इति।

घटप्रासादप्रदीपकल्पं संकोचविकाशि चित्तं शरीरपरिमाणाकारमात्रमित्यपरे प्रतिपन्नाः, तथा चान्तराभावः संसारश्च युक्त इति। वृत्तिरेवास्य विभूनः संकोच-

विकाशिनी इत्याचार्यः। तच्च धर्मादिनिमित्तापेक्षम्। निमित्तं च द्विविधं वाह्यमाध्यात्मिकं च, शरीरादिसाधनापेक्षं वाह्यं स्तुतिदानाभिवादनादि, चित्तमात्राधीनं श्रद्धाद्याध्यात्मिकम्। तथा चोक्तम्, 'ये चैते मैत्र्यादयो ध्यायिनां विहारास्ते वाह्यसाधननिरनुग्रहात्मानः प्रकृष्टं धर्ममभिनिर्वर्तयन्ति'। तयोर्मानसं बलीयः, कथं, ज्ञानवैराग्ये केनातिशय्येते, दण्डकारण्यं चित्तबलव्यतिरेकेण कः शारीरेण कर्मणा शून्यं कर्तुमुत्सहेत, समुद्रमगस्त्यवद्वा पिबेत्॥ १०॥

**Desire For Self-Welfare Being Everlasting It Follows That The Subconscious Impression From Which It Arises Must Be Beginningless. 10.**

In every creature there is a desire for self-welfare such as 'I may not be non-existent, let me live for ever.' This desire cannot be spontaneous, *i.e.* without a cause. How can a creature just born, which has not experienced death before, have fear of death, which is due to a memory of aversion and sorrow regarding death ? What is natural does not require a cause to come into being (1). This shows that the mind is filled with eternal Vāsanās. Being impelled by an appropriate situation, the mind becomes manifest, following one such Vāsanā, for experience of the individual. Some (2) hold that mind is shaped by the dimensions of the body like the light of a lamp which contracts if the lamp is placed in a pot and spreads if placed in a palace (hall). In their opinion this explains how there may be a middle state or how the mind gives up one body, takes up another and fills up the gap between them (between death and rebirth). It also explains Saṁsāra or the cycle of births. Āchārya (sage) says that it is the modification of the all-pervading mind (and not the mind itself) which contracts and expands and the cause of such contraction and expansion is virtue and its other similar attributes. This exciting cause is twofold, *viz.* external and internal (or relating to the self). The external ones presuppose actions by the body etc., *e.g.* worship, charity, adoration, etc. The internal ones depend only on the mind. Reverence etc. illustrate them. It has been said by Āchārya in this connection : "Friendliness etc., which the contemplative (Yogins) cherish as congenial pursuits, are not contingent on the achievement of something outside, and they are productive of the highest merit." Of the two causes, the mental ones (3) are stronger, because nothing can be superior to true knowledge and renunciation. Whoever can by physical force alone, without the help of will-power, empty out Daṇḍakāraṇya (a forest) or drink off a sea like sage Agastya ?

(1) What is natural does not require a cause to arise. It is seen that fear is caused through recollection of sorrows. Horror of death is a sort of fear. There must be a cause for it. Therefore, it cannot be a natural occurrence. To explain fear of death, previous experience of sorrow at the time of death must be admitted. Thus previous births have also to be admitted. The knower, instruments of reception and the knowables are inherent in any creature. They are not produced by any cause during its life-time.

'Āśīḥ'or desire for self-welfare is a feeling arising out of a desire to live and not to be non-existent. It is eternal and exists in all creatures, past, present and future. As 'Āśīḥ' is eternally present in all creatures without exception, Vāsanā is also eternal. As there was 'Āśīḥ' in the past, there must have been corresponding births, and we must therefore admit that the cycle of births and Vāsanā are eternal. Some people explain that fear of death is the result of an instinct. Instinct means untaught ability or a faculty which is noticeable from birth. But this does not say anything about the origin of instincts. Evolutionists hold that it is inherited. According to them in the beginning life takes the form of a unicellular creature called amoeba. After all, it is not denied that there is such a thing as instinct or untaught ability, but that does not explain whence it has come. This has been gone into in greater detail in connection with Sūtra II.9 (2).

(2) Incidentally, the magnitude of the mind has been spoken of. According to some, the mind is like a lamp in a pot or in a palace (hall). It assumes the form of the body it inhabits. Vijñāna-bhikṣu says that it is the view of some Sāṁkhya philosophers. Yogāchārya says that it is all-pervading as it has no spatial extent. Mind which has acquired super-

normal powers through knowledge of discernment can take in everything knowable at the same time and therefore it is regarded as all-pervading. Mind is not all-pervading like the sky, because the sky is only external space. Mind on the other hand is only power of knowing without any extension in space. Since its connection with innumerable external things which are potentially clearly knowable is ever existing, the mind and its faculty of knowing are limitless. Only the modifications of the mind contract and expand. That is why the mind appears as limited. With ordinary persons knowledge is acquired in small instalments while with Yogins of supernormal powers it dawns in its entirety. Thus it follows that mind itself is all-pervading, but its modifications admit of contraction and expansion.

(3) The causes which bring about the manifestation of Vāsanā have been analysed by the commentator. The cause in this case is the latent impression of actions. The actions produced by the effort, *i.e.* the activities of the sense-organs, of the organs of action and of the body, as also their latencies, are the external causes, while the activity of the internal organs and latent impressions thereof are the internal causes or mental acts. The commentator has emphasised the point that mental action is the stronger of the two.

———

हेतुफलाश्रयालम्बनैः संगृहीतत्वादेषामभावे तदभावः ॥ ११ ॥

भाष्यम्—हेतुः धर्मात् सुखमधर्माद् ुःखं सुखाद्रागो दुःखाद्द्वेषः, ततश्च प्रयत्नः, तेन मनसा वाचा कायेन वा परिस्पन्दमानः परमनुगृह्णात्युपहन्ति वा, ततः पुनः धर्माधर्मौ सुखदुःखे रागद्वेषौ इति प्रवृत्तमिदं षडरं संसारचक्रम्। अस्य च प्रतिक्षणमावर्त्तमानस्याविद्या नेत्री मूलं सर्वक्लेशानाम् इत्येष हेतुः। फलन्तु यमाश्रित्य यस्य प्रत्युत्पन्नता धर्मादेः, न ह्यपूर्वोपजनः। मनस्तु साधिकारमाश्रयो वासनानां, न ह्यवसिताधिकारे मनसि निराश्रया वासनाः स्थातुमुत्सहन्ते। यदभिमुखीभूतं वस्तु यां वासनां व्यनक्ति तस्यास्तदालम्बनम्। एवं हेतुफलाश्रयालम्बनैरेतैः संगृहीताः सर्वा वासनाः, एषामभावे तत्संश्रयाणामपि वासनानामभावः ॥ ११ ॥

**On Account Of Being Held Together By Cause, Result, Refuge And Supporting Object, Vāsanā Disappears When They Are Absent. 11.**

From a cause like virtue, pleasure or happiness results ; from impiety, pain or misery ; from happiness, attachment ; and from misery, hatred. Thence (from attachment and hatred) ensues effort ; and from effort results action of speech, mind or body, whereby creatures benefit or injure others ; from that again arise piety and impiety, happiness and misery, attachment and hatred. Thus revolves constantly the six-spoked wheel of births. Nescience which is at the root of all misery is the motive power of this perpetually moving wheel. Thus the process mentioned above serves as the cause. Result is the motive or purpose of an action which determines its moral value as virtuous or vicious. (In reply to a question, how it is possible for Vāsanā as cause to be held together by its effect, the commentator says—) Nothing which did not exist can come into being (*i.e.* effect is present in a subtle form in the cause and that is how the effect can be the receptacle of a cause). A mind prone to fluctuation is the refuge of Vāsanā, which for want of a supporting substratum, cannot reside in a Chitta in which this proneness is destroyed. The object which induces or calls forth Vāsanā, is its inciting cause. Thus the basic cause (Avidyā), result, refuge and inciting object together hold Vāsanā. When they disappear Vāsanās collected by them also disappear.

(1) Vāsanās are collected by or associated with cause, result, refuge and support. The fluctuations rooted in nescience, *i.e.* the wrong cognitions are the cause of Vāsanā. The latent impression of experience derived from the feeling created by being born in a particular species, living therein for a particular period of time, and the pleasure and pain experienced therein, is Vāsanā. The cause of birth, span of life and experience of pleasure and pain is good or evil action. The cause of actions is nescience in the shape of attachment, aversion, etc. Thus nescience is the root cause and this is how the root cause has kept together the Vāsanās. The consequence of Vāsanā is memory, *i.e.* some

modification of the mind. By being cast in the mould of Vāsanā it gives rise to pleasure or pain which leads to an effort towards good or evil actions. The commentator has stated earlier that the latent impression of the memory of a feeling is Vāsanā. Virtuous action or its opposite arises from memory shaped by Vāsanā of previous births, longevity and experience. Since memory gives rise to fresh Vāsanā, memory helps to sustain Vāsanā. For instance, memory of happiness leads to accumulation of Vāsanā of happiness. The expression 'Puruṣārtha' means that which serves the objective of Puruṣa. It may be the experience of pleasure or pain, or it may be liberation. This is not the outcome of Vāsanā alone, but of knowing the knowables as well. Birth, longevity and experience of pleasure and pain are the results of Karmāśaya and not of Vāsanā. Thus only memory results from Vāsanā.

Chitta prone to fluctuations is the abode of Vāsanā. When that proneness is destroyed through acquisition of discriminative enlightenment, the mind remains full of that knowledge alone and thus there is no room for Vāsanās of nescience. When the knowledge that Puruṣa is nothing but absolute Consciousness fills the mind, memory of such modifications as 'I am a man' or 'I am a cow' being impossible, all such Vāsanās are destroyed because they can no longer beget memory of wrong cognitions. Thus a mind which has finished its activity cannot be the abode of Vāsanā while an active mind with normal functions, *i.e.* a mind which has not acquired discriminative enlightenment is its abode.

Although Karmāśaya is the cause of appearance of Vāsanā, it appears with objects like light, sound, etc. and in the form of birth, longevity and experience ; that is why those objects are considered as the props of Vāsanā. Sound reveals the subconscious impression of hearing ; that is why sound is the prop of the Vāsanā of hearing. Thus Vāsanā is sustained by nescience, memory, an active Chitta and objects. When they disappear, Vāsanā also disappears. Uninterrupted discriminative knowledge is the cause of the cessation of nescience etc. With the dawning of discriminative knowledge, cognition of objects, inclination of the mind to Guṇa-induced activities, memory of Vāsanās and nescience disappear, consequently Vāsanā is destroyed. It might be questioned why it is necessary to mention all the other aspects such as Guṇas and the like when the destruction of nescience alone brings about their cessation. It should be understood in this connection that nescience is not destroyed outright. After shutting out knowables etc. one has to get to the root cause in the form of nescience and then destroy it. That is why it is necessary to know the different elements which sustain Vāsanā, and try to attenuate them from the very beginning.

*The six-spoked wheel of the round of birth and death, i.e. worldliness*

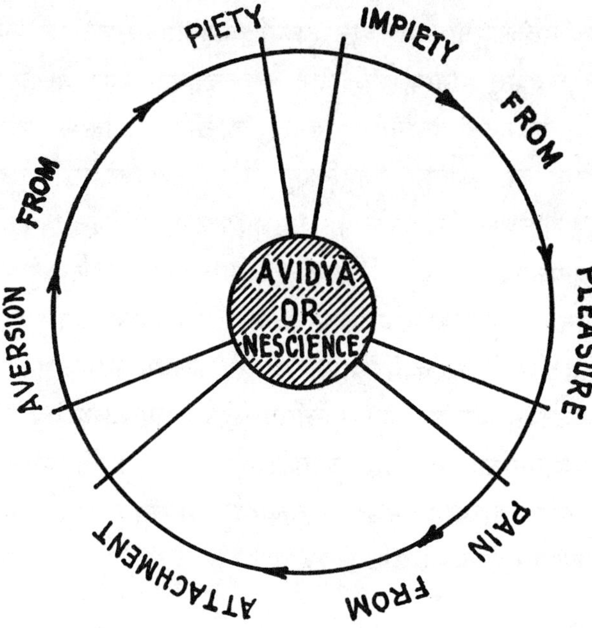


A creature does an act of piety or impiety prompted by attachment or aversion. From attachment to pleasure one does a pious act or an impious act in the form of oppressing others. Similarly, from aversion, seeking relief from pain, one does both pious and impious acts. From pious acts one gets more pleasure and less pain, while impious acts result in more pain and less pleasure. From pleasure arises attachment to objects which give pleasure and hatred towards things which hinder pleasure. Pain gives rise to hatred towards objects which cause pain and attachment towards objects which are antagonistic to pain. At the root of all is nescience or delusion in the shape of wrong knowledge. This is how the cycle of births is revolving.

———

भाष्यम्—नास्त्यसतः सम्भवो न चास्ति सतो विनाशः, इति द्रव्यत्वेन सम्भवन्त्यः कथं निवर्तिष्यन्ते वासना इति—

अतीतानागतं स्वरूपतोऽस्त्यध्वभेदाद्धर्माणाम् ॥ १२ ॥

भविष्यद्व्यक्तिकमनागतम् अनुभूतव्यक्तिकमतीतं स्वव्यापारोपारूढं वर्त्तमानम्। त्रयं चैतद्वस्तु ज्ञानस्य ज्ञेयं, यदि चैतत्स्वरूपतो नाभविष्यन्नेदं निर्विषयं ज्ञानमुदपत्स्यत, तस्मादतीतानागतं स्वरूपतः अस्तीति। किञ्च भोगभागीयस्य वापवर्गभागीयस्य वा कर्मणः फलमुत्पित्सु यदि निरुपाख्यमिति तदुद्देशेन तेन निमित्तेन कुशलानुष्ठानं न युज्येत। सतश्च फलस्य निमित्तं वर्त्तमानीकरणे समर्थं नापूर्वोपजनने, सिद्धं निमित्तं नैमित्तिकस्य विशेषानुग्रहणं कुरुते, नापूर्वमुत्पादयति। धर्मी चानेकधर्मस्वभावः, तस्य चाध्वभेदेन धर्माः प्रत्यवस्थिताः। न च यथा वर्त्तमानं व्यक्तिविशेषापन्नं द्रव्यतोऽस्त्येवमतीतमनागतं वा। कथं तर्हि, स्वेनैव व्यङ्ग्येन स्वरूपेण अनागतमस्ति, स्वेन चानुभूतव्यक्तिकेन स्वरूपेणातीतमिति वर्त्तमानस्यैवाध्वनः स्वरूपव्यक्तिरिति, न सा भवति अतीतानागतयोरध्वनोः। एकस्य चाध्वनः समये द्वावध्वानौ धर्मिसमन्वागतौ भवत एवेति, नाऽभूत्वा भावस्त्रयाणामध्वनामिति ॥ १२ ॥

Since anything positive cannot be produced out of nothing, nor can anything that exists be completely destroyed, how can subliminal impressions which exist as positive things be eliminated altogether ?

### The Past And The Future Are In Reality Present In Their Fundamental Forms, There Being Only Difference In The Characteristics Of The Forms Taken At Different Times (1). 12.

A thing which will appear later is said to be of the future. It is said to be of the past when its manifestation has already been experienced. The present is that whose functions are currently manifest. All the three aspects of a thing are objects of knowledge. Had the past and future things not existed in their special forms then the knowledge of the past and the future would have been contentless, but there can be no knowledge without content. Therefore the past and the future things are really in existence in a subtle form in the causes, of which they are the effects. Moreover, if the resultant effects of actions leading to experience (of pleasure and pain) or salvation were unreal, then nobody would be engaged in such pursuits. Cause can only bring forth to the present what is already in existence ; it can never produce what is altogether non-existent. Only a present, *i.e.* existent cause can bring out an effect in its present perceptible form, it cannot produce anything non-existent. An object has many characteristics, and they are situated, so to say, in the different periods of time. While the present characteristics are the particular manifestations (2) of the object, the past and future ones are not so. Then how do they exist? The future exists in its potential form, while the past exists in the cognitions and feelings experienced before. The present is manifest in its own true nature while the past and the future are not so. At the time of appearance of one phase, the characteristics of the other two phases lie unmanifest in the things. Thus there being no non-existence, the threefold aspect of a thing is proved, *i.e.* the threefold aspect exists because the individual aspects do exist, and are not non-existent.

(1) That the past and the future are real is proved by the fact of the knowledge of the past and the future. Apart from the case of Yogins, there are many examples of fore-knowledge of the future. There must be a content for knowledge. There is no instance of objectless knowledge, it is inconceivable or absurd. Thus if there is knowledge, there must be an object for it. Knowledge of the future has thus an object. It should therefore be admitted that a future object does exist. Thus it must be admitted that the past object also exists. Now it has to be demonstrated how the past and future states exist. There are three forms of existent things, *viz.* object, action or mutation, and potential. Of these, mutation changes things, thus mutation is the cause of change. It is to be admitted that although what we call an entity, *i.e.* an object, is

based on mutability yet there is something whose mutation it is. That something is the basic object or entity. Hardness etc. are attributes due to invisible actions of causal factors. Mutation is visible action. Visible action is the cause while manifestation due to unseen action or appearance as a steady object, is the effect. The mutation into effect through the action of the cause, is the characteristic of change pertaining to an object. The transfer from one potential state to another is the characteristic of the causal action. Visible gross activity is the collective knowledge of the subtle momentary ones. Light, sound, etc. are like that. Thus gross objects like (earthen) pot etc. are the collective knowledge of innumerable subtle activities taking place in quick succession as a rapidly revolving burning coal looks like a wheel of fire. From potentiality ensues activity which is the cause, from this cause ensues knowledge or a sentient state, and the sentient state relapses to a state of potentiality or latency—this continuous sequence of change is the basic nature of the phenomenal world. That is the subtlest form of all gross objects and the organs, which are manifestations of Sattva, Rajas and Tamas principles. (See next Sūtra.)

Conception of change is thus knowledge of an action or the manifest result of an action. As there is change in our internal organs of reception, so are there changes in the phenomenal world. According to the Sāṁkhya philosophy external things are basically the I-sense of particular beings, *i.e.* they are products of the mind. When latent impressions in their potency come up to our conscious level, they develop into an object as recollection and that process of development we call change; the changes in the phenomenal world are basically of the same nature.

The change arising out of interaction of external activity and mental action is knowledge of an object. In ordinary conditions our mind, due to its limited power of reception, cannot grasp either the subtle mutations taking place at imperceptible intervals or the totality of such innumerable changes. The perception in small quantities of momentary changes taking place around us, is the natural way of human perception which results in cognition of objects. Usually both the cause and the effect in the process of mutation are perceived in quanta. It has been stated before that the manifestation of mutation or action from the potential state is change. Since no estimate can be formed of all possible changes, they are innumerable. Although innumerable, we receive them in small instalments in a restricted manner by way of a cause and effect relationship. That is why we imagine that what we have taken in is past, what we are now taking in is present, and what is possible to be taken in later is future. When the limitations of the power of comprehension are removed by Saṁyama, all possible combinations of the momentary changes come within the purview of knowledge simultaneously, revealing both the cause and the effect, producing thereby knowledge of the past and the future. In other words, everything appears to be present.

What is stated above in respect of external objects is also applicable to internal states. That is why the author of the Sūtra has said that the past and the future really exist in a subtle form, but on the basis of the threefold aspect of time, we consider that they are not present, *i e.* they were present or will be present.

Ordinarily objects are perceived piecemeal. By the concept of time things are marked off as past and future and are considered non-existent. Time as such has no reality but the objects are real. Owing to our limited capacity of knowledge and subtleness of things we may not be able to perceive them fully in certain situations and thus impose temporal limitations on them as past and future, virtually making them non-existent. In an omniscient mind, however, there is no such limitation and things are intuited in their entirety, independent of any other considerations and hence they are ever present in their completeness.

In the last Sūtra reference has been made to the disappearance of Vāsanā ; that means only its submergence in a subtle from into its cause. When it submerges it does not come into the path of knowledge nor is it overseen by Puruṣa. This Sūtra has been enunciated to prove that what exists never becomes a non-entity, and what is non-existing can never become a real entity. It has just been demonstrated that change of state only gives the appearance of non-existence. [See I.7(1).] Absence of Vāsanā thus implies its existence for ever in an unmanifest state.

(2) The three states of past, present and future have been explained above in reference to the constituent principles. This can also be demonstrated by reference to ordinary objects. A clod of earth can be a pot or a pan as the potter may wish. Therefore the pot and the pan can be said to exist in the clod of earth in a subtle form. To bring forth the property of potness the efficient cause in the shape of the potter's will, industry, desire for money, energy and knowledge is necessary. That is why the commentator has said that a cause is able to render manifest an effect existing unmanifest in an object. It may be argued in this connection that since the formation of the pot means not the disappearance of the clod of earth of which it is made but a change in its shape in that it assumes a shape which it had not had before and that the unreal does not appear but there is taking in of a new form, it cannot be the object of future knowledge. It has been stated before that mutation is

nothing but potentiality made known. Modification of the ordinary intellect manifests the potential state slowly ; that is why the potter, by slowly exercising his will, gives expression to the shape which was in an unmanifest state. Thus the knowledge of the cause in the shape of the potter's will and of the potentiality of the clod of earth, coming into contact with each other is the manifestation of the pot or a knowledge of the presence of the pot. Change of form is also knowledge of energy in the form of action.

If the power of knowledge is so developed that the entire energy of the potter and all the properties of the clod of earth can be known, then the manifold contacts of these two can also be known, as well as all the sequences that are known to an ordinary intellect. It has been stated before that mind in itself is all-pervading, so it always has contact with everything, but its modifications being limited by its kinship with body, knowledge comes through a narrow channel. For example, when we look at the sky at night, the rays of all the stars and planets enter into our eyes but on account of our limited visual powers we do not see all of them, but only the bright ones. Similarly, when the grossness is removed from our intellect, and the Sāttvika or sentient faculty is cleared of dross and reaches its highest form, then all objects, past, present and future, would exhibit themselves before the mind's eye at the same time and everything will be present.

---

ते व्यक्तसूक्ष्मा गुणात्मानः ॥ १३ ॥

भाष्यम्—ते खल्वमी त्र्यध्वानो धर्मा वर्तमाना व्यक्तात्मानोऽतीतानागताः सूक्ष्मात्मानः षडविशेषरूपाः। सर्वमिदं गुणानां सन्निवेशविशेषमात्रमिति परमार्थतो गुणात्मानः, तथा च शास्त्रानुशासनं 'गुणानां परमं रूपं न दृष्टिपथमृच्छति। यत्तु दृष्टिपथं प्राप्तं तन्मायेव सुतुच्छकम्' इति ॥ १३ ॥

**Characteristics, Which Are Present At All Times, Are Manifest And Subtle, And Are Composed Of The Three Guṇas. 13.**

Of the three-phased characteristics, the manifest state is called the present. In the past and the future states they are in six non-specific (1) subtle forms. These phenomenal forms and their properties are but special combination (2) of the Guṇas, as basically they are nothing but the Guṇas. That is why it has been stated in the Śāstras : "The ultimate nature of the Guṇas is never visible; what is seen is extremely ephemeral like an illusion."

(1) The characteristics which are visible or present are said to be manifest. Objects which are cognised as manifest are the sixteen modifications of the Guṇas, *viz.* the five Bhūtas, the five sense-organs, the five organs of action, and the mind. Their previous state and what they will be hereafter, or in other words, their past and future states, are their subtle states. Therefore the subtle states would be the five Tanmātras and Asmitā or I-sense. Of course this is from the point of view of the ultimate nature of things. From a material point of view a clod of earth is the manifest or present state, while pot etc. would be its past or future subtle states.

(2) From the fundamental point of view, everything is made up of the three Guṇas—Sattva, Rajas and Tamas—which are respectively the sentient, the mutative and the static faculties. Looking at everything from this standpoint, liberation or extreme cessation of the threefold misery has to be attained. The state of equilibrium of the three Guṇas is their unmanifest state. Gross and subtle states are their unbalanced conditions. Although the manifest states are palpably visible, they should be shunned as they bring misery and are insignificant, transient and illusory. This proposition has been supported by a statement quoted from the Ṣaṣṭi-tantra-śāstra framed by Vārṣagaṇya.

———

भाष्यम्—यदा तु सर्वे गुणाः कथमेकः शब्द एकमिन्द्रियमिति—

परिणामैकत्वाद्वस्तुतत्त्वम् ॥ १४ ॥

प्रख्याक्रियास्थितिशीलानां गुणानां ग्रहणात्मकानां करणभावेनैकः परिणामः श्रोत्रमिन्द्रियं, ग्राह्यात्मकानां शब्दभावेनैकः परिणामः शब्दो विषय इति। शब्दादीनां मूर्त्तिसमानजातीयानामेकः परिणामः पृथिवीपरमाणुस्तन्मात्रावयवः, तेषाञ्चैकः परिणामः पृथिवी गौर्वृक्षः पर्वत इत्येवमादिः। भूतान्तरेष्वपि स्नेहौष्ण्यप्रणामित्वावकाशदानान्युपादाय सामान्यमेकविकारारम्भः समाधेयः।

नास्त्यर्थो विज्ञानविसहचरोऽस्ति तु ज्ञानमर्थविसहचरं स्वप्नादौ कल्पित-मित्यनया दिशा ये वस्तुस्वरूपमपह्नुवते ज्ञानपरिकल्पनामात्रं वस्तु स्वप्नविषयोपमं न परमार्थतोऽस्तीति ये आहुः ते तथेति प्रत्युपस्थितमिदं स्वमाहात्म्येन वस्तु कथमप्रमाणात्मकेन विकल्पज्ञानबलेन वस्तुस्वरूपमुत्सृज्य तदेवापलपन्तः श्रद्धेयवचनाः स्युः ॥ १४ ॥

But if all objects are products of the three Guṇas, then how can there be a single perception as 'one sound Tanmātra', 'one sense-organ (as ear, eye, etc.)' ?

**On Account Of The Co-Ordinated Mutation Of The Three Guṇas, An Object Appears As A Unit. 14.**

The Guṇas with the three properties of cognition, activity and retentiveness, mutate in the process of reception into one organ for reception of sound, *viz.* the ear. Similarly, the Guṇas serving as object, undergo modification to manifest as an object, *viz.* sound. The modifications of the various Tanmātras such as sound Tanmātra, smell Tanmātra, etc. into tangible states, form the various Bhūtas or elements such as Śabda-bhūta, Kṣiti-bhūta (1), etc. each according to the appropriate Tanmātra. In the same way from the mutation of those Bhūtas and their phenomenal conglomeration, are formed earth, cow, tree, hill, etc. In respect of the other Bhūtas (gross elements) according to their respective properties of fluidity, warmth, mobility and voidness, similar conclusions about their particular unified states may be made.

'An object prior or posterior to cognition is non-existent, but in dreams there can be cognition without the existence of any object'—there are thinkers who use such an argument and rule out the objective world, and hold that objects are produced from cognition only and like objects in a dream have no real existence. How can their views be respected since they dispute the existence of objects that appear by virtue of their very existence (2), and thus put trust on illogical wild imagination ?

(1) The three Guṇas are at the root of all things. How can a thing composed of these three be regarded as one ? To answer that query this Sūtra has been propounded. Guṇas though three in number are inseparable. Sattva-guṇa does not become cognisable without Rajas and Tamas. The same is the case with Rajas and Tamas. It has been said before that a modification is nothing but transformation of the potential state (which is inertia, *i.e.* Tamas) being activated (which is movement, *i.e.* Rajas) into perception (which is sentience, *i.e.* Sattva). Thus in all mutations the three constituent principles having sentient, mutable and static properties must be present. In other words, though different, the three act in unison and produce a change. Such is their nature. That is why the product of the change is regarded as one object. Take, for example, knowledge of sound. In it there are potentiality, activity and perceptibility, otherwise knowledge of sound would not be possible. But the sound is regarded as one and not as three different things. That is how on account of unification through mutation things are regarded as one.

Tanmātra-avayava—those whose component parts are the Tanmātras, *e.g.* Kṣiti-bhūta.

(2) The author of the Sūtra has admitted the existence of (extra-mental) substance. This controverts the theory of the Vaināśikas (a class of Buddhists). The commentator has elucidated this point, though the Sūtra does not go into this.

The Vijñānavādins or the Idealists (a Buddhist sect) argue that when there is no perception there is no awareness of the existence of external objects, but that when there is no external object, there may be knowledge of it, as, for example, in a dream one can have knowledge of colour, taste, etc. Therefore there is no substance outside perception and outside objects are figments of imagination. (That which is outside the sense-organs and whose action produces knowledge is the basic substance.) The fallacy in the above-mentioned argument is now being shown. It is true that knowledge of external objects is not possible without perception because without the power of perception there can be no knowledge. But it is not true that there can be knowledge of an external object which does not exist at all. In dream there is no perceptive knowledge of an outside object but the knowledge is that of the latent impressions of the external objects. There is no instance of such perception without once coming in contact with an activity external to the senses. For example, a person born blind can never dream of light. Imaginary concepts are the only proofs adduced by the Idealists. Sun, moon, earth, etc. which exist phenomenally and prove their existence by virtue of their presence are attempted to be disproved by them by merely semantic concepts. When they are asked how the phenomenal world came into being, they say that there is no reality in it, it is an illusion. In their view the cause is non-existent, so is the effect. Such are their delusions based only on the use of words.

Observing the worldly things from spiritual level one is bound to distinguish things eminently wholesome and desirable from those that are fit to be discarded. Sorrow and cause of sorrow are mutable objects and hence are to be discarded. What is permanent, pure, sentient and liberated is desirable. It is imperative for one to go through objects to be discarded and their annihilation so long as one is striving for salvation. Once salvation is attained, one does not need to look at things from such spiritual angle, and is no longer concerned with things to be discarded and their annihilation. Hence the commentator has stated that from spiritual standpoint impersonal objects that are to be discarded exist; what remains after the ultimate goal is reached is the Seer-abiding-in-Himself which is beyond ordinary comprehension.

———

भाष्यम्—कुतश्चैतदन्याय्यम्—

वस्तुसाम्ये चित्तभेदात्तयोर्विभक्तः पन्थाः ॥ १५ ॥

बहुचित्तावलम्बनीभूतमेकं वस्तु साधारणं, तत्खलु नैकचित्तपरिकल्पितं नाप्यनेकचित्तपरिकल्पितं किन्तु स्वप्रतिष्ठम्। कथं, वस्तुसाम्ये चित्तभेदात् धर्मापेक्षं चित्तस्य वस्तुसाम्येऽपि सुखज्ञानं भवति, अधर्मापेक्षं तत एव दुःखज्ञानम्, अविद्यापेक्षं तत एव मूढ़ज्ञानं, सम्यग्दर्शनापेक्षं तत एव माध्यस्थ्यज्ञानमिति। कस्य तच्चित्तेन परिकल्पितं—न चान्यचित्तपरिकल्पितेनार्थेनान्यस्य चित्तोपरागो युक्तः, तस्माद् वस्तुज्ञानयोर्ग्राह्यग्रहणभेदभिन्नयोर्विभक्तः पन्थाः। नानयोः सङ्कर-गन्धोऽप्यस्ति इति। सांख्यपक्षे पुनर्वस्तु त्रिगुणं, चलं च गुणवृत्तमिति, धर्मादि-निमित्तापेक्षं चित्तैरभिसंबध्यते, निमित्तानुरूपस्य च प्रत्ययस्योत्पद्यमानस्य तेन तेनात्मना हेतुर्भवति ॥ १५ ॥

Why is that (the statement controverted in the preceding Sūtra) illogical ?

**In Spite Of Sameness Of Objects, On Account Of There Being Separate Minds They (The Object And Its Knowledge) Follow Different Paths, That Is Why They Are Entirely Different (1). 15.**

There may be an object of common interest to many minds ; it is not figured by one mind, nor by many minds, but is grounded in itself. How do we illustrate this ? On account of there being different minds the same object evokes a feeling of pleasure in a virtuous mind, a feeling of misery in a vicious mind, a feeling of stupor in a mind full of nescience and an attitude of indifference in a mind with perfect insight. Then of which mind is the object a creation (assuming an object is a creation of the mind) ? Again it is not probable that the creation of one mind would influence another mind. That is why the paths of object and knowledge are demarcated by difference in the form of objectivity and receptivity, and there is no chance of confusion between the two. According to the Sāṁkhya philosophy all objects are made of the three Guṇas which are constantly mutating. They come into contact with the mind through an exciting cause such as virtue, vice, etc., when they produce corresponding impressions and thus become the cause of such impressions.

(1) In the previous Sūtra all phenomenal objects have been referred to. In this Sūtra the difference of mind and object is being shown. When from the same external object different feelings are roused in different minds, then that object and mind must be different. They are mutating in different directions.

As from the standpoint of feeling, difference between mind and matter has been shown, so from the point of view of perception of the objective world, the existence of different external objects common to all minds can be established. When the same object can produce the same perception in different minds, *e.g.* the sun and the perception of its light, then the mind and the object are different. If an object had been the creation of a mind, then there would have been difference in the conception of each, and there would have been no such thing as one perception common to all minds.

This is how the commentator has shown clearly that when the distinction between mind and matter is established, the views of Idealists become untenable. The perception of different objects, *e.g.* different colours etc., though modifications of the mind, is due to the existence of some external object as its source, on account of which the mind undergoes modification, because different perceptions do not arise out of the spontaneous mutation of the mind only.

———

भाष्यम्—केचिदाहुः ज्ञानसहभूरेवार्थो भोग्यत्वात् सुखादिवदिति, त एतया द्वारा साधारणत्वं बाधमानाः पूर्वोत्तरेषु क्षणेषु वस्तुरूपमेवापह्नुवते।

न चैकचित्ततन्त्रं वस्तु तदप्रमाणकं तदा किं स्यात् ॥ १६ ॥

एकचित्ततन्त्रं चेद् वस्तु स्यात्तदा चित्ते व्यग्रे निरुद्धे वा स्वरूपमेव तेनापरामृष्टमन्यस्याऽविषयीभूतमप्रमाणकमगृहीतस्वभावकं केनचित् तदानीं किन्तत्स्यात्, संबध्यमानं च पुनश्चित्तेन कुत उत्पद्येत। ये चास्यानुपस्थिता भागास्ते चास्य न स्युः, एवं नास्ति पृष्ठमित्युदरमपि न गृह्येत। तस्मात् स्वतन्त्रोऽर्थः सर्वपुरुषसाधारणः, स्वतन्त्राणि च चित्तानि प्रतिपुरुषं प्रवर्तन्ते, तयोः सम्बन्धादुपलब्धिः पुरुषस्य भोग इति ॥ १६ ॥

Some say that an object comes into being simultaneously with its perception because it is enjoyed by perception, *e.g.* happiness etc. are objects of experience and are co-existent with their experience ; so also sound etc., being objects of experience are simultaneously existent with their respective experience. Thus by refuting the general perceptibility of objects they try to establish the non-existence of a substance (substratum) in past or future. (Such a view is not supported by this Sūtra.)

### Object Is Not Dependent On One Mind, Because If It Were So, Then What Will Happen When It Is Not Cognised By That Mind (1) ? 16.

If an object were dependent on one mind, then what will happen to it when that mind is inattentive or is in an arrested state, and does not concern itself with the nature of the object ? Because then it will not be the object of any other mind, nor will it be noticed by any other mind. If it again comes into contact with the mind (from which it was said to have originated) wherefrom will it come ? On this line of argument there cannot be any unknown part (by a particular perceiver) of an object. For example, in ordinary parlance when we speak of the absence of the back the absence of belly is also implied. If, therefore, there is no unknown part, the known part and the perception thereof also become unrealities. That is why it must be admitted that an object has distinct existence common to all, and minds are also distinct and peculiar to each individual. The realisation arising out of the contact of these two is the experience of an object by a person.

(1) This aphorism has not been accepted by Bhojadeva ; it may perhaps be part of the commentary on the last Sūtra. This aphorism establishes that an object is common to all, whereas a mind is peculiar to each individual. A thing is an object of knowledge to many and is not conceived by the mind of one individual. Moreover, it is not conceived by many minds, but the mind and the object being separately established, both undergo mutations separately.

Granting that an object is dependent on one mind, the question that arises is what happens to the object when it is not being perceived by that mind. If it is the figment of a mind, naturally it would cease to exist when the mind is not directed to it. But it does not happen that way. It is also not a tenable argument that an object is the creation of many minds because there is no reason why many minds will conceive of the same thing.

Sāṁkhya philosophers do not need to resort to such hypotheses. They hold that the Draṣṭā (Seer) and the Dṛśya (seen or knowable) both exist. Of them the knowable or the world of phenomenal objects mutates as it exists while the Seer exists as an immutable entity. The discernment of the Seer and the seen through true knowledge leads to attainment of the spiritual goal. An object has two aspects : when it is being cognised and when it exists as an object of cognition without being cognised. The latter is known as its objectivity.

The first of the two aspects, *viz.* the actual cognition depends on and varies with each individual cogniser. But the second aspect, its knowability, can be cognised by all and is, therefore, commonly shared by them. When there is contact between the organ of reception and a knowable, cognition takes place.

———

तदुपरागापेक्षित्वाच्चित्तस्य वस्तु ज्ञाताज्ञातम् ॥ १७ ॥

भाष्यम्—अयस्कान्तमणिकल्पा विषयाः अयःसधर्मकं चित्तमभिसम्बध्योपरञ्जयन्ति, येन च विषयेणोपरक्तं चित्तं स विषयो ज्ञातस्ततोऽन्यः पुनरज्ञातः। वस्तुनो ज्ञाताज्ञातस्वरूपत्वात् परिणामि चित्तम् ॥ १७ ॥

**External Objects Are Known Or Unknown To The Mind According As They Colour The Mind. 17.**

Objects are like lodestones. They attract the mind as though it were a piece of iron, and influence it. The object with which the mind becomes related, comes to be known, while other objects remain unknown. On account of the knowability or unknowability of things, the mind is mutable (1).

(1) Objects attract the mind or modify it, as magnet does a piece of iron. The source of objects is the external actions of sound, light, etc., which entering into the proper place in the mind, through the sense-channels, modify the mind. Things do not bring the mind out of the body, but when the modifications relate to external objects, the mind is said to turn outward. Some hold that the mind goes out by the sense-channels and suffers fluctuation on contact with objects. This view is not correct. Mind, an internal organ of a being, cannot reside in an external object in the absence of a refuge. An object and the mind meet inside

the body and it is there that the mutation of the mind takes place. The place where the mutation takes place is called Hṛdaya (the heart or the affective centre). Perception of objects appears there and it disappears there also. Contact with, or influence of the activity of, an object is the cause of the mind being set in motion ; that is why an object is known or unknown according as it does or does not come into contact with the mind.

Objects cognised by the mind exist independently of it. Under suitable conditions they influence or shape the mind. Then the knowledge of the object appears in the mind ; otherwise the mere existence of the thing does not bring about its cognition by the mind. Thus a separate object is sometimes known by the mind and sometimes it remains unknown. From this is established that a mind suffers mutation in the shape of change in perception. In other words, the modification of the mind is caused by the action of a real (extramental) substance (see note to Sūtra II.20 in this connection). The significance of the subject has to be realised through introspection.

---

भाष्यम्—यस्य तु तदेव चित्तं विषयस्तस्य—

सदा ज्ञाताश्चित्तवृत्तयस्तत्प्रभोः पुरुषस्यापरिणामित्वात् ॥ १८ ॥

यदि चित्तवत् प्रभुरपि पुरुषः परिणमेत ततस्तद्विषयाश्चित्तवृत्तयः शब्दादिविषयवत् ज्ञाताज्ञाताः स्युः, सदाज्ञातत्वं तु मनसस्तत्प्रभोः पुरुषस्यापरिणामित्वमनुमापयति ॥ १८ ॥

Then again to whom the mind is an object—

**On Account Of The Immutability Of Puruṣa Who Is Master Of The Mind, The Modifications Of The Mind Are Always Known Or Manifest. 18.**

If like the mind, its master had been undergoing change, then the fluctuations of the mind which are manifest to him would have been known and unknown as objects like sound are. But the fact that the mind is ever manifest to its master, Puruṣa, establishes the latter's immutability (1).

(1) Objects are sometimes known and sometimes not known by the mind, but the mind as an object of Puruṣa, *i.e.* Grahītā, is always known by Him. It is not possible to have modifications of the mind without their being known. This has been explained fully in the notes to Sūtra II.20. Modifications of the mind, whether Pramāṇa or of any other kind, are felt as 'I am knowing', the 'I' being Grahītā or receiver. These are always witnessed by Puruṣa. There can be no knowledge or perception unseen by Puruṣa. Whenever there is perception it is seen or illumined by Puruṣa. As it is not possible to have perception which is not known, the mind as an object known by Puruṣa is always manifest as a modification.

If Puruṣa, the source of cognition, mutated, then this character of being perpetually known would have been vitiated. Mutation of Puruṣa implies that He is sometimes knower and sometimes non-knower. Had it been so the mind would not have been ever manifest, sometimes it would have been known and sometimes not known. But such a mind is inconceivable. Mutability of the mind and immutability of Puruṣa thus establish the distinction between the two.

The objectivity of the mind is its quality of being modified by (*i.e.* identified with) sound, colour, etc. Action of sound etc. excites the senses, which in turn activate the mind. That is how perception of objects takes place. It is not possible that modifications are there without being known or manifest to the Seer. If the fluctuations revealed to the Seer were sometimes unknown, then the Seer would not have been a perpetual absolute Seer but mutable. In other words, fluctuations become known through contact with the Seer. If it were seen that there was contact with Puruṣa but the fluctuations were not known, then Puruṣa would have been a Seer and a non-Seer, *i.e.* mutable.

———

भाष्यम्—स्यादाशङ्का चित्तमेव स्वाभासं विषयाभासं च भविष्यति अग्निवत्—

न तत्स्वाभासं दृश्यत्वात् ॥ १९ ॥

यथेतराणीन्द्रियाणि शब्दादयश्च दृश्यत्वान्न स्वाभासानि तथा मनोऽपि प्रत्येतव्यम्। न चाग्निरत्र दृष्टान्तः, न ह्यग्निरात्मस्वरूपमप्रकाशं प्रकाशयति,

प्रकाशश्चायं प्रकाश्यप्रकाशकसंयोगे दृष्टः, न च स्वरूपमात्रेऽस्ति संयोगः। किञ्च स्वाभासं चित्तमित्यग्राह्यमेव कस्यचिदिति शब्दार्थः, तद्यथा स्वात्मप्रतिष्ठमाकाशं न परप्रतिष्ठमित्यर्थः। स्वबुद्धिप्रचारप्रतिसंवेदनात्सत्त्वानां प्रवृत्तिर्दृश्यते क्रुद्धोऽहं भीतोऽहम्, अमुत्र मे रागोऽमुत्र मे क्रोध इति, एतत्स्वबुद्धेरग्रहणे न युक्तमिति॥१९॥

It may be argued that the mind is self-illuminating and also illuminator of objects like fire (but)—

**It (Mind) Is Not Self-Illuminating Being An Object (Knowable). 19.**

As the other organs and objects like light and sound, being knowable, are not self-illuminating, so is mind. In this case fire is not an appropriate example because fire does not illumine its own unmanifest self. The illumination caused by fire is the outcome of contact between the illuminer and the illuminated and has no connection with the true nature of the fire. Moreover, if it is said that the mind is self-illuminating, it will mean that the mind is not knowable by anything else ; as when we say that Ākāśa is self-supporting we mean that Ākāśa is not supported by anything else. But the mind is a knowable because from a reflection of the action in one's mind, one feels such modifications as 'I am angry', 'I am afraid', 'I like it'. This would not have been possible had there been no cognition of what was happening in one's own mind (1).

(1) The mind or cognition is not self-luminous, because it is knowable. That which is knowable is very different from the knower. There cannot be a seer of a Seer. That is why the Seer is self-luminous. One's 'I' is felt to be conscious but that which is knowable by one, such as knowledge of sound etc., or feeling of desire etc., is regarded as unconscious. What is felt as one's own self is the conscious part of the individual. Objects which are felt as 'mine' have no consciousness in them. They are knowables. Similarly the mind, being a knowable, is not self-luminous. Why is mind a knowable ? Because of the feelings : 'I have attachment', 'I have fear', 'I have anger', etc. Modifications of the mind like attach-

ment, fear, anger, etc. thus become knowables or objects. They are, therefore, not the Seer or Knower and because they are not the Seer, they are not self-luminous.

It might be asked why the mind should not be regarded as self-luminous since it knows the feelings arising in it. In reply, it can be said that one feels 'I know'. If you say that the feelings are known by the mind, then the 'mind' and 'I' would be the same. If 'I' am the knower then one part of the mind will be the knower and the other part knowable, such as feelings of attachment, fear, etc. Then again the question will arise : 'Who knows that I am the knower ?' The reply must be : 'I know that I am the knower.' Thus it must be admitted that there is in us a part, which knows itself, which is distinct from the unconscious part, *viz.* feelings etc. We must, therefore, admit the existence of a self-luminous, *i.e.* self-cognizant Knower. Moreover, that will be self-evident perception, while knowledge is acquired through the process of knowing. The act of knowing is perception, while that which perceives is pure Consciousness. Thus the distinction between the knowable and the Knower or Seer is established.

If the people, who hold that the mind is both self-luminous and illuminator of objects, are asked to cite something in which both the characteristics are present, they refer to the fire. But the illustration of fire is inappropriate. What is the meaning of the expression, 'fire is self-luminous' ? It means that another conscious Knower comes to know the light. What is the meaning of the expression, 'fire illumines other things' ? It means that a conscious person knows the object on which light falls. In either case the illuminer is the conscious Knower and the illuminable is the light *i.e.* Tejas-bhūta or light element. Like all other knowledge this is also the result of contact between the Seer and the object. Fire is thus not an example of self-luminosity and illumination of objects. If fire had been manifesting itself as 'I am fire' and also illuminating or knowing another object, then the analogy would have been apt ; but in this case there is no reference to the real nature of fire which, though described as sentient, is in reality insentient.

---

एकसमये चोभयानवधारणम् ॥ २० ॥

भाष्यम्—न चैकस्मिन् क्षणे स्वपररूपावधारणं युक्तम् । क्षणिकवादिनो यद् भवनं सैव क्रिया तदेव च कारकमित्यभ्युपगमः ॥ २० ॥

**Besides, Both (The Mind And Its Objects) Cannot Be Cognised Simultaneously. 20.**

Simultaneous cognizance of one's (mind's) own form and that of another (the object) is not possible (1). In the opinion of those who believe in the doctrine of universal momentariness, the result of an action, the action itself and its doer are all the same. (It would logically follow that cognition of both the agent or knower and the knowable or the effect produced by it on the mind, should take place at the same time. Since that is not the case, mind cannot be regarded as self-luminous.)

(1) That the mind is illuminer of objects is an established fact. To call it illuminer of self would be to regard it as both the subject and the object of knowledge. If it were illuminer of both then it would be cognizant simultaneously of its own nature, *i.e.* its cognising faculty ('I am the knower') and of the object. But that is not the case. They are separately cognised, one at a time. The mental process which brings about perception of a knowable, does not bring about perception of the knowing mind. The two operations are different. Since the two do not take place at the same time, the mind is not self-luminous.

To call the mind self-luminous is to regard it as a knower, implying thereby that it is cognizant of itself as both a knower and a knowable. The commentator has thus shown the fallacy of the believers in the doctrine of universal momentariness (a sect of Buddhists) who hold that the mental act, the subject, and the object of the act are not different. It is not logical to say that the object is known while the self is known, or that the self is known while the object is known. Moreover, in the doctrine of universal momentariness the mind being momentary and inclusive of the knower, the act of knowing and the object, there is no chance or possibility of knowing oneself (as 'I am the knower') and a knowable as distinct entities.

Therefore, the mind, not being the simultaneous illuminer of itself as the knower and the object, is not self-luminous. It is in fact a knowable and so it becomes an object and is cognised as such. As the cognitive principle is known by a process of reflection it is the result of an action, and so it is not self-luminous or absolute Consciousness, unrelated to action. If a self-luminous entity not subject to action or mutation is admitted, then it would mean admitting an immutable principle of Consciousness. The result of an operation cannot be self-established Consciousness.

The line of argument in this Sūtra is as follows : To call the mind (which is not self-illuminating) self-luminous, is to regard it as both the knower and the knowable. This would presuppose cognizance of two things at the same time, which is an impossibility. Hence the mind is not self-luminous.

---

भाष्यम्—स्यान्मतिः स्वरसनिरुद्धं चित्तं चित्तान्तरेण समनन्तरेण गृह्यत इति—

चित्तान्तरदृश्ये बुद्धिबुद्धेरतिप्रसङ्गः स्मृतिसङ्करश्च ॥ २१ ॥

अथ चित्तं चेच्चित्तान्तरेण गृह्येत बुद्धिबुद्धिः केन गृह्यते, साप्यन्यया साप्यन्ययेत्यतिप्रसङ्गः। स्मृतिसङ्करश्च यावन्तो बुद्धिबुद्धीनामनुभवास्तावत्यः स्मृतयः प्राप्नुवन्ति, तत्सङ्कराच्चैकस्मृत्यनवधारणं च स्यात्।

इत्येवं बुद्धिप्रतिसंवेदिनं पुरुषमपलपद्भिर्वैनाशिकैः सर्वमेवाकुलीकृतं, ते तु भोक्तृस्वरूपं यत्र क्वचन कल्पयन्तो न न्यायेन संगच्छन्ते। केचित् सत्त्वमात्रमपि परिकल्प्य अस्ति स सत्त्वो य एतान् पञ्च स्कन्धान् निःक्षिप्यान्यांश्च प्रतिसन्दधातीत्युक्त्वा तत एव पुनस्त्रस्यन्ति। तथा स्कन्धानां महानिर्वेदाय विरागायानुत्पादाय प्रशान्तये गुरोरन्तिके ब्रह्मचर्यं चरिष्यामीत्युक्त्वा सत्त्वस्य पुनः सत्त्वमेवापह्नुवते। सांख्ययोगादयस्तु प्रवादाः स्वशब्देन पुरुषमेव स्वामिनं चित्तस्य भोक्तारमुपयन्ति इति ॥ २१ ॥

(Admitting that the mind is not self-luminous) it may be argued that the mind, which is (momentarily) destroyable, is illumined by another mind (1) subsequently born. But

### If The Mind Were To Be Illumined By Another Mind Then There Will Be Repetition Ad Infinitum Of Illumining Minds And Intermixture Of Memory. 21.

If one mind is illumined by another, then what will illuminate the latter ? If the answer is : 'By another mind', then that other mind will be illumined by yet another and so on, resulting in infinite regress. There will also be intermixture of memory because there will be as many memories as there will be minds to illumine. Such intermixture of memories would render clear apprehension of any memory impossible. Thus the Vaināśikas have confused the issue by doing away with Puruṣa, the reflector of Buddhi. They are not logical in holding everything to be the experiencer (Knower). Others again hold that there is an entity which casts off the five earthly Skandhas or divisions of sense-objects, and in a liberated state enjoys the other Skandhas. Those who hold this view do not have the heart to pursue it. There are some who wish to eliminate the Skandhas completely, to cultivate the attitude of renunciation, to stop rebirth and to achieve peace ; for this purpose they approach their preceptor and take the vow to live the life of a Brahmachārin. But by denying the Self, they deny the very existence of what they aspire to attain. Sāṁkhya-yoga doctrine, on the other hand, demonstrates the existence of Puruṣa as the proprietor and experiencer of the mind by the use of the word Sva (one's own property) (2).

(1) Knowledge of the distinction between Buddhi and Puruṣa is the means of avoiding sorrow. One learns of the distinction first through inference and Āgama (traditional precepts), and then realises it fully (Viveka-khyāti) through concentration. That is why the author of the Sūtras has logically brought out the distinction between the mind and the Knower. Even admitting that the mind is not self-luminous one can still argue that the seer of the mind is another mind and thus eliminate the necessity of admitting the existence of Puruṣa. For example, the

mental modification 'I was angry', would mean the present mind seeing the previous mind. The author of the Sūtra has shown that this proposition is not correct. If it is said that the previous mind and the present mind are only two states of the same mind then it would not be correct to say that one mind is the seer of the other mind, because the mind being one and not self-luminous, it will always be a knowable and not a knower.

The question mentioned above can only be raised if it is assumed that the mind is distinct and separate at different times. But that will be a grave error. If one mind is said to be the knower of the previous different mind then it will involve infinite repetition of the knowing mind, because as soon as the present knowing mind is seen by another mind, that also will be a mind. But how can a future mind be the knower of the present one? The process will involve imagining the existence of an infinite number of knowing minds.

That again will bring about confusion of memory, because in such condition it will be difficult to have clear recollection of any particular experience. The Sāṁkhya doctrine appears to be the most cogent as we get clear and distinct recollection of experiences, one at a time. The doctrine admits of external and internal substances. The object which comes into contact with the faculty of knowing overseen by Puruṣa is experienced. Power of cognizance is inert in itself, because its constituents, the three Guṇas, are all knowables. It appears as conscious on being reflected by Puruṣa, *i.e.* the power of cognizance affected by a knowable, is reflected by Puruṣa.

(2) Puruṣa, the absolute Consciousness, is the experiencer according to the Sāṁkhya school. This view easily explains the desire for salvation. According to the Vaināśikas there is nothing beyond cognition; or besides cognition there is mere voidness, which cannot justify the endeavour to arrest the flow of modifications of the mind. An object that can convert itself into a void or render itself unreal is unknown. So it is not possible that a piece of cognition will convert itself into a void.

And the nihilists, with a view to achieving annihilation of the five Skandhas (*viz.* Vijñāna, Vedanā, Saṁjñā, Rūpa and Saṁskāra) go to their preceptors and take the vows of (learners') self-discipline. But the goal for the attainment of which they make so much ado, is in their opinion mere voidness, and this renders their view absurd.

Even if it is admitted, however illogically, for the sake of argument that there is no such thing as one's self, feelings such as 'I want to be free', 'I want to become void' cannot be avoided. So these hypotheses negating 'I' or self are empty talks. Mokṣa or liberation or Nirvāṇa really means separation from sorrow. Separation connotes two things—sorrow, and dissociation of the sufferer therefrom. It is, therefore, more correct to say that on liberation, sorrow, *i.e.* mind containing sorrow, and the sufferer therefrom are separated. This apparent sufferer is the Self or Puruṣa mentioned in the Sāṁkhya philosophy. That is the ultimate goal of the pure 'I' freed of all egoism.

———

भाष्यम्—कथम् ?—

चितेरप्रतिसंक्रमायास्तदाकारापत्तौ स्वबुद्धिसंवेदनम् ॥ २२ ॥

'अपरिणामिनी हि भोक्तृशक्तिरप्रतिसंक्रमा च, परिणामिन्यर्थे प्रतिसंक्रान्तेव तद्वृत्तिमनुपतति, तस्याश्च प्राप्तचैतन्योपग्रहस्वरूपाया बुद्धिवृत्तेरनुकारमात्रतया बुद्धिवृत्त्यविशिष्टा हि ज्ञानवृत्तिराख्यायते।' तथा चोक्तम् 'न पातालं न च विवरं गिरीणां नैवान्धकारं कुक्षयो नोदधीनाम्। गुहा यस्यां निहितं ब्रह्म शाश्वतं बुद्धिवृत्तिमविशिष्टां कवयो वेदयन्ते' इति ॥ २२ ॥

How (do the Sāṁkhyaites establish Puruṣa denoted by the word Sva) ?

**(Though) Untransmissible The Metempiric Consciousness Getting The Likeness (1) Of Buddhi Becomes The Cause Of The Consciousness Of Buddhi. 22.**

"The supreme entity to which experiences are due is not mutable, nor transmissible. It appears to be transmitted and follow the mutative modifications of Buddhi, which thereby seems to be endowed with consciousness, and thus pure Awareness appears to be identical with them." (Vide II.20.) It has been said in this connection : "The cave where the eternal Brahman resides, is situated neither in the nether world, nor in the mountain chasm, nor in darkness, nor in the cavern of deep sea. The sages know it (the cave) to be the modification of Buddhi indistinguishable from metempiric Consciousness."

(1) Metempiric Consciousness is not really transmitted to Buddhi, but through misapprehension appears as having been transmitted *e.g.* in the expression 'I am conscious', the inert portion of the mutative ego also appears as conscious on account of the presence of Consciousness. This is due to the untransmissible Consciousness appearing as having been transmitted to, *i.e.* infused in Buddhi, *i.e.* Consciousness appearing as having assumed the form of Buddhi. If it were untransmissible, it would be also immutable. Buddhi is always sentient, *i.e.* is always known. I-sense is a manifested idea like cognition of blue, red, etc. Pure I-sense is the irreducible form of cognition. Pure I-sense is sentient but mutable and is manifested under the influence of the immutable Knower. On analysing this I-sense we arrive at two entities—the pure Knower and the knowable which mutates. The I-sense being revealed by the immutable Knower, egotistic forms like 'I am the knower,' 'I am the enjoyer,' 'I am conscious,' etc. arise. That is how metempiric Consciousness assumes the form of Buddhi, which is cognition of the empiric self, *i.e.* the revelation of Buddhi by Consciousness. On account of this reflex action, some are apt to think that the absolute Knower is mutable. That it is not so, has been explained before.

———

भाष्यम्—अतश्चैतदभ्युपगम्यते—

द्रष्टृदृश्योपरक्तं चित्तं सर्वार्थम् ॥ २३ ॥

मनो हि मन्तव्येनार्थेनोपरक्तं तत्स्वयं च विषयत्वाद् विषयिणा पुरुषेणात्मीयया वृत्त्याऽभिसम्बद्धं तदेतच्चित्तमेव द्रष्टृदृश्योपरक्तं विषयविषयिनिर्भासं चेतनाचेतनस्वरूपापन्नं विषयात्मकमप्यविषयात्मकमिवाचेतनं चेतनमिव स्फटिकमणिकल्पं सर्वार्थमित्युच्यते। तदनेन चित्तसारूप्येण भ्रान्ताः केचित्तदेव चेतनमित्याहुः। अपरे चित्तमात्रमेवेदं सर्वं नास्ति खल्वयं गवादिर्घटादिश्च सकारणो लोक इति। अनुकम्पनीयास्ते। कस्मात्, अस्ति हि तेषां भ्रान्तिवीजं सर्वरूपाकारनिर्भासं चित्तमिति, समाधिप्रज्ञायां प्रज्ञेयोऽर्थः प्रतिविम्बीभूतस्तस्यालम्बनीभूतत्वादन्यः स चेदर्थश्चित्तमात्रं स्यात् कथं प्रज्ञयैव प्रज्ञारूपमवधार्य्येत,

तस्मात् प्रतिविम्बीभूतोऽर्थः प्रज्ञायां येनावधार्य्यते स पुरुष इति। एवं ग्रहीतृ-ग्रहणग्राह्यस्वरूपचित्तभेदात् त्रयमप्येतत् जातितः प्रविभजन्ते ते सम्यग्दर्शिनः, तैरधिगतः पुरुष इति ॥ २३ ॥

It follows from this (the previous Sūtra) that

**The Mind-Stuff Being Affected By The Seer And The Seen, Is All-Comprehensive (1). 23.**

The mind is coloured by the thing thought of; and it being itself a knowable (*i.e.* an object), comes into relationship through its own fluctuations with Puruṣa, the subject. Thus the mind affected by the Seer and the objective world, appears to be both subject and object while it is an object itself; though unconscious it seems to be both conscious and unconscious. Thus it behaves like a (reflecting) crystal and is known as all-comprehending. Seeing this likeness to Consciousness, the ignorant regard the mind itself as the conscious entity. There are others who hold that the mind alone is real and the world of objects containing cows and pots and the like along with their causes does not exist. They are objects of pity, because in their opinion only the mind, which is capable of taking the shape of everything and where lies the root of all illusion, exists. In Samādhi or concentration the object cognised is reflected in the mind and is different from the mind. If that object were nothing but mind, then how could a cognition cognise (2) itself as a cognition? Therefore, that which cognises the object reflected in the mind, is Puruṣa. That is why those who regard the knower, the organs of reception and the knowable to be of different categories and consider them as distinct on account of their disaffinity have true knowledge and by them is Puruṣa realised.

(1) What is implied by Consciousness illumining Buddhi has been explained in the previous Sūtra. Consciousness is untransmissible, consequently Consciousness assuming the form of the intellect is really a modification of Buddhi itself. Thus Buddhi is affected by Consciousness in the same way as it is affected by an object. That is what is being demonstrated in this aphorism. Chitta or mind is all-comprehensive ; in other words, it is able to take in both the seer and the seen. Both the modifications, 'I am the knower' and 'I am the body' arise in the mind. Similarly we know 'There is sound' as well as (through reflection), 'There is Puruṣa.' Since we have instances of both these ideas, Chitta or mind can be said to comprehend everything.

(2) The commentator has demolished the theory propounded by some that only cognition exists and there is no Puruṣa beyond it. In the opinion of those theorists mind does not cognise anything and the mind is not cognised. Mind when excited manifests itself as a knowable and as a knower. Mind and the knowing self being not different, persons with distorted vision regard the self as possessed of the three different characteristics of knowable, knower and knowledge. Looking upon the world from that standpoint, *i.e.* only as knowledge divorced from all knowables, one can escape the clutches of sorrow and attain Nirvāṇa. This view is not entirely correct. What will happen when through Samādhi the Puruṣa-like modification of Buddhi is cognised and what will then be the prop of that cognition ? Cognition alone cannot be the support of cognition. Therefore, for the cognisability (through Samādhi) of Puruṣa-like Buddhi, *i.e.* of reflection of Puruṣa in Buddhi, there must be a Puruṣa. If there is a Puruṣa, then only there would be His reflection.

Pauruṣa-pratyaya (literally, cognition of Puruṣa) has been explained before in Sūtra III.35. Puruṣa is not the prop of Buddhi, *i.e.* not an object of contemplation as a pot is. Pauruṣa-pratyaya is the Pratyaya or realisation that Buddhi has been illumined by the self-luminous Consciousness. In Samādhi indelible memory of that remains. That memory relating to Puruṣa is the object of knowledge acquired in such concentration and by analogy it is spoken of as the reflection of the absolute Consciousness. That is how it is made intelligible to others in a gross form.

The commentator has concluded his observations by stating what he means by correct knowledge acquired through study and contemplation. Those who regard the knower, the instrument of reception and the knowables as different on account of their being the objects of different cognisability, have the correct vision. Through such vision is established the existence of Puruṣa, and then on attainment of Viveka-khyāti (discriminative enlightenment) by means of concentration, knowledge about Puruṣa is acquired. After that, when the mind is dissolved by supreme renunciation, Kaivalya or liberation is attained.

———

भाष्यम्—कुतश्चैतत् ?—

तदसंख्येयवासनाभिश्चित्रमपि परार्थं संहत्यकारित्वात् ॥ २४ ॥

तदेतच्चित्तमसंख्येयाभिर्वासनाभिरेव चित्रीकृतमपि परार्थं परस्य भोगापवर्गार्थं न स्वार्थं संहत्यकारित्वाद् गृहवत्। संहत्यकारिणा चित्तेन न स्वार्थेन भवितव्यम्, न सुखचित्तं सुखार्थं, न ज्ञानं ज्ञानार्थम्, उभयमप्येतत्परार्थं—यश्च भोगेनापवर्गेण चार्थेनार्थवान्पुरुषः स एव परः। न परः सामान्यमात्रं, यत्तु किञ्चित्परं सामान्यमात्रं स्वरूपेणोदाहरेद्वैनाशिकस्तत्सर्वं संहत्यकारित्वात्परार्थमेव स्यात्। यस्त्वसौ परो विशेषः स न संहत्यकारी पुरुष इति ॥ २४ ॥

From what else is this (identity of Puruṣa as separate from the mind) established ?

**That (The Mind) Though Variegated By Innumerable Subconscious Impressions Exists For Another Since It Acts Conjointly. 24.**

The mind though diversified with countless Vāsanās, works for another, *i.e.* for the experience or emancipation of another, not for itself, because like a house (1) it is the result of assemblage of many components. A mind which is essentially an assemblage cannot act on its own to serve its own interests. A happy mind does not enjoy the happiness. In a wise mind the wisdom is not for the emancipation of the mind. Both these are for serving somebody else. He, to whom the experience (of pleasure and pain) and emancipation are ascribed, is someone different. This someone different is not of the nature of momentary perceptions. That other, which the Vaināśikas mention in general terms as the perceiver, must also be serving the interest of another, because it behaves like an assemblage. The particular entity, which is beyond momentary perceptions and is not a name only nor an assemblage, is Puruṣa.

(1) The all-embracing mind is coloured with countless Vāsanās. They are the outcome of the latent impressions of feelings derived from countless previous births, which lie stored up in the mind. That mind is working in the interest of another, because it acts conjointly with others. Anything that is not simple or is the outcome of the general action of several forces acting in unison, cannot work in the interest of any one of the forces working together. They serve the interest of a superior director who sets them to work together. Similarly the mind which is the result of the joint action of sentience, activity and retentiveness, *i.e.* of the sentient, mutative and static principles, is the conjoiner and serves the interest of someone else. That someone, for whose enjoyment or liberation the mind acts, is Puruṣa.

The commentator has given several examples of an assemblage. A house is the result of the combination of several parts and is meant for residence, not of its own self, but of someone else. Likewise when the mind is happy, no constituent part of the mind is made happy thereby, but it is the 'I' who is made happy. In the ego there is a meeting of two entities, one the seer and the other, the seen or knowable. The knowable part is the mind, and happiness etc. are states of the mind. This knowable part is being cognised by the other part. From that, the feeling 'I am happy' arises. Thus something different from the happy mind is made happy. Therefore, states of the mind like happiness, misery or peace (*i.e.* liberation) are for the benefit of another or made manifest by another. That other is Puruṣa, the reflector of the mind. The commentator has thus controverted other theories. According to the Sāṁkhya philosophy the enjoyer is something beyond perception and empirical knowledge—an entity which is Consciousness itself. The Knower is not a complex assemblage like knowledge, as He is One without component parts. That is the real Self within our ego, the rest are His objects.

———

विशेषदर्शिन आत्मभावभावनाविनिवृत्तिः ॥ २५ ॥

भाष्यम्—यथा प्रावृषि तृणाङ्कुरस्योद्भेदेन तद्बीजसत्तानुमीयते तथा मोक्षमार्गश्रवणेन यस्य रोमहर्षाश्रुपातौ दृश्येते तत्राप्यस्ति विशेषदर्शनबीजमपवर्गभागीयं कर्माभिनिर्वर्त्तितमित्यनुमीयते। तस्यात्मभावभावना स्वाभाविकी प्रवर्तते, यस्याभावादिदमुक्तं 'स्वभावं मुक्त्वा दोषाद् येषां पूर्वपक्षे रुचिर्भवति अरुचिश्च निर्णये भवति।' तत्रात्मभावभावना कोऽहमासं, कथमहमासं, किंस्विदिदं, कथंस्विदिदं, के भविष्यामः, कथं वा भविष्याम इति। सा तु विशेषदर्शिनो निवर्तते, कुतः? चित्तस्यैष विचित्रः परिणामः, पुरुषस्त्वसत्यामविद्यायां शुद्धश्चित्तधर्मैरपरामृष्ट इति ततोऽस्यात्मभावभावना कुशलस्य निवर्तते इति ॥ २५ ॥

**For One Who Has Realised The Distinctive Entity, i.e. Puruṣa (Mentioned In The Previous Aphorism), Inquiries About The Nature Of His Self Ceases** (1). **25.**

As the existence of seeds is inferred from the sprouting of vegetation in the rainy season, so from the tears falling from the eyes and hair standing on end on the body of a person (due to ecstasy) on hearing about the path of liberation, it is inferred that there is rooted in him the seed of previously acquired distinctive knowledge which leads to liberation. His reflections regarding his own self come about naturally. It has been said about its absence (*i.e.* absence of reflections on self) : "They (those in whom this absence is noticeable) give up pondering on the self, and on account of their defect (arising out of latencies of past actions) are inclined to the opposite view (that there is no after-life and the like) and do not feel disposed to ascertain the truth (relating to the twenty-five ultimate principles) (2)." The reflections regarding the self referred to, are like this : 'Who was I? What is this (body etc.)? How did it come into being? What shall I be and how?' Such queries cease for one who has the distinctive knowledge of the Self, Puruṣa. How do they cease? They are mutative modifications of the mind. If there is no nescience (Avidyā), Puruṣa who is pure, would not be affected by the attributes of the mind. Thus for the spiritually proficient person (one who has attained discriminative enlightenment) inquiry about the Self would disappear.

(1) After having established fully the distinction between the mind and Puruṣa, the author in this Sūtra, in order to explain what liberation is, indicates the type of mind conducive to it.

One who realises the existence of Puruṣa—the 'another' mentioned in the previous Sūtra—ceases pondering on the self. Queries about the self means pondering on matters relating to self. Persons ignorant about Puruṣa, who is beyond the mind, are incapable of resolving such queries. It is stated in the Muṇḍaka Upaniṣad : "For him who has seen the supreme Brahman and the manifest Brahman and is engrossed in their thought, his heart-strings of attachment and bondage are snapped, his doubts are removed and the results of his previous actions are eliminated."

(2) Special distinction (between the mind and Puruṣa) can be realised only if the seed of that knowledge has been carefully nurtured in numerous previous births. This can be conjectured by observing one's inclination towards the philosophy of liberation. If concentration is practised with the aid of that taste (or reverence), energy and carefully cultivated memory, one gains knowledge of the special distinction. After the Puruṣa-principle is realised, it becomes clear through discriminative enlightenment that the ordinary conceptions about the self are but modifications of the mind and that the mind appears to be related to Puruṣa on account of nescience. Therefore, all queries about the self cease and nothing remains obscure about it. 'What I am' and 'what I am not' become perfectly clear. Of course, in the initial stage misgivings about the self are allayed by true knowledge derived through inference and from the study of scriptures. Once the truths are realised through concentration, the doubts cease for ever.

———

तदा विवेकनिम्नङ्कैवल्यप्राग्भारञ्चित्तम् ॥ २६॥

भाष्यम्—तदानीं यदस्य चित्तं विषयप्राग्भारम् अज्ञाननिम्नमासीत्तदस्यान्यथा भवति, कैवल्यप्राग्भारं विवेकजज्ञाननिम्नमिति ॥ २६ ॥

**(Then) The Mind Inclines Towards Discriminative Knowledge And Naturally Gravitates Towards The State Of Liberation (1). 26.**

At that time (when it is filled with knowledge of the special distinction) the mind of the devotee, which was so long occupied with the experience of objects of senses and roaming along paths of ignorance, takes a different turn. Then it directs itself towards liberation and moves in the path of discriminative knowledge.

(1) When through a knowledge of the special distinction self-questionings cease, the mind starts flowing along the channel of discriminative knowledge. The flow terminates in liberation. When a canal inclining downwards terminates at the foot of a mound, the water flowing in that channel disappears on being sucked in under the mound. Similarly, the mind flowing downwards along the channel of discrimination disappears on reaching the foot of the mound of liberation.

———

तच्छिद्रेषु प्रत्ययान्तराणि संस्कारेभ्यः ॥ २७ ॥

भाष्यम्—प्रत्ययविवेकनिम्नस्य सत्त्वपुरुषान्यताख्यातिमात्रप्रवाहिणश्चित्तस्य तच्छिद्रेषु प्रत्ययान्तराणि अस्मीति वा ममेति वा जानामीति वा न जानामीति वा, कुतः ? क्षीयमाणबीजेभ्यः पूर्वसंस्कारेभ्य इति ॥ २७ ॥

**Through Its Breaches (i.e. Breaks In Discriminative Knowledge) Arise Other Fluctuations Of The Mind Due To (Residual) Latent Impressions. 27.**

In a mind full of discriminative knowledge, such thoughts as 'I' and 'mine', 'I am knowing' or 'I am not knowing', arise through breaks in that knowledge. Where do these come from ? From previous latent impressions which are being eliminated (1).

(1) On the attainment of discriminative enlightenment, the mind treads primarily the path of discrimination, yet other modifications born of nescience arise therein at times until the latencies are completely attenuated through attainment of the ultimate stage of enlightenment. All latent impressions born of nescience do not die out as soon as discriminative knowledge is acquired, but they are gradually thinned. From the residual latent impressions of wrong cognition which still linger, modifications born of nescience arise occasionally.

---

हानमेषां क्लेशवदुक्तम् ॥ २८ ॥

भाष्यम्—यथा क्लेशा दग्धवीजभावा न प्ररोहसमर्था भवन्ति तथा ज्ञानाग्निना दग्धवीजभावः पूर्वसंस्कारो न प्रत्ययप्रसूर्भवति। ज्ञानसंस्कारास्तु चित्ताधिकारसमाप्तिमनुशेरते इति न चिन्त्यन्ते ॥ २८ ॥

**It Has Been Said That Their Removal (i.e. Of Fluctuations) Follows The Same Process As The Removal Of Afflictions. 28.**

Kleśas burnt as roasted seeds become unproductive; similarly latencies burnt out by the fire of (true) knowledge, do not cause any fluctuation of the mind, *i.e.* they do not emerge into a state of knowledge. The latent impressions of (true) knowledge, however, wait for the termination of the functioning of the mind (*i.e.* they automatically die out when the mind ceases to act), and no special effort is necessary for this (1).

(1) The emergence of disturbing fluctuations fully ceases only when both contra-discriminative modifications and latencics thereof are destroyed. When the mind inclines to discriminative knowledge, nescience etc. become infructuous like roasted seeds. Further accumulation of afflictive latencies cannot take place as they are overpowered by discriminative knowledge as soon as they are formed (see II.26). But even then the undestroyed latent impressions give rise to contra-discriminative modifications such as, 'I', 'mine', etc. To stop that, the latent impressions responsible for such modifications have to be rendered infructuous. This

can be done through latent impressions of the ultimate insight which is the highest form of knowledge.

Latent impressions of the sevenfold ultimate stage of knowledge (see II.27) such as 'I have come to know all the knowables, there is nothing more to know,' etc. render infructuous the latent impressions of contra-discriminative knowledge. When no more contra-discriminative knowledge is gathered through fresh actions or through impressions of previous actions, it can be held that all grounds for formation of fluctuations have been destroyed. When causes of fluctuations are destroyed, the fluctuations cannot rise again. Cognition or modification is a function or manifestation of the mind. When cognition ceases altogether and there is no more chance of its resurgence, the mind ceases to exist as such, *i.e.* gets dissolved. That is the end of the play of the Guṇas—the three constituent principles. Thus do latent impressions of knowledge terminate the activities of the mind. Therefore, for the permanent disappearance of the mind, no means other than gathering latent impressions of knowledge need be thought of. If the functioning of the mind can be stopped by one's becoming averse to all its actions, then the mind will cease to work, or disappear. According to the Sāṁkhya philosophy mind does not then become non-esse, but merges into its causal substance and remains there unmanifest. Everything undergoes change through adequate cause. Cause in the form of knowledge destroys nescience. Mind similarly reverts from the manifest to the unmanifest state but does not become non-existent.

———

प्रसंख्यानेऽप्यकुसीदस्य सर्वथा विवेकख्यातेर्धर्ममेघस्समाधिः ॥ २६ ॥

भाष्यम्—यदायं ब्राह्मणः प्रसंख्यानेऽप्यकुसीदः—ततोऽपि न किञ्चित्प्रार्थयते, तत्रापि विरक्तस्य सर्वथा विवेकख्यातिरेव भवतीति संस्कारबीजक्षयान्नास्य प्रत्ययान्तराण्युत्पद्यन्ते । तदास्य धर्ममेघो नाम समाधिर्भवति ॥ २६ ॥

**When One Becomes Disinterested Even In Omniscience One Attains Perpetual Discriminative Enlightenment From Which Ensues The Concentration Known As Dharmamegha (Virtue-Pouring Cloud). 29.**

When the discriminating Yogin is disintersted even in Prasaṁkhyāna (1), *viz.* omniscience, *i.e.* does not want anything therefrom, he attains perpetual discriminative enlightenment. Thus on account of the destruction of the seeds of latent impressions, no other cognition arises in his mind. He then attains the concentration called Dharmamegha (cloud that pours virtue).

(1) Prasaṁkhyāna here means omniscience resulting from knowledge of discernment (see III.54). When the Yogin who has realised Brahman becomes indifferent even to omniscience, perpetual discriminative enlightenment prevails and the Samādhi that follows is called the Samādhi of the highest knowledge. It is so called because it renders easy the realisation of the Self, and because it keeps the mind fully saturated in that cognition it is known as virtue-pouring cloud. As cloud pours rain so this Samādhi pours the highest virtue, *i.e.* success is then attained without effort. That concentration is the highest achievement through devotional practice and constitutes perpetual discriminative enlightenment. It marks complete stoppage of all activities.

———

ततः क्लेशकर्मनिवृत्तिः ॥ ३० ॥

भाष्यम्—तल्लाभादविद्यादयः क्लेशाः समूलकाषं कषिता भवन्ति, कुशलाकुशलाश्च कर्माशयाः समूलघातं हता भवन्ति। क्लेशकर्मनिवृत्तौ जीवन्नेव विद्वान् विमुक्तो भवति, कस्मात्, यस्माद् विपर्य्ययो भवस्य कारणं, न हि क्षीणविपर्य्ययः कश्चित् केनचित् क्वचिज्जातो दृश्यत इति ॥ ३० ॥

**From That Afflictions And Actions Cease. 30.**

On attainment of that, afflictions arising out of nescience are uprooted and all Karmāśayas of virtuous and vicious actions are eradicated. On the cessation of those afflictive actions, the enlightened person is liberated even in his lifetime. Erroneous knowledge being the cause of rebirth, no one with attenuated nescience (*i.e.* nescience reduced to an unproductive state) is born again (1).

(1) When through Dharmamegha concentration, the Yogin is freed from afflictions and consequent actions, he is called Jīvanmukta, *i.e.* liberated though alive. Such proficient Yogin does not do anything, nor does he assume any corporeal form under the influence of previous latent impressions. If he does anything, he does it with a Nirmāṇa-chitta (constructed mind).

Yogins who have acquired discriminative enlightenment but have not fully attained an arrested state of mind can also be regarded as Jīvan-mukta. They continue to have bodily existence on account of residual latent impressions. They do not perform any new act but only wait for the disappearance of all latent impressions. They attain liberation on the cessation of those latencies which go out like a lamp without supply of fresh oil.

The word 'Mukti' means freedom from sorrows. He who can, at will, detach himself from his knowing faculty, is not touched by the miseries which exist only in the mind. The cycle of births of which nescience is the cause and which is responsible for all miseries comes to a stop in his case. It is impossible for a person who has acquired discriminative knowledge to be born again. Those who have been born are all (more or less) deluded. One who is free from delusion is not known to have been reborn.

According to the Sāṁkhya philosophy, a Jīvanmukta is one who has attained the highest stage of devotional practice. One who is not the least perturbed even by the severest sufferings, can be regarded as free from sorrow.

———

तदा सर्वावरणमलापेतस्य ज्ञानस्यानन्त्याज्ज्ञेयमल्पम् ॥ ३१ ॥

भाष्यम्—सर्वैः क्लेशकर्मावरणैर्विमुक्तस्य ज्ञानस्यानन्त्यं भवति। आवरकेण तमसाभिभूतमावृतज्ञानसत्त्वं क्वचिदेव रजसा प्रवर्तितमुद्घाटितं ग्रहणसमर्थं भवति। तत्र यदा सर्वैरावरणमलैरपगतमलं भवति तदा भवत्यस्यानन्त्यं ज्ञानस्यानन्त्याज्ज्ञेय-मल्पं सम्पद्यते, यथा आकाशे खद्योतः। यत्रेदमुक्तम् 'अन्धो मणिमविध्यत् तमनङ्गुलिरावयत्। अग्रीवस्तं प्रत्यमुञ्चत् तमजिह्वोऽभ्यपूजयद्' इति ॥ ३१ ॥

**Then On Account Of The Infinitude Of Knowledge, Freed From The Cover Of All Impurities, The Knowables Appear As Few. 31.**

Knowledge freed from the coating of all afflictions and actions, becomes limitless. Infinite knowledge (which is Sattva) gets covered by Tamas when overpowered by it but, sometimes, becomes capable of comprehension when uncovered by Rajas. When the mind-stuff is freed from all the impurities which cover it, knowledge becomes unlimited and the knowables become few like fireflies in the sky (1).

It has been said (to explain why rebirth does not take place after the afflictions have been uprooted) that (such a thing would be as absurd as) 'a blind man piercing pearls, a fingerless person stringing them, a person without a neck wearing the string, and a person without tongue praising it.'

(1) Rajas and Tamas are the coverings on knowledge, *i.e.* on Sattva-principle mutated as Chitta or mind. Restlessness and inertia hinder the full development of knowledge. The power of knowledge becomes inert when the ego is restricted through identification with the body and the organs, the activities of which, again, make it restless. That is why the power of knowledge cannot be fully applied to a knowable. The power of knowledge becomes limitless when perfect calmness is achieved and the ego is freed from its restriction to the body and the organs.

Through Dharmamegha-samādhi such limitless power of knowledge is acquired.

———

ततः कृतार्थानां परिणामक्रमसमाप्तिगुणानाम् ।। ३२ ।।

भाष्यम्—तस्य धर्ममेघस्योदयात्कृतार्थानां गुणानाम्परिणामक्रमः परिसमाप्यते, न हि कृतभोगापवर्गाः परिसमाप्तक्रमाः क्षणमप्यवस्थातुमुत्सहन्ते ।। ३२ ।।

**After The Emergence Of That (Virtue-Pouring Cloud) The Guṇas Having Fulfilled Their Purpose, The Sequence Of Their Mutation Ceases. 32.**

On attainment of that Dharmamegha-samādhi, the Guṇas having fulfilled their purpose, cease to have any further succession of changes. With the fulfilment of their twofold purpose, *viz.* experience and liberation of Puruṣa, and with the cessation of mutations, the Guṇas cannot remain manifest even for a moment (*i.e.* they disappear) (1).

(1) The results of Dharmamegha-samādhi are cessation of afflictions and actions, attainment of the highest development of knowledge, and the termination of the sway of the Guṇas, *i.e.* cessation of the sequence of mutations. Thus the Guṇas fulfil their purpose. All experiences cease for a Yogin who is completely indifferent to the results of his actions, *viz.* birth, longevity and pleasure or pain. By becoming cognizant of the *summum bonum, viz.* Puruṣa-principle, he attains liberation. Liberation ensues with the realisation of all that is attainable by the mind. The Guṇas which manifest themselves as Buddhi etc. fulfil their purpose when a Yogin attains liberation and so sequence of their mutations ceases. This happens because basically both experience and liberation from it are but succession of changes. With the termination of experience and the attainment of liberation, the mutations of the Guṇas disappear immediately. The Guṇas referred to in the aphorism relate to their mutations (*i.e.* Buddhi etc.) also.

———

भाष्यम्—अथ कोऽयं क्रमो नामेति—

क्षणप्रतियोगी परिणामापरान्तनिर्ग्राह्यः क्रमः ॥ ३३ ॥

क्षणानन्तर्य्यात्मा परिणामस्यापरान्तेन अवसानेन गृह्यते क्रमः। न ह्यननुभूतक्रमक्षणा नवस्य पुराणता वस्त्रस्यान्ते भवति। नित्येषु च क्रमो दृष्टः, द्वयी चेयं नित्यता कूटस्थनित्यता परिणामिनित्यता च। तत्र कूटस्थनित्यता पुरुषस्य, परिणामिनित्यता गुणानाम्। यस्मिन् परिणम्यमाने तत्त्वं न विहन्यते तन्नित्यम्। उभयस्य च तत्त्वानभिघातान्नित्यत्वम्। तत्र गुणधर्मेषु बुद्ध्यादिषु परिणामा-

परान्तनिर्ग्राह्यः क्रमो लब्धपर्यवसानः, नित्येषु धर्मिषु गुणेषु अलब्धपर्यवसानः। कूटस्थनित्येषु स्वरूपमात्रप्रतिष्ठेषु मुक्तपुरुषेषु स्वरूपास्तिता क्रमेणैवानुभूयत इति तत्राप्यलब्धपर्यवसानः शब्दपृष्ठेनास्तिक्रियामुपादाय कल्पित इति।

अथास्य संसारस्य स्थित्या गत्या च गुणेषु वर्तमानस्यास्ति क्रमसमाप्तिर्न वेति, अवचनीयमेतत्। कथम्, अस्ति प्रश्न एकान्तवचनीयः, सर्वो जातो मरिष्यति ओं भो इति। अथ सर्वो मृत्वा जनिष्यत इति, विभज्यवचनीयमेतत्, प्रत्युदितख्यातिः क्षीणतृष्णः कुशलो न जनिष्यते इतरस्तु जनिष्यते। तथा मनुष्यजातिः श्रेयसी न वा श्रेयसीत्येवं परिपृष्टे विभज्यवचनीयः प्रश्नः, पशूनुद्दिश्य श्रेयसी, देवानृषींश्चाधिकृत्य नेति। अयन्त्ववचनीयः प्रश्नः,—संसारोऽयमन्तवानथानन्त इति। कुशलस्यास्ति संसारक्रमसमाप्तिर्नेतरस्येति। अन्यतरावधारणेऽदोषस्तस्माद्व्याकरणीय एवायं प्रश्न इति ॥ ३३ ॥

What then is this sequence ?

**What Belongs To The Moments (1) And Is Indicated By The Completion Of A Particular Mutation Is Sequence. 33.**

Krama or sequence is of the nature of incessant flow of moments and is conceived only when a mutation becomes noticeable. A new piece of cloth does not become old unless it has passed through the sequence of moments which has caused its mutation, though not noticeable at the time (2).

This sequence of change is noticeable even in eternal entities. Eternalness is of two kinds—(a) immutably eternal and (b) mutably eternal. Of these, Puruṣa's eternalness falls in the first category, while the eternalness of the Guṇas falls into the second. That of which the essence is not destroyed even when it is mutating is called eternal (3).

Since the essence of both Puruṣa and the Guṇas is never disturbed, they are eternal. Sequence in respect of the modifications of the Guṇas, like Buddhi etc., which is noticeable after a complete mutation, comes to an end. But in the Guṇas, which are eternal, sequence never terminates. The existence of the liberated souls abiding in their own eternal immutable selves is conceived as a sequence; therefore, in their case also sequence does not cease. Such sequence is based on a semantic concept of time (as 'They were', 'They are' and 'They will be').

Is there or is there not an end to the sequence of mutation of the phenomenal world based on the Guṇas and manifest in the flow of creation and destruction? This question is unanswerable. There is a class of questions to which a straightforward answer can be given. 'Will all creatures who are born die?'—is an example of such a question. 'Yes' can be a reply to that question. But the question: 'Will all dead persons be born again?' can be answered only after analysis in this way: 'Persons who have attained discriminative enlightenment and whose desires have been attenuated will not be born again, others will.' Similarly, the question: 'Is mankind good?' can be answered in a comparative form, *e.g.* mankind is better than animals, but not better than the Devas and the Ṛṣis. The question: 'Does the cycle of births terminate in case of all persons?' cannot be answered categorically. It has to be split up and then answered: 'The sequence of births terminates in the case of liberated persons but not in case of others.' Of the two parts of the answer, each is established independently, hence such question is to be analysed and then answered.

(1) 'What belongs to the moments' means that which has the sequence of moments as its locus and stays there as the located, hence the momentary sequence is the continuity of momentary entities. These sequences are noticed on the termination of the changes. The flow of sequence in the mutation of attributes has no beginning. When through Yoga Buddhi disappears, the sequence of its mutation also ceases, but action in Rajas does not cease. With the cessation of the cause (*i.e.* witnessing by Puruṣa), Buddhi etc. cease to exist as such.

(2) This sequence is ordinarily inferred from the gross result as, being momentary, it is not perceptible. It is, however, directly revealed to an enlightened Yogin. There is no sequence of moments of time as

such, because time is a mere abstraction and has no plurality. Moments are distinguished as anterior and posterior on the basis of the change in characteristic of an entity. Therefore, sequence relates to mutations and not to moments of time. Sequence of moments implies mutation lasting for a moment and that is its minutest form.

Moments during which sequence of mutations has not occurred cannot be associated with the change of a new object into an old one. An object turning old is always associated with a perceptible sequence of moments, *i.e.* oldness of a thing is the end result of momentary mutations.

(3) The essence of Puruṣa and the Guṇas is never destroyed. That is why they are eternal. Though the Guṇas mutate their essential nature is never changed or destroyed. The three Guṇas are, therefore, called mutably eternal, while Puruṣa is immutably so. Yet we say that a liberated being or Puruṣa will continue to remain liberated for ever. In doing so, we conceive an entity which is beyond time by applying to it the concept of time because concept of mutation is unavoidably linked to our thinking process. That is why when we say that a liberated self-realised person will continue to exist for ever, we imagine that his existence will continue from moment to moment. An entity or principle which, in reality, does not mutate and to which mutation is imputed merely to signify its existence (in such words as 'was', 'is' and 'will be') is immutably eternal.

The Guṇas are changeably eternal. Therefore, their mutability never comes to an end ; but in the various evolutes like Buddhi through which the Guṇas manifest themselves, the sequence of moments comes to an end. Buddhi and other evolutes come into existence for serving as object of Puruṣa,and they go on changing on account of the mutable nature of their material cause—the three Guṇas. The real nature of Buddhi consists in mutation of the Guṇas witnessed by Puruṣa and is sometimes limited, sometimes unlimited. Unless witnessed by Puruṣa, the evolutes such as Buddhi stop functioning and merge in their causal substance. The natural mutation of the three Guṇas, however, continue and is experienced by other persons who are still in bondage, as knowledge and its objects. For liberated persons the Guṇas are without any purpose and so cease to function completely.

The absolute Knower, or Puruṣa, is immutably eternal. Any change attributed to Him is thus only a mental construct without any basis in reality. However, in common parlance, His eternal existence has to be described in words like 'was,' 'is,' and 'will be for ever'. But this is only an inadequate verbal description and has no bearing on the immutably eternal nature of Puruṣa.

---

भाष्यम्—गुणाधिकारक्रमसमाप्तौ कैवल्यमुक्तं तत्स्वरूपमवधार्यते—

पुरुषार्थशून्यानां गुणानां प्रतिप्रसवः कैवल्यं स्वरूपप्रतिष्ठा वा चितिशक्तिरिति ॥ ३४ ॥

कृतभोगापवर्गाणां पुरुषार्थशून्यानां यः प्रतिप्रसवः कार्यकारणात्मनां गुणानां तत् कैवल्यम्। स्वरूपप्रतिष्ठा पुनर्बुद्धिसत्त्वाऽनभिसम्बन्धात् पुरुषस्य चितिशक्तिरेव केवला, तस्याः सदा तथैवावस्थानं कैवल्यमिति ॥ ३४ ॥

इति श्रीपातञ्जले योगशास्त्रे सांख्यप्रवचने वैयासिके कैवल्यपादश्चतुर्थः।

It has been stated before that on the termination of the sway of the Guṇas, the state of liberation or the state of the Self-in-Itself is attained. Now the nature of that state is being determined.

**The State Of The Self-In-Itself Or Liberation Is Realised When The Guṇas (Having Provided For The Experience And Liberation Of Puruṣa) Are Without Any Objective To Fulfil And Disappear Into Their Causal Substance. In Other Words, It Is Absolute Consciousness Established In Its Own Self. 34.**

Kaivalya or liberation (of Puruṣa) is the state of permanent cessation of the Guṇas which work as cause and effect (1), and after having brought about experience and liberation (Apavarga), have no further service to render to Puruṣa*. In other words, Kaivalya is the state which is reached when

*There is a distinction between Apavarga and Kaivalya although both have been referred to as liberation. While Apavarga denotes the state of liberation in relation to the knowables [vide II.18(6)], Kaivalya denotes the same state in relation to Puruṣa (vide II.25).

the supreme Consciousness is established in Its own self, *i.e.* when It is unrelated to or unconcerned with Buddhi, and remains all alone for all time.

(Here concludes the chapter on the Self-in-Itself or Liberation which is the fourth part of the comments of Vyāsa known as the Sāṁkhya-pravachana on the Yoga-philosophy of Patañjali.)

(1) Guṇas working as cause and effect = The constituent principles becoming manifest as Mahaṭ or Buddhi and further mutations thereof in the shape of Liṅga-śarīra (sense-organs, organs of action and the Prāṇas). Through practice of Yoga, the Yogin's own organs of reception cease to function, but not so the objective world. The termination of the sequence of changes of the organs of reception is the cessation of their function, which is Kaivalya of Puruṣa.

From the point of view of absolute Consciousness established in Itself, Kaivalya is Its aloofness from everything else, *i.e.* It remains only as Consciousness, unrelated to Buddhi. 'Cessation of functioning of the Guṇas' refers to Buddhi's disappearance without subsequent resurgence. When Buddhi disappears Puruṣa remains alone for ever ; that is the state of liberation. We perceive objects either through our senses or from our feelings and then think of them with the help of words. But there are concepts which can be expressed in words but which have no corresponding real entities, *e.g.* space, time, void, infinitude, etc. Extension, existence, number, etc. are also words with no basis in reality but are only verbal concepts. This sort of idea (Vikalpa) rooted in words, which cannot be thought of in a concrete form, but is a vague ideation in respect of non-physical thing expressed in words for common use, is called Abhikalpanā or conception. Such conception may or may not be based on reason, and may or may not relate to real things. But the idea of Puruṣa and Prakṛti, or in other words, the metempiric Self and the constituent principle of the objective world has to be understood by cogent anticipatory conception since these cannot be thought of in any concrete form. In the Upaniṣads it is said that He is to be conceived in the heart of hearts by a subtle intellect with a tranquil mind. "He is to be conceived as only existing ; how else can He be realised ? " "He is not the subject of words (*i.e.* cannot ordinarily be described) as He is beyond the perception of the mind." 'Unperceivable', 'unusable', 'unthinkable', etc. are the negative adjectives through which we chiefly understand the Puruṣa-principle. He has to be described as existing and that existence is free from any trace of non-self and is the basis of the common experience of and the essence of non-dual I-sense. To conceive Him in this sort of logical terms is a rational conception. Starting with such rational conception of Puruṣa, one should later forsake even that, that is one should gradually shut out the fluctuations of the mind. This will lead to the direct apprehension of Puruṣa beyond attributes, which is realisation of the Self.

Puruṣa and Prakṛti have to be conceived in the following manner—Puruṣa is the basis of the sentient part of the ego of an individual. He is neither big nor small, and is minuter than the minutest, *i.e.* without any dimension. Puruṣa is the Consciousness of one's own self, *i.e.* one's Self in Its totality, and is, therefore, absolutely indivisible, distinct, that is without any admixture and is unitary. To imagine that He is existing somewhere will involve cognition of some external knowable object and will not be conducive to the conception of Puruṣa. Prakṛti, like Puruṣa, is minuter than the minutest in the matter of dimension, yet it constitutes the entire objective world. Although without dimension and any specific habitat , Prakṛti, being made up of the three Guṇas, is capable of infinite changes. Mutations of Prakṛti, which are subject to being witnessed by Puruṣa, are innumerable for each Puruṣa. Manifestation of Mahat in the form of pure I-sense takes place when there is predominance of the sentient character (Sattva) of Prakṛti. Although beyond space, Mahat is not free from the influence of time, because it mutates further into I-sense (Ahaṁkāra) etc. As soon as the I-sense is realised it is converted into latent impression by the operation of the principle of retentiveness. There being innumerable such latencies or Saṁskāras, the existence of 'I' from time without a beginning is apperceived and knowledge of its spatial extent is also gained by referring to the smallness or greatness of the knowable with which it is identified.

(Here concludes the annotations by Śrīmat Swāmī Hariharānanda Āraṇya on Vyāsa's comments on Yoga-philosophy.)

# APPENDIX

# APPENDIX A

# JÑĀNA-YOGA

## Or

## PRACTICE OF YOGA THROUGH SELF-CONSCIOUSNESS*

यच्छेद् वाङ्मनसी प्राज्ञस्तद् यच्छेज् ज्ञान आत्मनि ।
ज्ञानमात्मनि महति नियच्छेत् तद् यच्छेच्छान्त आत्मनि ॥

(The following translation of an article on Jñāna-yoga by the revered Āchārya Swāmiji suffers, of course, from the imperfections that result from the absence of exact equivalents of Sanskrit terms. It is hoped, however, that the candid reader will be able to supply what is lacking and to give precision to what is vague or obscure by a reference to the foregoing work. It sums up the experience of one who is a practical Sāṁkhya-yogin and not merely an academic student of the system. A free rendering of it is given below along with a paraphrase of the verse in the Kaṭhopaniṣad which forms the text of the dissertation.)

"The wise man, by inhibiting speech or ideation by language, should retreat to and stay speechless at the speech centre of the brain or mind. Then by inhibiting the conative impulses he should stay (by thus quieting involuntary and voluntary activities of the mind) in the (remaining) cognitive element—the knowing Self or I-know-feeling. Quieting next (by practice) the effort involved in knowing he should merge in the Great Self or pure I-sense which is knowing *par excellence.* After that by abolishing all phenomenal knowing he should realise the metempiric Self."

He is wise who after laying to heart the instruction imparted by a preceptor, reflects on it and thus acquires an abiding insight into reality. It is assumed that he has already abstained from those overt acts wherein desires and resolutions usually express themselves. But physical composure, the preliminary step, is not completed by such abstention, as all ordinary thinking and not merely willing is done with the aid of words and so involves some movement of the organ of speech. This has to be

*Translated by J. Ghosh M.A., Ph.D.

inhibited, therefore, by a grim resolution to renounce all longing for objects external to him, to abjure all forms of activity and even the futile processes of thought that have their origin in ignorance or misapprehension. When the resolution is effective, there is a sense of relaxation in all the organs of voluntary activity due to the disappearance of their functional tone or readiness to energise, and, above all, a stiffness like that of inanimate objects is experienced in the organ of speech. This is the first stage in Jñāna-yoga and is technically known as resolution of speech into the will. If difficulty is experienced at the outset in thus inhibiting speech, the neophyte should mentally repeat without intermission the sacred syllable OM and thus shut out all other thoughts and their expressions.

After practice has perfected the habit of keeping them out of the mind, the resolution to exclude them vanishes as being needless. There remains then the consciousness of external reality attended by a more or less distinct consciousness of the Ego as apprehending it. For, with the disappearance of desires and resolutions and their verbal accompaniments, attention comes naturally to be focussed on the Ego and the mental processes that are felt to belong to it. The Yogin finds it easy and helpful at this stage to conceive the Ego as enthroned in the back of the head and enjoying a comprehensive outlook of the finer mental processes that still continue and of which the afferent nerve-system is regarded as the seat. Here too sustained and strenuous practice is needed for perfection. And when it is attained, all sense-impressions bring to the fore the consciousness of the knower—the Ego, and of its cognising activity. An attempt has to be made now to keep the attention chained to the apperception so that the perceptions that furnish the occasions for it may recede always to the background. The consequent decline in cerebral activity has its counterpart in the feeling that the Ego descends, as it were, to the region of the thorax or has its seat all over the space between it and the brain. Success in this process of concentration completes the second stage of Jñāna-yoga which is technically called the absorption of the Will in the cognising Ego. The Yogin may associate the process at first with the mental repetition of some suitable word (preferably unbroken nasal *m* of OM) though he has to give up this linguistic aid as he advances.

The next step is marked by the disappearance of perceptual consciousness, so that the ego-sense has complete and uninterrupted possession of the field. The Ego is then felt to illuminate or reveal boundless space from its home of light in the region of the heart. There is, of course, no delusion about its nature as an immaterial and, therefore, dimensionless entity, and all that the feeling imparts is that there is no longer any obstacle to its capacity for apprehension as there was so long as the Ego was particularised or limited by the nature of its experience. Still the idea that it radiates light in all directions and reveals whatever may be in them, is foreign to it, suggestive as the idea is, of measure and location. And so the Yogin should give up this adventitious feature as he advances and contemplates it as a self-centred light that is neither here nor there and can be neither more nor less. If he succeeds in the attempt, he experiences an unalloyed joy the like of which cannot be found in any other state in empirical existence. It arises out of the absence of all longings and efforts and is intimately related to the subtle principle of pure self-consciousness. The Yogin lives immersed in it and apart, therefore, from the distraction and uneasiness that are inseparable from ordinary experience. Pain, dislike and fear vanish altogether from his mind, as the objects which might cause them are no longer within his ken. Hence it is unqualified bliss that he enjoys ; and if ever anything likely to disturb or impair it obtrudes on his consciousness, it is transformed at once into a new source of delight by the dominant mood of his mind. Contemplation of this sort is known by the significant name of Viśokā, which means untainted by the slightest measure of pain.

It is possible in its perfection only to those who have not skipped over the earlier forms of concentration. And even they may require at first a verbal symbol like the sacred OM to prevent the mind from flitting to other things, though, as in previous exercises, the mechanical aid of this verbal accompaniment must be dispensed with as soon as practice has confirmed the habit of resting on the object contemplated to the exclusion of all other things This, however, is not the acme of Yogic achievement, for the horizon widens as it is reached, the pure Ego being itself recognised now as an object in spite of its surpassing excellence. A subject, therefore, which is never an object, a Self that never lapses from its intrinsic virtue to be a part of the non-self or an item of experience, has to be sought, for of such an immaculate and changeless Self, the Ego or self of experience is at this stage felt to be a reflection. But feeling is not enough ; analytical enquiry of the highest order is needed for realising the subtle difference between the two with all the certitude and distinctness of perception so that it may never be lost sight of. This is the final stage of Jñāna-yoga, and it may be roughly said to consist of the reflection that what appears as mine like the body or the senses, is not the genuine Self, nor what poses as the recipient of experience but is all the same determined by it, nor again the pure Ego which in spite of its simplicity is yet an appearance. The perfection of this discriminating knowledge has the complete cessation of physical and psychical activity as its natural and necessary outcome on the practical side. And it is in this wise that perpetual cessation of effort and suffering, or the liberation of Puruṣa is effected.

A clear comprehension of what has been just said is hardly possible without direct instruction from an adept. But it may give some idea of the line of progress and of the goal aimed at by the Sāṁkhya-yogin, if taken along with the following observations about the higher principles that have to be visualised.

The Ego is particularised when, owing to association with different aspects of the non-ego, it acquires a definite and, therefore, limited character in keeping with them or regards any of them as belonging to itself. Particularisation of this sort is present, for instance, whenever the Ego is given a local habitation like the body or is regarded as the initiator of any kind of mental or physical activity or as the knower of any form of cognition. The pure Ego has no such attachments and is transformed, therefore, by being related to the psycho-physical apparatus and its various mutations. When, on the other hand, will and effort and also the consequent physical movements are inhibited, the faculty that controls the organs of activity is resolved into the principle that is the passive recipient of impressions, the Ego losing thus some of those accretions which adhere to it in ordinary empirical existence. When, again, its connection is cut off from all sorts of impression including those that originate in the body, it becomes pure self-consciousness or consciousness of the self by the self because everything that is obviously a part of the non-ego has disappeared from the field of vision. But after the Ego has been simplified in this manner by successive steps of discrimination, it stands out clearly as an object of experience itself. We have, indeed, a vague notion always of the combination of heterogeneous elements in it. But we imagine that they are compatible somehow. This Avidyā is the plague-spot in empirical consciousness. But as our insight into reality develops with the aid of the process just described, we clearly discern their incompatibility. And then it becomes impossible to find intellectual or spiritual repose in this complex and shifting principle of pure I-sense. So the earnest seeker after ultimate truth advances necessarily beyond the Ego and finds the ineffable bliss of the Absolute in the subject to which I-sense must be traced or of which it is an imperfect copy.

It has to be observed that the full-fledged mind or organ of empirical consciousness is present in the analytical process up to the apprehension of the pure Ego, and that it visualises the successive stages reached through this analysis. But when the Ego comes to be focussed in its simplicity, the psychical modifications like the perceptive faculty and the will are reduced to their simplest forms, as they converge on what is the subtlest or finest of phenomena. This has been termed, indeed, the Great One in view of its illimitable capacity or potentiality. But it lapses at once into the unmanifest or indiscrete as soon as the other developments of the mind are completely inhibited, for the self must posit itself against a non-self, however vague or shadowy, to be what it is. So this nucleus of empirical existence disappears along with everything else in it, leaving unconditioned Awareness, in whose light they appeared for a time, to shine forth in solitary grandeur.

## APPENDIX B

# TATTVAS AND THEIR REALISATION*

The principles or Tattvas are twenty-five in number. They are the five gross elements (Bhūtas), *viz.* (1) Kṣiti, (2) Ap, (3) Tejas, (4) Vāyu and (5) Ākāśa ; the five subtle monads (Tanmātras), *viz.* (1) smell (Gandha), (2) taste (Rasa), (3) light (Rūpa), (4) thermal (Sparśa) and (5) sound (Śabda) ; the five organs of action, *viz.* (1) vocal organ (Vāk), (2) manual organ (Pāṇi), (3) organ of locomotion (Pāda), (4) excretory organ (Pāyu) and (5) genital organ (Upastha) ; the five sense-organs, *viz.* (1) the auditory sense (Karṇa), (2) the thermal sense (Tvak), (3) the visual sense (Chakṣu), (4) the gustatory sense (Jihvā) and (5) the olfactory sense (Nāsā) ; besides these (6) mind (Manas), (7) the mutative ego (Ahaṁkāra or Asmitā), (8) the pure I-sense (Buddhi-tattva) and (9) Prakṛti or Pradhāna or the three Guṇas which are the ultimate constituent cause of all the above twenty-three principles.

These twenty-four principles and beyond them the absolute Knower or Puruṣa, the efficient cause of all phenomena, make up the twenty-five principles or Tattvas of the Sāṁkhyaites.

We shall now discuss the *modus operandi* of the realisation of the principles or Tattvas as enumerated in the Sāṁkhya philosophy. Dhāraṇā or fixation of mind implies concentrating the mind on any desired object. By practising Dhāraṇā over and over again the mind can, with ease, hold on to one Vṛtti (mental modification) continuously. In the ordinary state, the Vṛtti that arises in the mind at one particular moment, may at the next moment be followed by a different Vṛtti ; thus a flow of diverse mental modifications continues. In Dhāraṇā, however, the flow of transient mental modifications occurs but they tend to be of identical nature, the succeeding Vṛtti being the same as the preceding one. In Dhyāna the same modification seems to stay continuously in the mind for a long time—it is the continuity of the same cognition. Dhāraṇā is like the succession of droplets of water while Dhyāna is continuous like the uninterrupted flow of honey or oil. There is nothing implausible about this—anyone can apprehend it after a little practice. Initially the

*Translated by Dip Kumar Sen

flow of one modification (mind fixed on the desired object) may continue for a brief period only, but by repeated practice its duration can be gradually prolonged. This is an established truism in psychology. The longer the duration of the continuous flow, the deeper grows the knowledge, *i.e.* all other objects recede from the mind and the object contemplated upon remains fixed in it. With continued practice the continuous flow of a single modification becomes so intense that the Yogin becomes completely absorbed, as it were, in the object of contemplation, forgetting even his own self. This is called the state of Samādhi. Getting established in Samādhi is, however, extremely difficult. Very rarely does a person succeed in doing so, because to attain Samādhi one must be totally free from all cravings for material objects and possess extraordinary zeal and knowledge. The expression 'realisation' has been used in this essay to denote the keeping of any object, internal or external, in a state of direct cognition through Samādhi. Realisation of Puruṣa and Prakṛti is, however, of a special kind which cannot be achieved through direct apprehension. To attain it one has to stop the flow of all modifications arising in the mind.

During Samādhi concept of everything except that of the object contemplated upon fades away. The Yogin completely forgets even his bodily existence ; that is why his body becomes like an inanimate object. Total relaxation and effortlessness of the body through Āsana (posture) and Prāṇāyāma (control of breath) are therefore essential for success in Samādhi. When the body becomes perfectly still, sense-organs and organs of action, so long working through the body, work independently of it. In hypnotic clairvoyance, one finds that the hypnotic's power of vision etc. work independently of the seats of the physical organs, when his sense-organs are stilled by the power of the hypnotist. It is therefore easy to understand that when a person becomes established in Samādhi his mind, being quite detached from the body, comes fully under his control and his supernormal power of cognition becomes unimpeded.

We normally concentrate our mind to apprehend any subtle object. In the same way we fix our eyes for visualising any minute object. So on the attainment of Samādhi, the acme of concentration, the knowledge that dawns on the Yogin's mind is the ultimate insight on any object. That is why the author of the Yoga aphorisms has stated : 'Tajjayāt Prajñālokaḥ', III.5. One does not necessarily have to concentrate only on external objects ; one can also fix one's mind on any desirable mental concept or one's own internal organs as long as one likes. The object can thus be distinguished from all others and apprehended in its completeness. One can, in this way, realise the constituent principles underlying the mind, the I-sense, or the organs of the body. Once these are realised, one can develop them to perfection, transforming their basic nature. Thus one can even attain omniscience in the long run.

Let us now examine how Tattvas are realised through concentration. Suppose our object is to realise the Tejas-bhūta. One has now to fix one's eyes on the visual form of a specific object, *e.g.* on the red colour of a flower. Normally the mind is undergoing continual modification. Therefore even when the red colour (of the flower) is kept before one's eyes hundreds of fluctuations may arise in the mind in the course of a few minutes. Besides the usual form, knowledge of other characteristics of the flower would arise and get mixed up in the mind. A material object is one whose various characteristics can be known simultaneously in a blended form. But in Samādhi, with the mind being concentrated only on the red colour, all other perceptible characteristics like sound, touch, etc. will fade away and it would appear as if only the red colour exists. The knowledge of the flower, *i.e.* the knowledge of the diverse perceptible characteristics blended into one, *viz.* the flower, will disappear and the Tejas-bhūta Tattva will be realised. External source emitting continuous sound not being available, one has to concentrate in the first instance on the spontaneous Anāhata-nāda or unstruck sound to realise the sound element. Various types of sound arising out of the internal functioning of the body that are heard, when the mind is calm and no external sound assails the ears, constitute Anāhata-nāda.

Continuous stimulation by an external object is no longer required once a person is established in Samādhi. Then the mind can hold on to the object cognised momentarily and attain concentration thereon. It is like the persistence of a glow within felt by many who shut their eyes after gazing once at the light. Vāyu, Ap, and Kṣiti-bhūtas are also realised in this manner. At the time when any of these is realised, the world appears to be filled with it. This knowledge is superior to ordinary one. In the ordinary process of knowing, the cognition of a characteristic remains for a fleeting moment, while knowledge acquired through Samādhi is retained in a very distinct form for a long time.

The procedure for realisation of the Tanmātras, which come next, is now being described. Let us consider the realisation of Rūpa-tanmātra. If even a minute object is observed with a serene mind and if it is the only item to be cognised to the exclusion of everything else, then it would appear to fill the entire field of vision, because then knowledge of any other object would not exist. When after being hypnotised, the hypnotic gazes at the eyes of the hypnotist, those eyes tend to grow in size as he comes under the spell and ultimately when he is completely hypnotised, those eyes seem to cover his entire field of vision. Same thing occurs at one's own will in Samādhi. Suppose the mind is fixed on a tiny mustard seed, the constituent principle underlying its dark colour (Tejas-bhūta) would first be apprehended. Then the mind will be filled with vivid cognition of its colour, extending over his entire field of vision.

Next, concentrating the mind further, the internal power of vision will have to be focussed on a fraction of that extensive vision. That fraction, in its turn, would then appear to grow and fill the entire field of vision. With the repetition of the process, the power of vision will be progressively calmed. When it will become perfectly still, that is, when there will not be the faintest trace of optical activity, the sense of vision will come to a stop. Cognition of any visual form arises out of the sense-organ of vision being stimulated by some external cause. When the power of vision becomes still and cannot be activated by even the subtlest stimulation, there cannot be any cognition of Rūpa or visual form just as during deep, dreamless sleep, a person completely loses knowledge of all objects, owing to inertness of the sense-organs.

Immediately before the fading out of all knowledge of any of the five Bhūtas, resulting from the quietude of the mind attained through Samādhi, the sense-organs can transmit only the subtlest trace of sensation necessary for cognition. This subtle knowledge of any of the Bhūtas produced by the minutest stimulation and received as such by the mind is Tanmātra of that particular Bhūta. Thus the subtle knowledge received by the mind in the aforesaid manner from the minutest stimulation emanating from the mustard seed is the realisation of the Rūpa-tanmātra. Ordinary light, when subjected to such scrutiny would decompose into seven primary colours like blue, yellow, etc. With greater concentration of the mind in Samādhi, the distinction between different colours like blue, yellow, etc. will vanish because the aggregated sensation produced by them would be perceived in the subtle form as an undiversified single light element.

Any one of the colours like blue, yellow, etc. which is the aggregate of a larger number of subtlest stimulations will produce the sensation of Rūpa-tanmātra (light atom) for a much longer period (compared to that in connection with the realisation of gross Tejas-bhūta), but every one of them will produce a visual sensation of identical nature. Gross stimulations are the aggregate of subtle ones. Rūpa-tanmātra is therefore the basic cause of the gross Tejas-bhūta such as blue, yellow, etc. Tanmātra is also called undiversified (Aviśeṣa) as it is devoid of diversities like blue, yellow, etc. Other Tanmātras like those of sound etc. are also realised in a similar manner. Such subtle states of light, sound, etc. are called the atoms in the Sāṁkhya philosophy. The realised Tanmātra is not spatial; it exists in time only.

Next comes the realisation of the external organs (Indriyas). Just as, after the realisation of the Bhūtas, a person apprehends the Tanmātras by further quietening the corresponding sense-organs, so by relaxing them, *i.e.* making them more receptive to gross stimulation, he can apprehend the Bhūtas again.

During the realisation of the Tanmātras there remains the subtlest form of receptive activity in the respective sense-organs. If that again is made still all knowledge of the external world is shut out. A person is able to realise the sense-organs after he has mastered the art of shutting out knowledge of the external world and also of reviving the cognition of the Tanmātras and the Bhūtas by relaxing the Indriyas (thus increasing their receptivity).

Common people perceive the outer world as full of animate and inanimate objects. This false cognition comes to an end in a person who has directly apprehended the Bhūtas and the Tanmātras. To him the world then appears as an object devoid of all diversities and fit to be merely apprenhended *per se.* He then realises that the cognition of the external objects is due to the stimulation of the sense-organs (by outside agents). If the mind is directed further inward, *i.e.* towards his ego, he can clearly comprehend that the cognition of objects rests entirely on ego, and emanates from the mutation of the ego underlying the various sense-organs. Once the sense-organs become absolutely still, the ego withdraws from them, and with the slackening of the effort to keep them completely inactive the close connection between ego and the respective sense-organs surfaces itself and along with it comes knowledge of the external world. When the Yogins can realise this they can directly apprehend that external organs are permeated by one's ego and all knowledge is due to the specific mutations of that ego.

Meditating further on the Indriyas after directly apprehending them, one perceives that all external organs are similar from the point that they consist essentially of, and rest on, one's ego and that diversities like sound and colour are only differences in the mutations of the ego. The I-sense common to all organs is the sixth undiversified principle called Asmitā or Ahaṁkāra.

When one apprehends that with the withdrawal of the I-sense from it the body becomes completely still as during Samādhi and that the bodily senses reappear as soon as the ego descends on them, one comes to realise that organs of action and the vital Prāṇas have also one common root (base), *viz.* Asmitā. A sentient effortless state is conducive to happiness. One derives supreme happiness from concentration associated with the realisation of the Indriyas. That is called Sānanda-samādhi. When one apprehends through Samādhi that sense-organs, organs of action and the Prāṇas are nothing but specific channels of the ego by which it comes into contact with the external world, one is said to have realised the Indriya-tattva. Proficiency in the realisation that the Indriyas are nothing but evolutes of Asmitā, leads to the direct apprehension of the internal organ, the basic causal principle from which the Indriyas originate. It has been mentioned before that one can specifically realise not merely external objects but also internal states through concentration. Chitta or the internal organ is to be realised by concentrating on the internal state attained after apprehending the Indriyas. It may sound paradoxical that Chitta or the internal organ is to be realised through Chitta itself. To become aware of and to abide in this active I-sense after completely stopping the mental processes like volition etc. is to realise Ahaṁ-tattva (the principle of ego). On the next higher plane lies Buddhi-tattva or Mahat-tattva (the principle of awareness) which is the ultimate 'knower', 'doer' and 'retainer'. It is the I-sense alone which is at the bottom of ego and is the root of all physical and mental activities. By reflecting on I-sense alone one can reach Buddhi-tattva. Vyāsa has quoted Pañchaśikhāchārya as saying: "By reflective meditation on the self or self in its pure atomic (*i.e.* non-spatial) form, there arises the pure knowledge of 'I am'." After direct apprehension of the Indriya-tattva it is realised that 'I' or Buddhi is connected with the organs by ego. The activities of the Indriyas are constantly giving rise to knowledge or making 'I' the knower. If one transfers one's reflective attention from the 'knowables' to the 'knower', one realises the Buddhi-tattva or Mahat-tattva. The pure state of knower or cogniser is the most sentient principle and is the cause of all sentience in the organs. If one achieves control of that pure state through Samādhi one attains omniscience. Knowledge then is not derived through the narrow channels of Indriyas alone as it happens ordinarily. That is why Bhagavān Patañjali has said that the knowables then appear to be few on account of the infinitude of knowledge which is freed from the cover of all impurities. This is the reverse of the ordinary position in which the knowables seem to be innumerable and knowledge limited. Correct understanding of many important Sāṁkhya propositions depends on proper realisation of the exact nature of Mahat-tattva. Although the Mahat-tattva is of the nature of 'I', that 'I' is tempered by the character of the knowables. It is not free from dualism. That is why there may be a sense of all-pervasiveness in the realisation of Mahat since omniscience is concomitant with all-pervasiveness. Veda-vyāsa, the commentator, has described the nature of Mahat thus : 'It is resplendent, like the boundless void,...waveless ocean, placid and limitless.' Those who realise this Mahat-tattva are like Saguṇa-īśvaras (Gods with attributes) and are found in Satyaloka, the highest level of existence according to the Vedas. Prajāpati Hiraṇyagarbha is one such God.

Realisation of Mahat-tattva, among all states related to non-self, makes one enjoy perfect bliss, and is therefore called Viśokā (*i.e.* where all types of miseries are non-existent). It is also called Sāsmita-samādhi. A foretaste of that perfect bliss can be had, even before complete realisation through Samādhi, by converging one's mind to, or contemplating on, Mahat.

How is it possible to realise Mahat-tattva in the extant body with the ego attached to it ? Or if on the complete withdrawal of the ego from the body the I-sense ceases to exist, how does it become possible to apprehend Mahat ? Despite the ego-sense pervading the sense-organ of vision in a general way, if we concentrate in Samādhi on the sense-organ of hearing we receive sensation of sound and not of vision. In the like manner it is possible to realise Mahat-tattva in the extant body by diverting the mind from all feelings of attachment to the body and concentrating it on I-sense alone.

Mahat is mutable since it is constantly undergoing modification into ordinary I-sense or ego, and since its manifestation is stimulated by conditions related to non-self. In the ordinary state of the mind those mutations are excessively gross and assume simultaneously various forms. Even after Mahat is apprehended through Samādhi, its mutation in the subtlest form remains and does not disappear. That mutation serves as a break in the immutable awareness of the absolute Self. The Yogin having identified himself with the inner self in Samādhi becomes completely detached even from the stimulations of the senses which produce omniscience. He then becomes established in the absolute Self, unbounded by space and time, and therefore immutable and stripped of everything related to non-self. And that is Puruṣa-tattva. Puruṣa being the absolute Knower cannot be perceived as a knowable. Hence realisation of Puruṣa is attained in the following manner : 'All mental and physical activities being completely immobilised by supreme renunciation, only the Absolute remained.' Recollection of this experience is the realisation of Puruṣa. The knowledge, acquired through Samādhi, of this distinction between the immutable Self and the mutable Mahat is the highest form of discriminative knowledge (*i.e.* discriminative enlightenment).

Discriminative enlightenment is the highest form of Sattva-modification. Supreme renunciation denotes severance of all connections related to non-self and the effort to do it is the highest form of Rajas-modification. To totally arrest the Chitta as well as the external organs and to remain in that state is Nirodha-samādhi. This is the ultimate form of Tamas-modification. By these three conjoint processes equilibrium of the three Guṇas is attained. The Sāṁkhyaites describe the unmanifest state marked by the equilibrium of the three Guṇas as Prakṛti or the basic cause of the phenomenal world. When one is established in that state wherein the senses become totally inactive and the Chitta ceases to cognise the knowables, one is said to have 'realised' the Prakṛti-tattva. Thus the realisations of Puruṣa and Prakṛti are identical. Puruṣa or Prakṛti is not an object to be directly apprehended. Both of them are to be realised in the aforesaid manner.

Only complete immobilisation of all mental and physical activities does not bring about Kaivalya-mokṣa or liberation for all time to come. There are persons who having attained Sāsmita-samādhi consider Mahat as the ultimate principle and remain absorbed in that state full of bliss and happiness. Later, on discerning the mutative character of Mahat and the knowables, if they practise renunciation, all objects related to non-self become totally non-existent and the three elements forming the internal organ (Antaḥ-karaṇa) *viz.* Mahat, Ahaṁkāra and Manas becoming quiescent, they attain a state similar to that of Kaivalya-mokṣa. But their minds are liable to re-emergence since they have not attained the discriminative knowledge, *i.e.* distinction between Buddhi and the absolute Awareness, Puruṣa. In liberation there is no possibility of re-emergence as that state is attained with the help of discriminative knowledge. When, as a result of the Yogin stopping repeatedly the mental fluctuations by means of supreme renunciation and discriminative knowledge, it becomes natural for Chitta to remain in the arrested state, permanent liberation from all miseries ensues. That is Kaivalya-mokṣa or eternal quiesence. It should be remembered that Kaivalya-mokṣa is far more desirable than the achievement of omniscience and omnipotence.

APPENDIX C

## THE DOCTRINE OF KARMA*

The activities of the body for its sustenance, its span of life, its mutations and its death are directly perceivable phenomena. So are the mental processes such as volition and imagination, feelings of attachment and aversion, and of pleasure and pain. Had all these been due to external causes alone, the natural sciences could have explained them away. But it is a fact established by experience and direct observation that mutations of the body and mind are due as much to internal as to external causes.

Of how many types are these internal causes ? Where are they to be found ? How do they produce the effects ? Do we have any control over them ? If we have any, how is it exercised ? To discuss the nature of these fundamental queries and to furnish answers to them is the subject matter of the doctrine of Karma (action).

One cannot regulate or modify an occurrence unless one knows its cause. Fever is directly experienced by all. But no step to cure it can be taken unless its cause is known. From a study of the doctrine of Karma we come to know of the basic causes of the mutations of our body and mind. We also have evidence to prove that all the experiences of an individual, be it suffering in hell or the attainment of Nirvāṇa, are entirely due to his own actions.

A distinctive feature of the doctrine of Karma is to establish, with cogent reasons, that the law of cause and effect holds good as much in its case as it does in the case of the natural sciences. That is why blind faith or agnosticism or fatalism has no place in it. It should be borne in mind that like the natural sciences, the doctrine of Karma enunciates general laws governing actions and their effects. The physical science gives us the general law that cloud is formed out of water vapour and that rain is produced by clouds. It will, however, be well-nigh impossible to determine exactly how many inches of rainfall a particular spot will have at a particular time. To ascertain this an enquirer will have to take into account and examine so many factors that the exercise will not be worth

*Translated by Tarit Kumar Mukherji

his while. Similarly the doctrine of Karma lays down some general principles from which we can derive sufficient knowledge to enable us to lead a balanced life. The aspirant for Mokṣa (liberation), who has firmly grasped the principles of Karma, can truly control his self and acquire, in the words of the Upaniṣad, the competence of being the 'master of his self'.

## Definition Of Karma

Continuous activities of the mind, the sense-organs, the organs of action and the vital forces of the body, *e.g.* cognition, volition, maintenance of body etc., which bring about their mutations are called Karma. Karma is of two kinds : (a) acts done by an individual out of his own free will or those that he performs being induced by the impulse of some particular organ, there being some amount of resistance on his part to the impulse, and (b) acts done by an individual either unconsciously or being under the complete control of some dominant organ or some exciting cause. Karma of the first kind is called Puruṣakāra. Karma of the second type is called Adṛṣṭaphala Karma (not caused by Karma of present life) and Yadṛchchhā Karma (regulated by chance or fortuitous assemblage of external causes). The act which an individual may or may not perform at a particular moment is Puruṣakāra. On the other hand the activities which are innate within us and which we are destined to perform are Adṛṣṭaphala Karma. Many of our mental activities are Puruṣakāra while most of the actions of the animals fall under the category of Adṛṣṭaphala Karma. Puruṣakāra is the attempt to overcome one's innate tendencies.

Will is the basic or principal Karma. It can arise from cognition of a knowable (in the form of a new cognition or recollection). Desire that is related to definite mental ideation is Saṁkalpa or volition. Will may, in turn, give rise to cognition and Saṁkalpa. All the actions of the body and the different organs are also caused by will. Of them cognition is the association of the mind with the sense-organs. Will, in association with the organs of action and the vital forces, is Kṛti (efferent impulse) that activates the organs of action. The activities of the vital forces in the subconscious or unconscious level also occur in association with the mind as stated in the Upaniṣad : "Kṛti or the efferent impulse reaches the body when excited by the mind."

Since the will of a Yogin can stop the flow of thoughts (cognition, imagination, etc.) arising spontaneously in the mind, they may be said to have been caused by will. Any voluntary will repeatedly translated into action changes into an involuntary one and arises spontaneously in the mind. Automatic activities of the vital forces and organs of action can be stopped by means of Haṭha-yoga by conscious effort. Hence although they are involuntary, yet basically they are not independent of the will. Thus will is the principal Karma. Volition which acts, and to the extent it acts, independently of us, being entirely under the control of Saṁskāras or latencies, is Adṛṣṭa or Bhogabhūta Karma (Karma arising out of previous latencies). Similarly will, which acts (and to the extent it acts) under our control, overcoming the latencies, is Puruṣakāra.

Just as earth is the material of which earthen pots etc. are made, so is will the ingredient of Karma or Karma itself. Will, though continuously being transformed into activity, exists as all living beings do from time without a beginning.

The term Bhoga or experience denotes (a) all involuntary actions, and (b) experience of pleasure and pain. All actions, entirely subservient to Saṁskāras (previous latencies), constitute experience or Bhoga. Although Bhoga is called Karma, it is Puruṣakāra or action prompted by free will that is acknowledged as the principal Karma. All involuntary actions (*e.g.* actions of the heart etc.) are part of the inherent physical functions that commence with birth and are concomitant with experience associated with the fruition of Karma.

The three Guṇas (Sattva, Rajas and Tamas) are always in a state of flux—one overwhelming the other two. This is the root cause of the mutations which the Bhūtas and the organs (both internal and external) constantly undergo. All the organs including the mind are nothing but particular combinations of the three Guṇas. Mutation implies change in those combinations. Inherent mutation not under one's control is called Bhoga or Karma due to previous latencies. The voluntary but compulsive activities which an individual has to perform owing to his physical existence are examples of Bhoga.

With the help of Puruṣakāra an individual can accelerate, control or divert into a different channel this flow of inherent modifications of the faculties. As the line of demarcation between light and darkness is indiscernible, so is it between Puruṣakāra and the innate and involuntary activities, but their extremes are distinct and different.

The aforesaid activities are again of two kinds according to the time taken by them to fructify : (a) activities which are performed and which fructify during the same life and (b) Karma that will fructify in a future life. The latter may belong to the present life or to any previous life.

According as it gives us pleasure or pain, Karma is divided into four kinds : (a) white, (b) black, (c) white-and-black and (d) neither white nor black. Karma that begets happiness is white ; that which produces pain is black ; that which gives us both happiness and misery is white-and-black, and that which leads to neither happiness nor sorrow is neither white nor black.

Karma is further classified under the following heads : (a) fruit bearing Karma, the results of which are already manifest, (b) fresh Karma that are being performed in the present life and (c) accumulated Karma, the results of which have not become manifest.

## Saṁskāra Or Latent Impressions Of Karma

The impression of every act or feeling is retained in our mind by its retentive faculty. Having seen a tree we can go on thinking about it after shutting our eyes. This proves that after looking at an external object (the tree in this case) we can retain its impression in our mind. The impressions of the activities of the hand and other organs of action are similarly retained. The subtle impression of a thing stored up in the mind is its latency. The impressions of all things seen, done or felt are retained as Saṁskāras and it is for this reason that we can recall them later on. The latency of Karma is also usually referred to as Karma.

It is true that certain events or things cannot sometimes be properly recalled, but this is an exception which proves the rule. In cases in which they cannot be properly recalled, there exist reasons for such lapse of memory. The reasons for lapse of memory are : (a) perception or conception not being very keen, (b) lapse of considerable time, (c) change of condition or environment, (d) confused ideation and (e) absence of proper exciting cause. If these causes hampering recollection are absent and if all or any one of the following factors, *viz.* keenness of perception, the intervening period being not very long, like condition of the mind, distinct (especially made clear by Samādhi) cognition, presence of suitable exciting cause, are or is present, all impressions retained in the mind can be recollected.

Like living beings, latencies exist from time without a beginning. They are of two kinds : (a) those which result in recollection alone and (b) those which produce three types of consequences, *viz.* birth, longevity and experience. Saṁskāras by which birth, longevity and experience are given particular shapes and forms, are latencies of past recollection or memory. Latencies which are so modified as to become the force behind the organs, internal and external, leading to manifold activities and modifying more or less the nature of the organs as well, are Trivipāka (capable of producing three consequences). The latencies which result in recollection alone are called Vāsanā. They originate from the feelings of physical existence, span of life and experience (of pleasure and pain). The Trivipāka Saṁskāras are called Karmāśaya. Both Puruṣakāra Karma and Bhogabhūta Karma (Karma not associated with free will) belong to the category of Trivipāka Karma.

### Karmāśaya

All organs, external and internal, have a natural tendency to act. An individual's present actions are to some extent modified by latencies of his previous actions. This latent force behind the organs is Karmāśaya. It is three-fold and is what (a) manifests itself in birth, (b) determines the body's span of life and (c) produces experiences of pleasure and pain. If an individual acts in a certain life according to his previous experience or performs fresh acts, the impressions of both of these go to form the latencies from which follow similar activities. Thus only the power to act is not Karmāśaya ; it is innate in us. In each life, however, this power is modified by latencies of fresh acts and thus the Karmāśaya (potential energy) is formed. If we pour water into a pitcher or a glass, the water takes the shape of the container. Karmāśaya may be likened to water and Vāsanā to the container which gives the ultimate shape to our Karma.

The Trivipāka Karmāśaya manifests itself in a particular birth of an individual with the help of some of the Vāsanās which have accumulated from time without a beginning till that particular birth. Karmāśaya is uni-genital, *i.e.* formed in one life and that too mainly in the life immediately preceding the present one. The latencies of Karma performed in a particular life, being more prominent than those of previous lives, form the seed of the next life. This seed is Karmāśaya. That Karmāśaya is uni-gential is the general rule ; in actual practice, however, some of the active latencies of previous lives may be incorporated in the present Karmāśaya, while some of the latencies of Karma done in that particular life during which the Karmāśaya is formed may, being dissimilar in nature, be left out and remain stored up.

Latent impressions of Karma normally performed by an adult do not fructify in the case of those who die in their childhood. They remain as such and therefore go to form the Karmāśaya for the next birth. This is another exception to the rule that Karmāśaya is uni-genital.

Karmāśaya is the aggregate of manifold latencies of Karma. They may be Puṇya (those attended by pleasurable consequences) or Apuṇya (those leading to painful consequences), or Miśra, *i.e.* mixed (those leading to consequences both pleasurable and painful). Among those latencies some are primary and others secondary and supplementary to them. The dominant Karmāśaya which takes effect first and marks off the broad outlines of the next existence is the primary one. The weaker Karmāśaya which functions as supplementary to the dominant Karmāśaya is the secondary one. Primary or dominant Karmāśaya is formed out of acts repeatedly done or out of the intensity of feelings arising out of them. Other Karmāśayas are secondary ones.

Karmāśaya in its entirety reveals itself at the time of one's death. Immediately before the soul leaves the body, latencies of all Karma done during lifetime flash at once, as it were, across the mind. All primary and secondary latencies appear, at that moment, properly arranged according to their character and strength. Latencies of previous lives which are similar in nature also join the main stream, while some latencies of acts done during that lifetime, being dissimilar in nature, remain subdued. Since they appear simultaneously in a single moment they are formed, as it were, into a lump (the whole and the parts being cognised in one and the same moment). Thus concreted, the latencies form the potential energy or Karmāśaya. Formed immediately before death, this Karmāśaya, or the aggregate of Saṁskāras, becomes, on the dissolution of the existing body, the cause of the construction of a new body conforming to its nature. Thus Karmāśaya becomes the cause of the next birth.

At the time of death cognizance, being withdrawn from external things, is turned entirely inward. And on its being concentrated on internal objects, the individual gets a clear and distinct knowledge of them. Cognition of internal objects means recollection of all past deeds and feelings. During one's lifetime the power of knowledge is limited by the feeling 'I am the body'. With the disappearance of that feeling at the time of death, the power of cognition becomes unlimited. This explains why and how an individual is able to recollect, at the time of finally relinquishing his body, all the events of his life in one and the same moment. One should remember that memory of whatever one is doing now*, will arise in one's mind at the time of death. Vyāsa's commentary on the subject is given in Sūtra 13 of Book II. If latencies of beastly acts predominate in the Karmāśaya, Vāsanā for a beastly life will be revived and the individual will be born a beast. Similarly he will get a celestial or a purgatorial body according as the divine or the evil impul-

*Here the actions include both the mental and the physical activities done conjointly with the mind.

ses predominate in the Karmāśaya. One should therefore remain absorbed as far as practicable in meditation on God and His attributes in order that high and noble impulses may be dominant in the Karmāśaya at the time of one's death.

## Vāsanā

The feelings of pleasure and pain of an individual, like all his actions, leave lasting impressions in his mind. Impressions of the nature of the body he is invested with and its duration are also formed. All these latent impressions are Vāsanā.

We recollect experience of pleasure and pain. The Saṁskāras which give shape to feelings of pleasure and pain are their Vāsanās. Through the activities of the organs of the body latent impression is formed of the indistinct cognition of the shape and nature of those organs as also that of the duration of life. These three types of subliminal imprints are called Vāsanā.

Vāsanā results only in Smṛti (memory). Smṛti shaped by Vāsanā becomes the matrix, out of which through Karmāśaya, evolves fresh Karma and fruits thereof. From our experience of a particular feeling of pleasure emanates Vāsanā for that kind of pleasure. And although it does not create any new object of pleasure it shapes anew a feeling of pleasure quite similar to what was experienced before. Inherent attachment following recollection of that pleasure induces further action.

Vāsanā is of three kinds, being related to birth, span of life, and experience. Vāsanā of experience can again be experience of either pleasure or pain. There is another type of feeling which is neither pleasurable nor painful, *e.g.* feeling of health or of stupefaction. In a healthy state there is no distinct feeling of either pleasure or pain, but the state is desirable to the individual. In an inert state of the mind also there is no feeling of either pleasure or pain, but the state is undesirable. The mould-like impression of all the components of the body is the Vāsanā of birth, while impressions of the duration of the body in each life constitute the Vāsanā of span of life. Vāsanās of pleasurable and painful experiences can be explained in this way : pleasure and pain are the outcome of special types of activities of our body and mind. Such activities are moulded by subliminal imprints or Vāsanās and are cognised as either pleasurable or painful feelings in the conscious level. Imprint may imply either an ordinary impression or a mould-like impression ; it should be borne in mind that Vāsanā is the mould-like imprint of our experiences.

Broadly speaking, Vāsanās relating to birth are of five types : (a) celestial, (b) purgatorial, (c) human, (d) animal and (e) vegetal. If a living being or Jīva is born successively in each of the five classes, his mind comes to cognise in turn the nature and characteristics of all the organs belonging to each particular body. The subliminal mould-like imprint of such cognitions is Vāsanā relating to birth.

Vāsanās relating to span of life may be innumerable ranging from the life-span of Hiraṇyagarbha, the Lord of the universe, to that of a micro-organism which exists for an infinitesimally small period.

As the mind exists from time without a beginning so do the Vāsanās. On account of this they are also countless. It may therefore be taken for granted that Vāsanās relating to all types of existence, longevity and experience exist in the mind of every living being.

Vāsanā is revived by appropriate Karmāśaya. It is with the support of Vāsanā so stimulated that Karmāśaya manifests itself, *i.e.* becomes productive. Vāsanā may be likened to the mould and Karmāśaya to the molten metal poured into it. Alternatively, one may look upon Vāsanā as the channel through which, like water, flows the Karmāśaya.

How is it that a man, because of bestial acts performed in his previous life, is born a beast ? A man is incapable of performing all the activities of an animal body ; he can only perform some of the major bestial acts. The latencies of such acts revive the inner Vāsanā relating to the animal body. With the aid of such Vāsanā Karmāśaya manifests itself in an animal body. Otherwise, the latent impressions of a human body cannot ever produce an animal body.

## Fruits Of Karma

When the latent impression of certain action comes up to the manifest state and begins to fructify, the resultant changes in the body and its organs are regarded as the fruits of that action. Of these, Vāsanā results in moulding of the recollection, and Trivipāka Karma becoming manifest, produces the body, its longevity and the experience of pleasure and pain. As mentioned earlier, some of the fruits of Karma become manifest in the same birth and others in a future birth. A portion of skin if repeatedly rubbed becomes hard and a corn is formed. In other words, the nature of the skin changes owing to the act of rubbing. This is an example of Karma fructifying in the same birth. The fruits of Karma which are prevented from becoming manifest in the present life by fruits of other Karma (which have already started fructifying) are examples of the other type, *i.e.* they become manifest in a future birth.

The external and internal organs of the body originate from their respective underlying forces, the power of cognition is modified by the latency of cognition and the body is maintained by the vital forces pervading all the organs. The organs, the power of cognition and the body that become manifest are but given different shapes and character by the latencies of Karma ; they are not actually 'created'. Like the wind which does not create the cloud but changes its shape continuously, latency of Karma merely transforms and gives shape to the body and its organs when they come into being.

As mentioned before, fruits of Karma or manifestations of the Karma Saṁskāras are of three kinds, *viz.* birth, span of life, and Bhoga or experience of pleasure and pain. Bodies of living beings, with differences in nature and form as determined by the manifestation of different organs, moulded by their Saṁskāras, constitute the fruit of the latency of birth. Span of life means the period of time during which a body exists and experiences pleasure and pain. This is regulated by the latency of longevity or by some external cause. The feelings of pleasure and pain and of stupefaction, which result from corresponding latencies, constitute Bhoga.

It has been mentioned earlier that both Puruṣakāra and Bhogabhūta Karma go to form the Karmāśaya. All efforts for the maintenance of the body, working of the mind without volition and in dreams, and all the activities of a subtle body are examples of Bhogabhūta Karma. The latencies of such actions form Karmāśaya which, in turn, reproduces similar actions.

### Jāti (Birth Or Assuming The Body In A Particular Species)

Jāti or assuming the body in a particular species is mainly the outcome of latencies of Karma which relate to the maintenance of the body and which are not associated with free will. If the quality of Karma of a Jīva is befitting the type of his species, its latencies will produce a similar body in his next birth. But if the Karma is modified by Puruṣakāra or by environment, its latencies will produce a different kind of body. Species are innumerable because of the fact that the worlds of living beings are varied and countless. It is, therefore, possible that innumerable types of living beings inhabit those different and countless worlds.

The body is basically of two types, *viz.* subtle and mundane. Inhabitants of heaven and hell have subtle bodies. The three earthly species of human, animal and vegetal beings have mundane bodies. Tamas Guṇa is predominant in the vegetal while Sattva Guṇa is dominant in the human species. The animal species extend over a wide range, bordering on the vegetal at the lower end and on the human at the higher.

Differences in the development of mind, sense-organs, organs of action and the vital forces (the Prāṇas) account for the difference in the species. The vital forces of the vegetals are the most developed. Among the animals certain organs of action and the lower sense-organs are more developed. In the human species the mind, the vital forces and all other organs are more or less equally developed. The mind and the sense-organs are more developed in subtle bodies.

When the underlying forces of the organs are so modified by the Karmāśaya as to partake of the nature of a particular class of body, the Jīva is born in that species. Latencies of specific acts, integrated in the Karmāśaya, modify and give particular shapes to the different organs. Karma is thus the cause of change from one class of body to another.

From time without a beginning there have been countless mutations of our mind and in the years to come there may be innumerable such mutations. In every mind lie hidden countless mould-like impressions of organs (Vāsanā) and impregnated by the dominant Karmāśaya they manifest themselves in a body akin to them. A block of stone contains material for many types of images that can be carved out of it. Similarly any one of the many types of Liṅgas (dispositions) which exist in our mind as subliminal imprints may manifest itself in a body when revived by an appropriate Karmāśaya. The example of a block of stone is fully applicable in the case of manifestations not experienced before, *e.g.* a person established in Samādhi, or a divine being, but not so much in the case of Vāsanā. A book, on the other hand, is a better illustration of Vāsanā. A closed book containing, say a thousand pages, appears at a first glance as a solid object, but when it is opened two pages of printed matters become visible. Here the opening of the book is the specific external cause. Similarly innumerable Vāsanās lie stored up in our mind, as it were, in a lump, yet each remaining distinct and separate, any one of which may be revived by a suitable Karmāśaya. A mind established in Samādhi is, however, something which could not have been realised in a previous birth (because the person attaining it would not have been born again). As an image has to be carved out of a block of stone by chipping off the superfluous parts, so also has the liberated mind to be attained by discarding the afflictive impediments. Freedom from afflictions is its chief characteristic ; to attain it one has to acquire nothing new, he has only to discard all worldly attachments.

If the organs through which the Karmāśaya reproduces itself be similar to the preceding body, the individual is born in the same species. If, however, a human being makes excessive use of those organs which are dominant in an animal and makes minimum use of the organs which are undeveloped in such animal body, then he is born an animal.

After the dissolution of the material body, the Jīva usually assumes a subtle body for the following reason. In dream as well as in wakefulness one's mind can carry on its activities independently of one's body. Such activities are different from those that activate the body. Mental activities like volition etc. can go on even when the body is inert, and they being entirely mental their latencies produce just after death a subtle body in which the mind predominates.

The subtle body is of two kinds : (i) celestial and (ii) purgatorial. If Sattva Guṇa predominates in the Karmāśaya, the Jīva assumes a subtle body which is pleasurable. That is celestial. Predominance of Tamas Guṇa leads to a purgatorial subtle body which is painful. After having experienced the pre-determined quantum of pleasure or pain in a subtle existence, the Jīva is born again with a material body.

Among the subtle celestial bodies are the Devas of the higher category, who on account of having attained Samādhi do not assume the mundane body. They attain liberation on completion of the residual work of purifying the mind in the course of their subtle existence. For this reason their bodies are described as a combination of Bhoga and Puruṣakāra and not of Bhoga alone.

Unbalanced development of the difierent organs is the reason why a Jīva assumes a body in which he experiences pleasure and pain but has no free will. With some of his organs more dominant than the others, all his activities are performed in complete subordination to those dominant organs, and as explained earlier such activities fall in the category of Bhogabhūta and not of Puruṣakāra.

The mind is dominant in the subtle bodies residing in heaven and hell. It is mentioned in the Śāstras that whenever a will arises in the mind of a celestial being it is at once fulfilled. If one of them wishes, for example, to go to a place a hundred miles away, his subtle body would immediately be there. This does not happen in the case of human beings in whom mental powers and the powers of locomotion are evenly balanced. Even when the desire is there, a man would ponder and may or may not act as he thinks fit. But one with a celestial body being subject to unbalanced mentation (the wish getting fulfilled as soon as it arises in the mind) has no such power to refrain from an act. In accordance with the rule mentioned before, his efforts will be involuntary or Bhoga.

Compared to the celestial or the animal body, the human body is found to possess an evenly balanced set of organs and this enables it to combine both experience and free will.

## Āyus Or Span Of Life

The period during which a body exists and experiences pleasure and pain is called Āyus or span of life. Since Āyus determines the period of time during which the other two fruits of antecedent Karma (*viz.* Jāti and Bhoga) are experienced one may argue that it should be included in them. What, then, is the reason for treating it as a separate item ? We have seen that fruits of Karma follow from the accumulated latencies of such Karma. Latencies of birth result in birth and latencies of acts relating to experience (of pleasure and pain) produce only experience. But whether the body of the Jīva will last for a short or a long duration depends on the latencies of a special kind of Karma relating to Āyus, which is determined at the time of birth. The fruit of such latencies is the span of life.

Span of life of a subtle body may be much longer than that of a mundane body. Manifestation of the latency of sleep marks the end of a subtle body. Mind being dominant in the subtle body, mentation is its life and its end comes as soon as mentation drops below the conscious level, mind becoming inert as in a dreamless sleep.

As already mentioned, Āyus is generally determined at the time of birth. This may, however, be varied by one's subsequent Karma. The practice of Prāṇāyāma etc. prolongs the duration of one's life, while the shortening of the life span is also caused by one's own Karma in that very life. Ignorance or negligence of rules of health leads very often to prolonged sickness. On the other hand, persons suffereing from chronic illness often perform acts which are favourable to long life. These may bear fruit in a future life if prevented from fructifying in the present existence.

A multitude of persons may perish simultaneously in a shipwreck or in an earthquake. A cosmic catastrophe would lead to the death of all living beings on the earth. Such universal destructions have occurred in different ages in the past. Death of large number of persons in a single moment, in the same manner and as a result of the same calamity may make one wonder as to how this happens. We are all living in this universe and as such we are governed by its laws. Our activities are, to some extent, regulated by them. In us lie dormant latencies which may cause all sorts of suffering and all forms of death. Afflictions such as the identification of self with the body, passion, hatred etc., which are the root causes of all our misery and pain, are also ever present in our mind. To give an example, a person dies as a result of his own Karma, but that event will excite the latency of attachment in his parents and cause them misery and suffering. In such cases the feelings of pleasure and pain that are experienced are really the fruits of the individual's own Karma. The only difference is that the latency lying dormant does not fructify by itself unless and until it is excited by a powerful external factor. External factors are obviously not regulated by our Karma.

Discriminative knowledge acquired by Puruṣakāra annihilates latencies of all Karma and the individual can thereby transcend the laws of the universe. When all the fluctuations of the mind are stopped by Samādhi, the knowledge of the universe disappears and the individual is no longer governed by its laws.

Many hold the view that all activities cease for ever once their fruits have been fully experienced. But they fail to realise that the individual continues to perform fresh activities while experiencing the fruits of antecedent latencies. Fresh Karmāśaya and Vāsanā are thus formed which keep the cycle of Karma ever on the move. It is only by stopping all mental fluctuations through Yoga that Karma including its latencies can be totally destroyed.

## Bhoga Or Experience

Experience of feelings of pleasure and pain constitutes the result of latencies of Karma called Bhoga. Events that are desirable produce in us feelings of pleasure and those that are disagreeable give us pain.

Every living being desires happiness. Therefore acquisition of what one desires and being spared from what one detests, are the two causes of pleasure. Its opposites give us pain. Acquisition here means conjunction of the desired object with the I-sense. Such acquisition may be either inborn or manifested later, and may be brought about either by self or by external causes. It is of the first kind when we get what we desire by virtue of our own superior intelligence, discrimination and proper effort ; or fail to do so owing to our imperfect intelligence, error in judgement or wrong effort. It is of the second type when our inherent qualities like godliness, absence of envy, non-injury, etc. inspire feelings of amity, benevolence and the like in others ; or the opposite qualities like envy, violence, etc. induce feelings of hatred, non-co-operation, etc. in others. This explains why some persons are universally liked while others fail to arouse any sympathy in their fellow men.

Adequate power is a prerequisite for fulfilment of one's desires. As mentioned earlier, every effort of the organs is Karma. Every Karma has its latency, and accumulated latencies of Karma repeatedly done become potential energy which enables the individual to do it proficiently. For example, inscribing the alphabet repeatedly makes perfect the art of handwriting. Modifications of the power of organs arising out of Karma are of three kinds, *viz.* Sāttvika, Rājasika and Tāmasika.

Mind being the master of all external organs is superior to them. The sense-organs are superior to the organs of action, which in turn are superior to the vital forces. Excellence of a species varies with the degree of development of the superior sense-organs. The more developed the superior faculties of a Jīva, the subtler is their power of reception. Hence a Jīva born in an advanced species can enjoy greater happiness.

As the states of mind such as wakefulness, dream and (dreamless) sleep, caused by the three Guṇas, move in a cyclic order, so move constantly and cyclically different types of fluctuations of mind caused by the Guṇas. The period of manifestation of Sāttvika fluctuations can be extended and more pleasure derived therefrom by performing many acts of the Sāttvika type. Preponderance of Sāttvika manifestations can be brought about by regular practice ; it cannot be gained at once.

Efforts of the organs of the body engaged in various activities result in feelings of pleasure and pain. Latencies acquired from activities of previous lives also produce such feelings, mostly in an indirect way. Adequate strength to attain what one desires, or the lack of it, stems from such latencies and fresh acts following therefrom produce feelings of pleasure and pain.

If from an event or a circumstance a person experiences pleasure or pain, then only can he be said to have experienced the fruit of Karma and not otherwise. Suppose we remain unmoved when a certain person abuses us, in that case we do not experience the fruit of Karma, only the person who has abused us commits a nefarious act. The fruit of Karma cannot therefore affect one who can rise above feelings of pleasure and pain. If an individual can immobilise all organs including the vital forces by Samādhi, he transcends the other two fruits of Karma as well, *viz.* birth and span of life.

## Virtuous And Vicious Acts

In Yoga-sūtra IV.7, Karma has been divided into four classes according as its fruits are pleasurable and / or painful. They are : (a) black, (b) white, (c) black-and-white and (d) neither black nor white. Black Karma is unalloyed sin or Adharma, and the remaining three are generally called Puṇya Karma or meritorious acts.

Karma that results in excessive pain is black Karma. Karma that produces both pleasure and pain is called black-and-white. White Karma results in great pleasure. And Karma which leads to neither happiness nor sorrow and which goesa gainst the flow of mutation caused by the three Guṇas, is neither black nor white.

The activities which bring prosperity here and hereafter or those which lead to liberation of the soul are Dharma (virtuous acts). This is the accepted definition of Dharma. Of these, acts which are conducive to prosperity here and hereafter are white and black-and-white, and those that lead to Nirvāṇa are neither white nor black. The last named are called Parama Dharma (acme of virtuous acts). It has been said that the realisation of Puruṣa by Yoga is Parama Dharma.

As mentioned in Yoga-sūtra II.3, five-fold false cognition or Avidyā is the root of all our afflictions. From this point of view Karma may be classified under two categories : that which is opposed to Avidyā (and which thereby destroys our afflictions) is Dharma and that which strengthens and maintains Avidyā (thereby adding to our afflictions) is Adharma.

Commendable virtuous practices enjoined by all creeds, if scrutinisd, will be found to be opposed to Avidyā and include (1) devotion to God or to a great soul, (2) redressing others' distress, (3) self-restraint, (4) eschewing passions like anger, attachment etc. Worship brings about calmness of mind. Calmness means getting rid of the fluctuations, *i.e.* weakening the effect of Rajas. This leads to turning inward and gradually cutting off all connections with the phenomenal world for realisation of Self. Constant meditation on God as a repository of all virtues also enables one to imbibe those divine qualities. Relieving others' distress can be brought about by charity, voluntary service, etc. These proceed from self-abnegation and elimination of attachment to wealth and are thus contrary to Avidyā. Anger, attachment, etc. are constituents of Avidyā, and eschewing them amounts to an anti-Avidyā act. So also is self-restraint as it means severing connections with the external world. Thus anti-Avidyā is the one common trait in all acts of Parama Dharma. Manu, the ancient law giver, has thus enumerated the ten fundamental acts of merit : contentment, forgiveness, self-restraint (practice of non-injury by body, mind and speech, is the principal restraint), non-covetousness, cleanliness (physical and mental), subjugation of all organs, clear intellect, Vidyā (self-knowledge), truthfulness and absence of anger.

He who possesses these qualities is said to be established in Dharma and is always happy. But one who is advancing on the path of Dharma, *i.e.* engaged in observing the practices with a view to imbibing them is not happy in all respects. Devotion to God does not find a place in the list probably because Manu considered it as the best means to imbibe all the virtues, or, it may have been included in Vidyā.

Yama, Niyama, compassion and charity have also been designated as acts of merit. Going through the list of Yama and Niyama as given in Yoga-sūtras II.30 and II.32, it is apparent that all of them together with kindness and charity are opposite to Avidyā and lead to one's happiness here and hereafter. Their opposites strengthen and support Avidyā and result in misery and sorrow.

Practices like austerity, meditation on God, non-injury, amity, etc. do not require any external materials for their observance and they do not inflict any harm on others. They are white acts and their outcome is unmixed happiness. Acts like ritual sacrifices, in which doing harm to others is inevitable, produce pleasure mixed with pain. The elements of restraint, charity, etc. in ritual sacrifices constitute Dharma.

According to the Śāstras performance of certain ordinary commonplace acts is supposed to yield exceptional results. For instance, it is stated that if an individual takes a dip at a particular place of pilgrimage he is not reborn. These cannot obviously be true, for they are contrary to the law of cause and effect and in this particular instance it goes against the basic teachings of the Upaniṣads. Some seek to justify them by saying that the law of cause and effect is subservient to the will of God, who is the ultimate dispenser. The correct attitude should be not to take them literally but only as exaggerated eulogies.

Samprajñāta and Asamprajñāta Yogas and all the practices that are conducive to their attainment are neither white nor black. Their performance yields the highest result, *viz.* permanent peace (*i.e.* cessation of all mental fluctuations for all time to come) and for this reason they are called the acme of virtue.

Latencies of the first three kinds of Karma incite our organs and activate them, but latency of Karma of the Yogins, which is neither white nor black, brings about cessation of all activities of the mind and external organs. As explained under Yoga-sūtras I.1 and I.2, Yoga is of two kinds : Samprajñāta and Asamprajñāta. Ordinarily the mind is distraught or stupefied or restless. But if one constantly practises the habit of recollecting one and the same subject, the mind develops the power of remaining fully occupied with it. Such fixity of mind is the state of one-pointedness. The cognition of the principles or Tattvas by direct perception or inference attained in a fluctuating mind, does not last for long owing to the inherently distracting nature of the mind. So long as that disposition remains intact the individual once behaves wisely in an enlightened manner, at other times he acts differently like a person with false cognition. But the wisdom attained by a person with a one-pointed mind remains manifest as long as he wishes it to be so. For in that state the mind acquires the habit of ever remaining fixed on the thing it wants to cognise. Realisation of the Tattvas by the one-pointed mind in which recollection of them has been established is called Samprajñāta-yoga. That Prajñā, which culminates in discriminative knowledge, destroys the latencies of all afflictive Karma in the following manner. Suppose an individual has latency of anger hidden in his mind. Though ordinarily he may realise that anger is a thing to be discarded, yet at times its latency results in emotions of anger. If, however, he cognises in a one-pointed state of mind that anger is fit to be discarded, then that cognition remains permanently ingrained in his mind. That is, if there be any cause of anger, that cognition being immediately recollected will not allow the emotion of anger to be roused. And if that emotion can never become manifest, then it must be admitted that its latency has been destroyed by true knowledge. In this way all evil and harmful latencies are destroyed by Samprajñāta-yoga.

Since sleep is a Tāmasa manifestation of the mind, it makes one oblivious of one's own Self. A Yogin, established in Samprajñāta-yoga, is therefore above both (dreamless) sleep and dream (which is a kind of involuntary thinking). The body, however, needs some rest. This is provided by keeping the body at rest and the mind engaged continuously on recollection of Self. It is said that Lord Buddha used to take rest in this manner for an hour or so. And if they so wish, Yogins can remain without sleep for days together in the state of Nirodha-samādhi.

When all latencies, even those of Samprajñāta-yoga, are destroyed by discriminative enlightenment (Viveka-khyāti) and when by supreme detachment the Yogin does not want cognition of even the pure I-sense to remain, mutation is completely stopped by the cessation of all modifications. That is called Asamprajñāta-yoga. Then the mind merges into the unmanifest and liberation is attained. In the mind wherein the arrested state is firmly established, even the latencies of the Karma which is being done cannot fructify, not to speak of accumulated latencies of previous Karma. As a wheel set in motion keeps on rotating for some time out of its own inertia, so also the Karma of such a person having started fructifying, gradually becomes attenuated and then vanishes for ever.

## Fructification Of Karma—Internal And External Factors

We have so far dealt with the subject of Karma primarily from the point of activities performed by the living being, why and how he acts under the impulse of his past latencies and by exercising his own free will, and how he is affected by their consequences. These are the natural fruits of his Karma. At the root of almost all acts, however, there are both intrinsic and external factors. Activities of living beings may be caused by favourable or unfavourable external events and the environment ; and the feelings of pleasure and pain that are experienced as their consequence are called fruits of Karma caused by external factors. Fruits of Karma are therefore divided into the above two heads. This is explained with the help of the following illustration. Let us take the case of an individual becoming angry. Manifestation of the emotion of anger in accordance with previous latency is a natural fruit of his Karma. Being angry he hurts another person. That is also a natural fruit of Karma. But the reaction he meets with from the person whom he hurts (who may abuse him, beat him up, or even kill him or simply let him go) is an example of consequence of Karma caused by an external factor. It is not a direct fruit of the individual's Karma and is beyond his control. Consequences arising out of the application of social rules and statutory regulations are examples of this type of fruits of Karma. Social rules and penal laws vary from country to country and from age to age. For instance, an act of stealing may be punishable by imprisonment, cutting off the hands of the thief, etc.

Following the rule of cause and effect, three consequences (*viz.* birth, span of life and experience of pleasure and pain) are produced by our Karmāśaya. They are the real and distinct fruits of Karma. It has been shown earlier that external factors activate some of our bodily organs and produce certain results. In some cases the effects caused by the efforts of our organs are influenced and modified by external factors. But the view that all external phenomena are caused by our own Karma and they occur only to enable us to enjoy or suffer their good or bad effects is contrary to the doctrine of Karma. Such a view has no rational basis.

Fruits of Karma caused by external factors are not fully within our control. Feelings of pleasure and pain are cognised by one's 'I'. One part of the 'I' stands for the inner instruments of reception ( the mind, mutative ego, pure I-sense) taken collectively and the other part is the body. It is because of the dual character of the 'I' that we use expressions like, 'I am fat' or 'I am lean' on the one hand, and 'I have a feeling of attachment', 'I am peaceful', 'I am restless', on the other,

The mind in association with appropriate latencies is the root cause of the body. But the body is physically made of the five gross elements. For this reason, just as the mind can control the body, so also its material constituents, the five gross elements, have the power to control and modify it. And because of the existence of the 'I am the body' feeling, external factors, *viz.* the gross elements acting on the body, influence the mind as well. Since the external factors cannot be entirely controlled or modified by an individual, their results are unpredictable.

From the standpoint of an individual's latencies, such consequences are irregular in as much as they are not the natural fruition of Karma. External factors that produce the consequences, however, follow their own law of cause and effect. To cite an example, soil having been washed away from the side of a hillock, a boulder becomes loose and topples down. This is clearly in terms of the laws of nature. A certain person may happen to be underneath the toppling boulder and get knocked down by it. From the point of his latencies, this effect is abnormal. As a result of the accident, he may die or lie bedridden for the rest of his life and prolonged sickness may gradually change his disposition. Chronic, incurable diseases may similarly produce such effects. Effects brought about by external factors are therefore abnormal and irregular.

Sufferings caused by ailments are to a large extent beyond our control. If an individual suffers for not observing the rules of health, his suffering is his own doing. But there are certain ailments which are caused by external factors over which we have no control. Persons leading a pious life may also suffer such ailments. All bodies are prone to disease and decay ; assumption of a mundane body and its continued maintenance is the effect of the affliction called Asmitā. One who has invested himself with a mundane body cannot claim immunity from them, even if one practises virtues like non-injury, truthfulness etc. But a virtuous man with a Sāttvika bent of mind will not be perturbed like the common man.

In order that we may not be unduly disturbed by external factors, we deliberately take certain well thought out measures which are also Karma of the precautionary type. By that, effects caused by external factors may, to some extent, be regulated. Most of us do take some such precautionary measures.

A storm in the sea is not caused by an individual's Karma but the decision to sail or not to sail in such storm lies with him alone. Similarly, the desire to assume the mundane body and to experience concomitant feelings of pleasure and pain undergoing the cycle of births in a world in which almost everything is left to chance, is the result of our own Karma.

From this standpoint it may be said that all our internal and external experiences follow directly or indirectly from our own acts and permanent deliverance from them can also be attained by efforts of our own. That effort is nothing but the practice of Yoga accompanied by a strong Puruṣakāra or free will.

## Application Of The Rules Of Karma

Much, however, remains to be said about the application of the rules mentioned before. A popular conception of fruition of Karma is : 'As we sow, so we reap.' That is, if an individual commits theft, murder, etc. these recoil on him in the same form. The natural fruition of Karma is, however, not so straightforward. This can be apprehended if we examine each of the virtuous and sinful acts enumerated before.

Let us first take up Ahiṁsā (non-injury) and its opposite. Non-injury means not to hurt any living being. By simply not hurting others one does not perform any act as such, one merely refrains from the particular type of act that causes injury to others. Feelings like amity, compassion, non-anger, etc. lie at the root of the practice of non-injury. Latencies of those feelings in the person who practises amity will accumulate and in the long run bring him happiness by inducing reciprocal feelings in others.

One's antecedent Karma is not the only factor responsible for one's being wronged, met with violence or killed. The pigeon often falls a prey to the hawk. This does not mean that the pigeon has committed an act of killing in its previous life. Its weakness and inability to defend itself account for its being overpowered by the hawk. To cite another example, a burglary is committed in the house of a particular person ; from this it does not follow that he committed a similar act of dacoity in his previous life. Amassing of wealth, inadequate security measures etc. are the main reasons for its occurrence Most cases of theft occur because of negligence. Many so called well meaning persons suffer insult and ill treatment because they cannot properly defend themselves.

Lord Buddha observed : 'Those who are shameless, dare-devil, arrogant, roguish and who declaim the good qualities in others live in comfort, while modest, non-attached and wise persons suffer.' How is it that sinners live in comfort and the good and the pious suffer ? In order to understand the significance of the above statement it will be necessary to have a clear idea of the following concepts.

Besides the specific acts of piety constituting it, Dharma in its broad sense includes knowledge, power and detachment. Adharma similarly includes false cognition, lack of power and attachment. Knowledge means right cognition of true things and principles. Power means adequate strength to attain one's desired object. Renunciation implies non-attachment. It is clearly seen that happiness results from these qualities. But all of them are not present at the same time in all persons. For instance, the burglar has adequate physical strength and proper knowledge of the art of stealing. If, on the other hand, lack of power in the form of inadequate physical strength and false cognition in the form of unwariness exist in the householder, he is easily overpowered by the burglar. A person attains his objective in those directions in which his powers are excellently developed. Some person may have mental strength but may lack physical power. This explains why all persons are not happy in all respects.

It has been explained before that owing to the effects of Karma caused by external factors, persons treading the path of virtue (but not as yet established in it) suffer in many cases while others engaged in sinful acts appear to be happy. How then do we justify the well known saying 'Dharma triumphs over everything ?' It is like this. Triumph of Dharma implies its triumph in the psychic sense, *i.e.* triumph over false cognition or Avidyā, which lies at the root of all miseries. From the material standpoint, however, this may mean failure in many respects. For instance, it is not possible for a man treading the path of virtue to triumph over his enemy by killing him in the battlefield. He may also be deprived by others of an inherited kingdom. A person established in virtue will, however, remain unperturbed at such a turn of events. To acquire wealth and power or to lord over others is against his ideal. His aim is to renounce all wealth and worldly power. In the eyes of common people he may appear as a failure but in fact he will remain invincible. Victory means depriving the opponent of his desired object. In this case, his desired object is renunciation and nobody can deprive him of it.

If an individual can combine qualities such as sufficient knowledge, power, devotion to duty, courage, etc. with a desire for enjoyment, hankering after fame and some amount of selfishness, he is likely to win success in the material world and enjoy pleasure for some time. It is not possible to achieve that kind of success by means of unalloyed white (virtuous) acts. But such acts help the individual in eradicating the root cause of all miseries, the consequence of which is permanent elimination of all sorrow. That is the ***summum bonum*** of life for everybody, be he virtuous or vicious. And this proves that Dharma ultimately triumphs.

## APPENDIX D

# COLLECTION OF YOGA APHORISMS

## BOOK I

### ON CONCENTRATION

1. Now then Yoga is being explained.
2. Yoga is the suppression of the modifications of the mind.
3. Then the Seer abides in Itself.
4. At other times the Seer appears to assume the form of the modification of the mind.
5. They (modifications) fall into five varieties, of which some are 'Kliṣṭa' and the rest 'Akliṣṭa'.
6. (They are) Pramāṇa, Viparyaya, Vikalpa, (dreamless) sleep and recollection.
7. (Of these) Perception, inference and testimony (verbal communication) constitute the Pramāṇas.
8. Viparyaya or illusion is false knowledge formed of a thing as other than what it is.
9. The modification called 'Vikalpa' is based on verbal cognition in regard to a thing which does not exist. (It is a kind of useful knowledge arising out of the meaning of a word but having no corresponding reality.)
10. Dreamless sleep is the mental modification produced by the condition of inertia as the state of vacuity or negation (of waking and dreaming).
11. Recollection is mental modification caused by reproduction of the previous impression of an object without adding anything from other sources.
12. By practice and detachment these can be stopped.
13. Exertion to acquire Sthiti or a tranquil state of mind devoid of fluctuations is called practice.
14. That practice when continued for a long time without break and with devotion becomes firm in foundation.
15. When the mind loses all desire for objects seen or described in the

scriptures it acquires a state of utter desirelessness which is called detachment.

16. Indifference to the Guṇas or the constituent principles, achieved through a knowledge of the nature of Puruṣa, is called Para-vairāgya (supreme detachment).
17. When concentration is reached with the help of Vitarka, Vichāra, Ānanda and Asmitā, it is called Samprajñāta-samādhi.
18. Asamprajñāta-samādhi is the other kind of Samādhi which arises through constant practice of Para-vairāgya which brings about the disappearance of all fluctuations of the mind, wherein only the latent impressions remain.
19. While in the case of the Videhas or the discarnates and of the Prakṛtilayas or those subsisting in their elemental constituents, it is caused by nescience which results in objective existence.
20. Others (who follow the path of the prescribed effort) adopt the means of reverential faith, energy, repeated recollection, concentration and real knowledge (and thus attain Asamprajñāta-samādhi).
21. Yogins with intense ardour achieve concentration and the result thereof, quickly.
22. On account of the methods being slow, medium and speedy, even among those Yogins who have intense ardour, there are differences.
23. From special devotion to Īśvara also (concentration becomes imminent).
24. Īśvara is a particular Puruṣa unaffected by affliction, deed, result of action or the latent impressions thereof.
25. In Him the seed of omniscience has reached its utmost development which cannot be exceeded.
26. (He is) The teacher of former teachers because with Him there is no limitation by time (to His omnipotence).
27. The sacred word designating Him is Praṇava or the mystic syllable OM.
28. (Yogins) Repeat it and contemplate upon its meaning.
29. From that comes realisation of the individual self and the obstacles are resolved.
30. Sickness, incompetence, doubt, delusion, sloth, non-abstention, erroneous conception, non-attainment of any Yogic stage, and instability to stay in a Yogic state—these distractions of the mind are the impediments.
31. Sorrow, dejection, restlessness of body, inhalation and exhalation arise from (previous) distractions.

32. For their stoppage (*i.e.* of distractions) practice (of concentration) on a single principle should be made.
33. The mind becomes purified by the cultivation of feelings of amity, compassion, goodwill and indifference respectively towards happy, miserable, virtuous and sinful creatures.
34. By exhaling and restraining the breath also (the mind is calmed).
35. The development of higher objective perceptions called Viṣayavatī also brings about tranquillity of mind.
36. Or by perception which is free from sorrow and is radiant (stability of mind can also be produced).
37. Or (contemplating) on a mind which is free from desires (the devotee's mind gets stabilised).
38. Or by taking as the object of meditation the images of dreams or the state of dreamless sleep (the mind of the Yogin gets stabilised).
39. Or by contemplating on whatsoever thing one may like (the mind becomes stable).
40. When the mind develops the power of stabilising on the smallest size as well as on the greatest one, then the mind comes under control.
41. When the fluctuations of the mind are weakened, the mind appears to take on the features of the object of meditation—whether it be the cogniser (Grahītā), the instrument of cognition (Grahaṇa) or the object cognised (Grāhya)—as does a transparent jewel, and this identification is called Samāpatti or engrossment.
42. The engrossment, in which there is the mixture of word, its meaning (*i.e.* the object) and its knowledge, is known as Savitarkā Samāpatti.
43. When the memory is purified, the mind appears to be devoid of its own nature (*i.e.* of reflective consciousness) and only the object (on which it is contemplating) remains illuminated. This kind of engrossment is called Nirvitarkā Samāpatti.
44. By this (foregoing) the Savichāra and Nirvichāra engrossments, whose objects are subtle, are also explained.
45. Subtlety pertaining to objects culminates in A-liṅga or the unmanifest.
46. These are the only kinds of objective concentrations.
47. On gaining proficiency in Nirvichāra, purity in the inner instruments of cognition is developed.
48. The knowledge that is gained in that state is called Ṛtambharā (filled with truth).
49. (That knowledge) Is different from that derived from testimony or through inference, because it relates to particulars (of objects).

50. The latent impression born of such knowledge is opposed to the formation of other latent impressions.
51. By the stoppage of that too (on account of the elimination of the latent impressions of Samprajñāna) objectless concentration takes place through suppression of all modifications.

## BOOK II

### ON PRACTICE

1. Tapas (austerity or sturdy self-discipline—mental, moral and physical), Svādhyāya (repetition of sacred Mantras or study of sacred literature) and Īśvara-praṇidhāna (complete surrender to God) are Kriyā-yoga (Yoga in the form of action).
2. That Kriyā-yoga (should be practised) for bringing about Samādhi and minimising the Kleśas.
3. Avidyā (misapprehension about the real nature of things), Asmitā (egoism), Rāga (attachment), Dveṣa (aversion) and Abhiniveśa (fear of death) are the five Kleśas (afflictions).
4. Avidyā is the breeding ground for the others whether they be dormant, attenuated, interrupted or active.
5. Avidyā consists in regarding a transient object as everlasting, an impure object as pure, misery as happiness and the non-self as self.
6. Asmitā is tantamount to the identification of Puruṣa or pure Consciousness with Buddhi.
7. Attachment is that (modification) which follows remembrance of pleasure.
8. Aversion is that (modification) which results from misery.
9. As in the ignorant so in the learned, the firmly established inborn fear of annihilation is the affliction called Abhiniveśa.
10. The subtle Kleśas are forsaken (*i.e.* destroyed) by the cessation of productivity (*i.e.* disappearance) of the mind.
11. Their means of subsistence or their gross states are avoidable by meditation.
12. Karmāśaya or latent impression of action based on afflictions, becomes active in this life or in a life to come.
13. As long as Kleśa remains at the root, Karmāśaya produces three consequences in the form of birth, span of life and experience.
14. Because of virtue and vice these (birth, span and experience) produce pleasurable and painful experiences.
15. The discriminating persons apprehend (by analysis and anticipa-

tion) all worldly objects as sorrowful because they cause suffering in consequence, in their afflictive experiences and in their latencies and also because of the contrary nature of the Guṇas (which produces changes all the time).

16. (That is why) Pain which is yet to come is to be discarded.
17. Uniting the Seer or the subject with the seen or the object, is the cause of that which has to be avoided.
18. The object or knowable is by nature sentient, mutable and inert. It exists in the form of the elements and the organs, and serves the purpose of experience and emancipation.
19. Diversified (Viśeṣa), undiversified (Aviśeṣa), indicator-only (Liṅgamātra), and that which is without any indicator (Aliṅga) are the states of the Guṇas.
20. The Seer is absolute Knower. Although pure, modifications (of Buddhi) are witnessed by Him as an onlooker.
21. To serve as objective field to Puruṣa, is the essence or nature of the knowable.
22. Although ceasing to exist in relation to him whose purpose is fulfilled, the knowable does not cease to exist on account of being of use to others.
23. Alliance is the means of realising the true nature of the object of the Knower and of the owner, the Knower (*i.e.* the sort of alliance which contributes to the realisation of the Seer and the seen is this relationship).
24. (The alliance has) Avidyā or nescience as its cause.
25. The absence of alliance that arises from lack of it (Avidyā) is the freedom and that is the state of liberation of the Seer.
26. Clear and distinct (unimpaired) discriminative knowledge is the means of liberation.
27. Seven kinds of ultimate insight come to him (the Yogin who has acquired discriminative enlightenment).
28. Through the practice of the different accessories to Yoga, when impurities are destroyed, there arises enlightenment culminating in discriminative enlightenment.
29. Yama (restraint), Niyama (observance), Āsana (posture), Prāṇāyāma (regulation of breath), Pratyāhāra (withholding of senses), Dhāraṇā (fixity), Dhyāna (meditation) and Samādhi (perfect concentration) are the eight means of attaining Yoga.
30. Ahiṁsā (non-injury), Satya (truth), Asteya (abstention from stealing), Brahmacharya (continence) and Aparigraha (abstinence from avariciousness) are the five Yamas (forms of restraint).

31. These (the restraints), however, become a great vow when they become universal, being unrestricted by any consideration of class, place, time or concept of duty.
32. Cleanliness, contentment, austerity (mental and physical discipline), Svādhyāya (study of scriptures and chanting of Mantras) and devotion to God are the Niyamas (observances).
33. When these restraints and observances are inhibited by perverse thoughts, the opposites should be thought of.
34. Actions arising out of perverse thoughts like injury etc. are either performed by oneself, got done by another or approved ; performed either through anger, greed or delusion ; and can be mild, moderate or intense. That they are the causes of infinite misery and unending ignorance is the contrary thought.
35. As the Yogin becomes established in non-injury, all beings coming near him (the Yogin) cease to be hostile.
36. When truthfulness is achieved, the words (of the Yogin) acquire the power of making them fruitful.
37. When non-stealing is established, all jewels present themselves (to the Yogin).
38. When continence is established, Vīrya is acquired.
39. On attaining perfection in non-acceptance, knowledge of past and future existences arises.
40. From the practice of purification, aversion towards one's own body is developed and thus aversion extends to contact with other bodies.
41. Purification of the mind, pleasantness of feeling, one-pointedness, subjugation of the senses and ability for self-realisation are acquired.
42. From contentment unsurpassed happiness is gained.
43. Through destruction of impurities, practice of austerities brings about perfection of the body and the organs.
44. From study and repetition of the Mantras, communion with the desired deity is established.
45. From devotion to God, Samādhi is attained.
46. Motionless and agreeable form (of staying) is Āsana (Yogic posture).
47. By relaxation of effort and meditation on the infinite (Āsanas are perfected).
48. From that arises immunity from Dvandvas or opposite conditions.
49. That (Āsana) having been perfected, regulation of the flow of inhalation and exhalation is Prāṇāyāma (breath control).
50. That (Prāṇāyāma) has external operation (Vāhya-vṛtti), internal

operation (Ābhyantara-vṛtti) and suppression (Stambha-vṛtti). These, again, when observed according to space, time and number become long and subtle.

51. The fourth Prāṇāyāma transcends external and internal operations.
52. By that the veil over manifestation (of knowledge) is thinned.
53. (Moreover) The mind acquires fitness for Dhāraṇā.
54. When separated from their corresponding objects, the organs follow, as it were, the nature of the mind, that is called Pratyāhāra (restraining of the organs).
55. That brings supreme control of the organs.

## BOOK III

### SUPERNORMAL POWERS

1. Dhāraṇā is the mind's (Chitta's) fixation on a particular point in space.
2. In that (Dhāraṇā) the continuous flow of similar mental modifications is called Dhyāna or meditation.
3. When the object of meditation only shines forth in the mind, as though devoid of the thought of even the self (who is meditating), then that state is called Samādhi or concentration.
4. The three together on the same object is called Saṁyama.
5. By mastering that (Saṁyama), the light of knowledge (Prajñā) dawns.
6. It (Saṁyama) is to be applied to the stages (of practice).
7. These three are more intimate practices than the previously mentioned ones.
8. That also is (to be regarded as) external in respect of Nirvīja or seedless concentration.
9. Suppression of the latencies of fluctuation and appearance of the latencies of arrested state, taking place at every moment of blankness of the arrested state in the same mind, is the mutation of the arrested state of the mind.
10. Continuity of the tranquil mind (in an arrested state) is ensured by its latent impressions.
11. Diminution of attention to all and sundry and development of one-pointedness is called Samādhi-pariṇāma or mutation of the concentrative mind.
12. There (in Samādhi) again (in the state of concentration) the past and the present modifications being similar, it is Ekāgratā-pariṇāma, or mutation of the stabilised state of the mind.

13. By these are explained the three changes, *viz.* of essential attributes or characteristics, of temporal characters, and of states of the Bhūtas and the Indriyas (*i.e.* all the knowable phenomena).
14. That which continues its existence all through the varying characteristics, namely, the quiescent, *i e.* past, the uprisen, *i.e.* present, or unmanifest (but remaining as potent force), *i.e.* future, is the substratum (or object chracterised).
15. Change of sequence (of characteristics) is the cause of mutative differences.
16. Knowledge of the past and the future can be derived through Saṁyama on the three Pariṇāmas (changes).
17. Word, object implied, and the idea thereof overlapping, produce one unified impression. If Saṁyama is practised on each separately, knowledge of the meaning of the sounds produced by all beings can be acquired.
18. By the realisation of latent impressions, knowledge of previous birth is acquired.
19. (By practising Saṁyama) On notions, knowledge of other minds is developed.
20. The prop (or basis) of the notion does not get known because that is not the object of (the Yogin's) observation.
21. When perceptibility of the body is suppressed by practising Saṁyama on its visual character, disappearance of the body is effected through its getting beyond the sphere of perception of the eye.
22. Karma is either fast or slow in fructifying. By practising Saṁyama on Karma or on portents, fore-knowledge of death can be acquired.
23. Through Saṁyama on friendliness (amity) and other similar virtues, strength is obtained therein.
24. (By practising Saṁyama) On (physical) strength, the strength of elephants etc. can be acquired.
25. By applying the effulgent light of the higher sense-perception (Jyotiṣmatī), knowledge of subtle objects, or things obstructed from view, or placed at a great distance, can be acquired.
26. (By practising Saṁyama) On the sun (the point in the body known as the solar entrance) the knowledge of the cosmic regions is acquired.
27. (By practising Saṁyama) On the moon (the lunar entrance) knowledge of the arrangements of stars is acquired.
28. (By practising Saṁyama) On the pole-star, motion of the stars is known.

29. (By practising Saṁyama) On the navel plexus, knowledge of the composition of the body is derived.
30. (By practising Saṁyama) On the trachea, hunger and thirst can be subdued.
31. Calmness is attained by Saṁyama on the bronchial tube.
32. (By practising Saṁyama) On the coronal light, Siddhas can be seen.
33. From knowledge known as Prātibha (intuition), everything becomes known.
34. (By practising Saṁyama) On the heart, knowledge of the mind is acquired.
35. Experience (of pleasure or pain) arises from a conception which does not distinguish between the two extremely different entities, *viz.* Buddhisattva and Puruṣa. Such experience exists for another (*i.e.* Puruṣa). That is why through Saṁyama on Puruṣa (who oversees all experiences and also their complete cessation), a knowledge regarding Puruṣa is acquired.
36. Thence (from the knowledge of Puruṣa) arise Prātibha (prescience), Srāvaṇa (supernormal power of hearing), Vedana (supernormal power of touch), Ādarśa (supernormal power of sight), Āsvāda (supernormal power of taste) and Vārtā (supernormal power of smell).
37. They (these powers) are impediments to Samādhi, but are (regarded as) acquisitions in a normal fluctuating state of the mind.
38. When the cause of bondage gets weakened and the movements of the mind are known, the mind can get into another body.
39. By conquering the vital force (of life) called Udāna, the chance of immersion in water or mud, or entanglement in the thorns, is avoided and exit from the body at will is assured.
40. By conquering the vital force called Samāna, effulgence is acquired.
41. By Saṁyama on the relationship between Ākāśa and the power of hearing, divine sense of hearing is gained.
42. By practising Saṁyama on the relationship between the body and Ākāśa and by concentrating on the lightness of cotton wool, passage through the sky can be secured.
43. When the unimagined conception can be held outside, *i.e.* unconnected with the body, it is called Mahāvideha or the great discarnate. By Saṁyama on that, the veil over illumination (of Buddhisattva) is removed.
44. By Saṁyama on the grossness, the essential character, the subtlety, the inherence and the objectiveness, which are the five forms of the Bhūtas or elements, mastery over Bhūtas is obtained.

45. Thence develop the power of minification and other bodily acquisitions. There is also no resistance by its characteristics.
46. Perfection of body consists in beauty, grace, strength and adamantine hardness.
47. By Saṁyama on the receptivity, essential character, I-sense, inherent quality and objectiveness of the five organs, mastery over them can be acquired.
48. Thence come powers of rapid movement as of the mind, action of organs independent of the body and mastery over Pradhāna, the primordial cause.
49. To one established in the discernment between Buddhi and Puruṣa come supremacy over all beings and omniscience.
50. By renunciation of that (Viśokā attainment) even, comes liberation on account of the destruction of the seeds of evil.
51. When invited by the celestial beings, that invitation should not be accepted nor should it cause vanity because it involves possibility of undesirable consequences.
52. Differentiating knowledge of the self and the non-self comes from practising Saṁyama on moment and its sequence.
53. When species, temporal character and position of two different things being indiscernible they look alike, they can be differentiated thereby (by this knowledge).
54. Knowledge of discernment is Tāraka or intuitional, is comprehensive of all things and of all times, and has no sequence.
55. (Whether secondary discriminative discernment is acquired or not) When equality is established between Buddhisattva and Puruṣa in their purity, liberation takes place.

## BOOK IV

### ON THE SELF-IN-ITSELF OR LIBERATION

1. Supernormal powers come with birth or are attained through herbs, incantations, austerities or concentration.
2. (The mutation of body and organs into those of one born in a different species) Takes place through the filling in of their innate nature.
3. Causes do not put the nature into motion, only the removal of obstacles takes place through them. This is like a farmer breaking down the barrier to let the water flow. (The hindrances being removed by the causes, the nature impenetrates by itself).

4. All created minds are constructed from pure I-sense.
5. One (principal) mind directs the many created minds in the variety of their activities.
6. Of these (minds with supernormal powers) those obtained through meditation are without any subliminal imprints.
7. The actions of Yogins are neither white nor black, whereas the actions of others are of three kinds.
8. Thence (from the other three varieties of Karma) are manifested the subconscious impressions appropriate to their consequences.
9. On account of similarity between memory and corresponding latent impressions, the subconscious impressions of feelings appear simultaneously even when they are separated by birth, space and time.
10. Desire for self-welfare being everlasting, it follows that the subconscious impression from which it arises must be beginningless.
11. On account of being held together by cause, result, refuge and supporting object, Vāsanā disappears when they are absent.
12. The past and the future are in reality present in their fundamental forms, there being only difference in the characteristics of the forms taken at different times.
13. Characteristics, which are present at all times, are manifest and subtle, and are composed of the three Guṇas.
14. On account of the co-ordinated mutation of the three Guṇas, an object appears as a unit.
15. In spite of sameness of objects, on account of there being separate minds they (the object and its knowledge) follow different paths, that is why they are entirely different.
16. Object is not dependent on one mind, because if it were so, then what will happen when it is not cognised by that mind ?
17. External objects are known or unknown to the mind according as they colour the mind.
18. On account of the immutability of Puruṣa who is master of the mind, the modifications of the mind are always known or manifest.
19. It (the mind) is not self-illuminating being an object (knowable).
20. Besides, both (the mind and its objects) cannot be cognised simultaneously.
21. If the mind were to be illumined by another mind then there will be repetition ***ad infinitum*** of illumining minds and intermixture of memory.
22. (Though) Untransmissible, the metempiric Consciousness getting the likeness of Buddhi becomes the cause of the consciousness of Buddhi.

23. The mind-stuff being affected by the Seer and the seen, is all-comprehensive.
24. That (the mind) though variegated by innumerable subconscious impressions, exists for another, since it acts conjointly.
25. For one who has realised the distinctive entity, *i.e.* Puruṣa, inquiries about the nature of his self cease.
26. (Then) The mind inclines towards discriminative knowledge and naturally gravitates towards the state of liberation.
27. Through its breaches (*i.e.* breaks in discriminative knowledge) arise other fluctuations of the mind due to (residual) latent impressions.
28. It has been said that their removal (*i.e.* of fluctuations) follows the same process as the removal of afflictions.
29. When one becomes disinterested even in omniscience one attains perpetual discriminative enlightenment from which ensues the concentration known as Dharmamegha (virtue-pouring cloud).
30. From that, afflictions and actions cease.
31. Then on account of the infinitude of knowledge, freed from the cover of all impurities, the knowables appear as few.
32. After the emergence of that (virtue-pouring cloud) the Guṇas having fulfilled their purpose, the sequence of their mutation ceases.
33. What belongs to the moments and is indicated by the completion of a particular mutation is sequence.
34. The state of the Self-in-Itself or liberation is realised when the Guṇas (having provided for the experience and liberation of Puruṣa) are without any purpose to fulfil and disappear into their causal substance. In other words, it is absolute Consciousness established in Its own Self.

APPENDIX E

## GLOSSARY OF SANSKRIT WORDS

*Note* :—The pronunciation and diacritical marks used are explained below.

| | | | | | |
|---|---|---|---|---|---|
| a | to | be | pronounced | as | *awe* |
| ā | ,, | ,, | ,, | ,, | *ah* |
| ī | ,, | ,, | ,, | ,, | *ee* |
| e | ,, | ,, | ,, | ,, | *eh* |
| ū | ,, | ,, | ,, | ,, | *oo* |
| ch | ,, | ,, | ,, | ,, | in *chosen* |
| chh | ,, | ,, | ,, | ,, | hard—midway between *ch* and *sh*—as in *chaw* |
| ḍ | ,, | ,, | ,, | ,, | *rh* (r hard) |
| ḥ | ,, | ,, | ,, | ,, | *Haw* |
| ṁ / ṅ | ,, | ,, | ,, | ,, | *ong* as in *Song* |
| Jñ | ,, | ,, | ,, | ,, | *gaw* with *g* nasal |
| ṇ | ,, | ,, | ,, | ,, | *naw* as in *gnaw* |
| ṛ | ,, | ,, | ,, | ,, | *rhi* |
| ś or ṣ | ,, | ,, | ,, | ,, | *sh* as in *Shilling* |
| t | ,, | ,, | ,, | ,, | *th* (soft) |
| ṭ | ,, | ,, | ,, | ,, | *Taw* (hard) |
| v | ,, | ,, | ,, | ,, | *wa* |
| y | ,, | ,, | ,, | ,, | *yaw* |

## GLOSSARY

### A

*Abhikalpanā* —Cogent anticipatory conception which is necessary in the initial stage for forming an idea of the principles which are beyond ordinary conception, *e.g.* Puruṣa and Prakṛti.

*Abhimāna* —I-sense ; mutative ego ; conception of one's ego which gives rise to feelings like 'I am the body', 'I am wealthy (or poor)', etc.

*Abhiniveśa* —Determination. Fear of death or of non-existence of self which is really immortal ; a type of affliction.

*Ābhoga* —Engrossed attachment of mind to one thing.

*Āchārya* —Preceptor ; teacher.

*Arāḍa-kālāma* —A Sāṁkhya philosopher who was the spiritual guide of Lord Buddha at one stage.

*Adarśana* —Non-awareness ; lack of discernment.

*Adharma* —Impiety ; vice.

*Adhibhautika* —Caused by living beings ; relating to animate objects.

*Ādhidaivika* —Brought on by nature.

*Ādhyātmika* —Relating to self ; spiritual.

*Adhyātma-prasāda* —Purity of the inner instruments of reception, especially of Buddhi.

*Adṛṣṭa* —Unseen. Fate.

*Adṛṣṭaphala* —Not caused by Karma of the present life or not fructifying in the present life.

*Āgama* —Written or verbal instruction or testimony of a trustworthy person directly transmitted to the mind of the listener ; traditional doctrine ; sacred knowledge ; Śāstras.

*Agastya* —A sage. He is said to have once drunk up a whole sea.

*Agryā Buddhi* —(Agryā = foremost) Buddhi (inner instruments of reception) which brings about realisation of the Puruṣa-principle ; highest form of intellect.

*Ahaṁkāra* —Mutative ego ; I-sense.

*Ahiṁsā* —Harmlessness ; non-injury ; abstaining from killing or giving pain to others by thought, word or deed.

*Ākāśa* —Vacuity ; free space ; void ; substratum of the property of sound. One of the gross elemental principles.

*Akliṣṭa* —Not marred ; unimpaired. Non-afflictive.

*Aliṅga* —That which has no cause ; Prakṛti.

*Ambarīṣa* —One of the hells.

*Anābhoga* —Opposed to Ābhoga. Not engrossed in an object.

*Anāhata-nāda* —Spontaneous unstruck sound heard by Yogins as emanating from within the body.

*Ananta* —Boundless ; infinite ; eternal, where time and space are not applicable, *e.g.* Puruṣa.

*Aṇimā* —Minification.

*Aniyata-vipāka* —Fruition of action not restricted to one life.

*Antaḥ-karaṇa* —Inner instruments of reception comprising Buddhi, Ahaṁkāra and Manas.

*Anuśāsana* —Instruction ; precept ; explanation. An explanatory treatise on what has been taught before.

*Ānuśravika* —Described in religious books or sacred tradition.

*Ap* —A gross elemental principle ; water.

*Apāna* —One of the five Prāṇas that governs excretion of wastes from the body.

*Aparigraha* —Abstinence from avariciousness ; not to possess more than what is required for bare subsistence.

*Apavarga* —Liberation (of Puruṣa) in relation to the knowables ; termination of functioning of Buddhi.

*Apsarā* —Celestial damsel.

*Āpta* —A person who is worthy of credence ; reliable ; trustworthy.

*Apuṇya* —Impiety ; with painful results (relating to action).

*Ārṣa* —Relating to Ṛṣis (sages).

*Artha* —Wealth. Meaning of words. Objectivity of the Guṇas in relation to Draṣṭā.

*Artha-śāstra* —The science of wealth. Political economy and finance.

*Asamprajñāta* —A kind of Samādhi (intense concentration) surpassing Samprajñāta.

*Asampramoṣa* —Non-acquistion of objects or ideas not one's own.

*Āsana* —Seat ; posture ; one of the eight accessories conducive to Yoga.

*Āśīḥ* —Desire for self-welfare.

*Asmitā* —I-sense ; mutative ego ; pure I-sense. Type of affliction.

*Asmitā-mātra* —(Mātra = only) Pure I-sense.
*Asteya* —Non-covetousness.
*Asura* —Demon.
*Āsuri* —A sage, disciple of Kapila.
*Atha* —A term expressing beginning, doubt, interrogation, condition.
*Ātman* —Soul.
*Avidyā* —Misapprehension ; wrong knowledge ; type of affliction.
*Avyasana* —Absence of attachment.
*Āyurveda* —Ancient Indian medical sciences.
*Āyus* —Span of life.

## B

*Bhagavān* —God. Revered person.
*Bhāṣya* —Commentary.
*Bhava* —State of being ; existence ; cause of birth ; latent impressions of nescience.
*Bhāvanā* —Contemplative thinking.
*Bhavapratyaya-nirodha*—A type of arrested state of the mind not conducive to liberation.
*Bhāvita-smartavya* —Recollection of an experience that is unreal or imagined.
*Bhoga* —Feelings of pleasure or pain experienced by living beings. Action arising out of latencies of previous actions ; involuntary action.
*Bhogabhūta* —Action arising out of latencies of previous actions ; involuntary action.
*Bhūrloka* —World ; universe.
*Bhūta* —Gross elemental principle (the five elements being Kṣiti, Ap, Tejas, Vāyu and Ākāśa).
*Bhūtādi* —The ego of the Creator, the cause of manifestation of elements.
*Bṛhadāraṇyaka* —One of the Upaniṣads.
*Brahmā* —One of the Indian trinity said to be the creator of the universe.
*Brahmacharya* —Continence, both physical and mental.
*Brahman* —The supreme Spirit regarded as impersonal.
*Brāhmaṇa* —The portion of the Vedas which contains rules for the employment of Mantras on various occasions. Highest caste among the Hindus.

*Brahma-vihāra* —Mental purification through cultivation of feelings of amity towards happy persons, compassion for those who are miserable, goodwill for the virtuous and benevolent indifference towards the sinful.

*Buddhi* —Intellect ; intelligence. The third of the twenty-five principles of the Sāṁkhya philosophy ; pure I-sense. Inner instruments of reception taken collectively.

*Buddhi-sattva* —Pure I-sense. Inner instruments of reception taken collectively.

*Buddhi-tattva* —Pure I-sense. Inner instruments of reception taken collectively.

## C

*Chaitanya* —Absolute Consciousness. The supreme Spirit regarded as the essence of all living beings. Puruṣa.

*Charitārthatā* —The state of having accomplished the end or desired object.

*Chit* —Pure Consciousness ; the Spirit ; Brahman.

*Chiti-śākti* —Supreme conscious power ; Puruṣa.

*Chitta* —Mind ; heart ; intellect ; reasoning faculty. The special sense in which it has been used in Yoga-philosophy is as follows—Chitta or mind-stuff is the internal power which creates the sensations of cognition, conation and retention. It comprises the three inner instruments of reception, *viz.* Buddhi, Ahaṁkāra and Manas.

## D

*Daṇḍakāraṇya* —Name of a forest.

*Darśana* —Seeing ; knowing. Science of knowledge, *i.e.* philosophy. Pure Consciousness. Discriminative knowledge.

*Deva* —Celestial being.

*Dhāraṇā* —Fixity ; steady abstraction of the mind.

*Dharma* —Religion. Virtue ; piety. Attribute ; property.

*Dharmamegha-samādhi*—The final state of concentration, when the devotee becomes disinterested even in omniscience and omnipotence.

*Dhyāna* —Meditation.

*Draṣṭā* —Seer. Puruṣa.

*Dṛśya* —Object seen or known. A knowable.
*Dvandva* —Opposite conditions like feelings of heat and cold.

**E**

*Ekāgra* —Intent on one object ; one-pointed.
*Ekendriya* —That which resides in only one sense-organ. A state of detachment.

**G**

*Garuḍa* —Mythical king of the birds.
*Gomaya-pāyasa* —(Gomaya = Cowdung ; Pāyasa = Milk pudding). Regarding cowdung and pudding as the same thing, both having a common source in the cow. Instance of fallacious reasoning.
*Grahaṇa* —Receiving ; apprehension. Instrument of reception.
*Grahītā* —Receiver ; recipient. One who apprehends, denoting both Puruṣa and Buddhi.
*Grāhya* —Thing received ; object apprehended ; knowable ; perceptible.
*Guṇa* —Any one of the three primary constituents of phenomenal world (Sattva, Rajas and Tamas). Quality. Property. Rope.

**H**

*Hāna* —Abandoning everything that is fit to be discarded. Liberation.
*Hānopāya* —Means of achieving liberation.
*Heya* —A thing fit to be abandoned or discarded.
*Heyahetu* —Cause of Heya.
*Hiraṇyagarbha* —Omniscient and all-prevading Creator.
*Hṛdaya* —Heart ; the psycho-physical centre where one feels pleasure and pain.

**I**

*Indriya* —Organ of action or perception.
*Īśvara* —God.
*Īśvarakṛṣṇa* —The philosopher who compiled the extant maxims of Sāṁkhya philosophy and versified them.
*Īśvara-praṇidhāna* —Devotion to God.

## J

*Janaka* —King of Mithilā in ancient India who was also a philosopher and led the life of a Yogin.

*Janma-kathantā* —Knowledge of past lives and apprehension of future existence.

*Jāti* —Birth ; species.

*Jīva* —Living being.

*Jivanmukta* —One who has attained liberation from sorrow but has not as yet given up one's body ; one purified by true knowledge while still living and therefore freed from the cycle of births.

*Jīvātmā* —Individual or personal soul.

*Jñāna-prasāda* —Highest wisdom when all coverings on knowledge are removed.

*Jyotiṣmatī* —A state of mind pervaded by Sattva-guṇa resulting in tranquillity. Effulgent.

## K

*Kaivalya* —Liberation of Puruṣa ; Self-in-Itself ; final emancipation or beatitude.

*Kapila* —The great sage who founded the Sāṁkhya-yoga philosophy. In the opinion of some he was Hiraṇyagarbha incarnate.

*Karma* —Action, both mental and physical ; deed ; religious rite ; performance of religious rites as opposed to spiritual practice or path of knowledge.

*Karmāśaya* —Latent impression of action which will eventually fructify.

*Khyāti* —The faculty of discriminating objects. Dominating knowledge. Modification of consciousness of Buddhi.

*Kleśa* —Pain ; anguish ; distress ; worry. Affliction.

*Krama* —Sequence.

*Kṛti* —Efferent impulse.

*Kṛṣṇa-dvaipāyana Vyāsa* —A great sage, author of the Mahābhārata.

*Kṣaṇa* —Moment ; minimal time.

*Kṣiti* —A gross elemental principle. Earth.

*Kṣipta* —Thrown ; scattered. Restless.

*Kuśala* —Proficient in Yoga ; one who has attained discriminative knowledge.

*Kūtastha* —Immovable ; immutably and eternally the same.

## L

*Liṅga* —Mark ; sign ; indicator ; symbol ; characteristic.

*Liṅga-śarīra* —The indestructible core of the gross or visible body.

*Loka* —The world ; a division of the universe.

## M

*Madhumatī* —A state of knowledge attained by Yogins through concentration.

*Mahābhārata* —The great historical epic containing also the ancient philosophical thoughts of India.

*Mahadātman* —The supreme Spirit. Buddhi-tattva ; pure I-sense.

*Mahāmoha* —Obsession. Great delusion.

*Manas* —Mind in a general sense.

*Mantra* —Sacred word symbolic of God or supreme Self. Vedic verse.

*Manu* —Ancient law-giver of India.

*Mauna* —Observance of silence. A type of Yogic discipline included in Tapas.

*Miśra* —Mixed. Action leading to both pleasurable and painful consequences.

*Moha* —Delusion which prevents the discernment of truth.

*Mokṣa* —Liberation ; final emancipation ; beatitude.

*Mūḍha* —Stupefied ; infatuated ; bewildered.

## N

*Nahuṣa* —A king who was transformed into a serpent through the curse of a sage.

*Nandīśvara* —An ancient prince who through pious action was transformed into a celestial being.

*Nidrā* —Dreamless sleep (as distinguished from sleep with dreams).

*Niraya* —Infernal region.

*Nirguṇa* —Attributeless.

*Nirguṇa Īśvara* —Attributeless Godhead.

*Nirmāṇa-chitta* —Created mind. Yogins may, if they desire, assume such a mind after the attainment of emancipation for propagating the gospel of liberation.

*Nirodha-bhūmi* —Arrested state of the mind.

*Niruddha* —Stopped ; obstructed ; checked ; curbed ; arrested.

*Nirupakrama* —Action which has not started producing result.

*Nirvāṇa* —Calmed ; liberated from corporeal existence ; final emancipation.

*Nirvichāra* —Relating to subtle objects without the help of words.

*Nirvīja* —Seedless. Objectless concentration.

*Nirvikalpa* —(Applied to concentration) An exclusive concentration upon an entity without distinct and separate consciousness of the knower, the knowable and the process of knowing.

*Nirvitarka* —Relating to gross objects without the help of words.

*Nivṛtti* —Suspension ; termination ; abstention ; renunciation.

*Niyama* —Observance as an accessory to Yoga comprising cleanliness, contentment, Tapas, Svādhyāya and Īśvara-praṇidhāna.

*Niyata-vipāka* —Fruition of action restricted to one life.

## P

*Pañchaśikha* —The Ṛṣi who first framed the Sāṁkhya aphorisms, having learnt the principles from Āsuri, a direct disciple of Kapila.

*Parama Dharma* —Acme of virtuous action ; realisation of the Puruṣa-principle through Yoga.

*Paramātman* —The supreme Spirit.

*Para-vairāgya* —Supreme and final renunciation ; ultimate state of detachment.

*Pariṇāma* —Result ; effect ; fluctuation ; transformation.

*Patañjali* —An ancient sage who compiled the Yoga aphorisms.

*Pauruṣa-pratyaya* —Highest knowledge of Puruṣa ; Puruṣa-like Buddhi.

*Piśācha* —Demon.

*Pradhāna* —Chief ; pre-eminent. The source of the material world ; the primary germ out of which all material appearances are evolved ; Prakṛti.

*Prajāpati* —The God presiding over creation. An epithet of Brahmā, the Creator.

*Prajñā* —Deep understanding. Insight derived from meditation.

*Prajñā-jyoti* —A type of Yogin.
*Prakhyā* —Sentience.
*Prakṛti* —Mutable constituent of phenomena commonly called nature ; collective name of the three Guṇas.
*Prakṛti-āpuraṇa* —Permeation of nature-innate.
*Prākṛtika* —Derived from Prakṛti.
*Prakṛtilaya* —Merger into Prakṛti.
*Pramā* —Accurate conception ; true knowledge.
*Pramāṇa* —True or accurate conception or notion. Source of true knowledge.
*Prāṇa* —Breathing. First of the five vital forces.
*Prāṇa* —(in plural form) Vital forces of the body.
*Praṇava* —Sacred syllable 'OM' symbolic of God.
*Prāṇāyāma* —Breath control ; one of the eight accessories conducive to Yoga.
*Prasaṁkhyāna* —Abstract contemplation ; ultimate knowledge of discrimination between Puruṣa and Prakṛti. Omniscience.
*Praśānta-vāhitā* —Continuity of the tranquil state of mind.
*Pratisaṁkrama* —Transmission.
*Pratyāhāra* —Restraining one's organs from their objects.
*Pratyak* —Peculiar to oneself. Individual personality of self.
*Pratyaya* —Knowledge or perceptible state of the mind. Cause producing an effect.
*Praviveka* —Height of wisdom.
*Pravṛtti* —Clear mode of mind ; inclination to worldliness (*e.g.* in Pravṛtti-mārga) ; conation ; supersensuous perception.
*Preta* —Departed spirit.
*Puṇya* —Piety or pious action leading to pleasurable consequences.
*Purāṇa* —Aged ; ancient. A class of Indian scriptures.
*Puruṣa* —The supreme Soul. Absolute Awareness. The first of the twenty-five principles of Sāṁkhya philosophy. Man.
*Puruṣakāra* —Action done under one's own freewill.
*Puruṣārtha* —The object of Puruṣa. Object known by Puruṣa.

## R

*Rāga* —Attachment.
*Rajas* —The mutative principle, the second of the three Guṇas. Dirt ; dust.
*Ratna* —Jewel.
*Ṛṣi* —Sage.
*Ṛta* —Unalloyed truth. Perceptual fact.
*Ṛtambhara* —Full of Ṛta.
*Rūpa* —Light as one of the five Bhūtas. Form ; colour.

## S

*Śabda* —The characteristic of Akaśa. Sound.
*Saguṇa* —With attributes.
*Samādhi* —Intense concentration.
*Samāna* —One of the five Prāṇas by which nourishment from food is evenly distributed to all parts of the body.
*Sāmānya* —General ; common ; universal.
*Samāpatti* —Engrossment.
*Saṁjñā* —A state of the mind. Consciousness. Definition.
*Saṁkalpa* —Volition ; resolution.
*Sāṁkhya-kārikā* —The tenets of Sāṁkhya philosophy in verse form composed by Īśvarakṛṣṇa.
*Sāṁkhya-pravachana* —Sāṁkhya principles in the form of aphorisms ; Yoga-sūtras.
*Samprajanya* —Watchfulness over the state of one's body and mind.
*Samprajñāna* —Knowledge of Tattvas gained through concentration and retained in a one-pointed mind.
*Samprajñāta-yoga* —Intense concentration in a one-pointed mind in which the Tattvas are revealed and permanently retained.
*Sampratipatti* —Similarity of usage ; tradition.
*Saṁskāra* —Latent impression of mental as well as physical actions.
*Saṁvega* —Intense ardour derived from long practice.
*Saṁyama* —Technical name of fixity, meditation and concentration ; application of Dhāraṇā-Dhyāna-Samādhi on the same object. Abstinence.
*Sānanda* —With blissful feeling.
*Sarva* —All.

*Sāsmita-samādhi* —Concentration on the pure I-sense.
*Ṣaṣṭitantra* —A name of the Sāṁkhya philosophy.
*Śāstra* —Scriptures.
*Sat* —That which always exists.
*Śatapatha Brāhmaṇa* —One of the Vedic subdivisions.
*Sattva* —The sentient principle ; the first of the three Guṇas.
*Sattva-saṁsevana* —Cultivation of self-cognition.
*Sāttvika* —Of the sentient principle. Virtuous.
*Satya* —Truth ; truthfulness ; conceptual fact.
*Savichāra* —Associated with reasoning.
*Savitarka* —Associated with words.
*Skandha* —The five forms of mundane consciousness (in Buddhist philosophy).
*Smṛti* —Recollection ; remembrance ; memory.
*Smṛti-sādhanā* —Watchfulness over one's own mind.
*Sopakrama* —Action which has started producing result.
*Śraddhā* —Reverential devotion.
*Śruti* —Words of sages ; the Vedas.
*Sthiti* —Inertia. Tranquillity.
*Suśruta* —A sage who propounded the medical sciences.
*Sūtra* —Terse maxim ; aphorism.
*Svādhyāya* —Study of scriptures or the repetition of Mantras.
*Svah-loka* —A heavenly region.
*Svapna* —Sleep with dreams (as distinguished from dreamless sleep).
*Svarūpa* —Essence ; substratum.
*Svavyañjakāñjana* —Coloured by one's own manifestation.

## T

*Tamas* —Retentiveness ; the third of the three Guṇas. Darkness ; obscurity ; insentience.
*Tanmātra* —Element in its subtle or monadic form. The smallest particle of elemental knowables.
*Tapas* —Devotional austerity.
*Tapasyā* —Devotional austerity.
*Tāraka* —Intuitive knowledge ; discriminative knowledge.
*Tattva* —Principle. Any one of the twenty-five principles enumerated in the Sāṁkhya philosophy.
*Tattva-samāsa* —One of the earliest extant collections of Sāṁkhya tenets.

*Trivipāka* —Capable of producing threefold consequence (*viz.* birth, span of life and experience of pleasure and pain).

U

*Upaniṣad* —Spiritual and theological scriptures being part of the Vedas.

*Uruvilva* —A place in Northern India (present name : Bodh Gaya) where Buddha attained salvation.

V

*Vāchaspati Miśra* —A philosopher, author of explanatory treatise on Vyāsa's commentaries on Yoga aphorisms.

*Vaikārika* —Relating to modification.

*Vaināśika* —A Buddhist sect ; nihilist.

*Vairāgya* —Renunciation ; detachment.

*Vārṣagaṇya* —A Sāṁkhya sage.

*Vāsanā* —Subliminal imprint of an experience but not producing direct result like Karmāśaya.

*Vaśīkāra* —Control. A state of detachment.

*Vichārānugata* —Relating to subtle objects following reasoning associated with words.

*Videha* —Merger into discarnate state.

*Vidyā* —Knowledge ; true knowledge.

*Vijñāna-bhikṣu* —A philosopher, author of explanatory treatise on Vyāsa's commentaries on Yoga aphorisms.

*Vikalpa* —Significant or useful verbal concept of ideas which has no corresponding reality, *e.g.* space, time etc.

*Vikāra* —Change ; modification ; mutation.

*Vikṛti* —Changed state.

*Vikṣipta* —Distracted.

*Vilaya* —Dissolution.

*Vipāka* —Fruition of Karma ; result.

*Viparyaya* —Erroneous knowledge.

*Vīrya* —Energy ; enthusiasm.

*Viśeṣa* —Peculiarity. Diversified form. A division of constituent principles.

*Vitarkānugata* —Relating to gross objects following reasoning associated with words.

*Viveka-khyāti* —Discriminative enlightenment. Discernment of

Puruṣa being distinct and separate from Prakṛti, *i.e.* Self from non-self.

*Vṛtti* —Occupation. Mental mode.

*Vyāna* —One of the five Prāṇas which controls the voluntary motor nerves and muscles all over the body.

*Vyāsa* —A sage, the original commentator on Yoga aphorisms. There were other sages of the same name.

*Vyasana* —Attachment.

*Vyatireka* —Exclusion ; exception. A state of detachment.

*Vyavadhi.* —Cover. Interposition. Shape.

## Y

*Yama* —Restraint as an accessory to Yoga comprising Ahiṁsā, Satya, Asteya, Brahmacharya and Aparigraha.

*Yatamāna* —Engaged in effort. A state of detachment.

*Yoga-sūtra* —Yoga aphorism.

## INDEX

It is not an exhaustive index. Selected words of greater significance have been included and only those places where these have been dealt with in detail have been cited. The first number in the citation refers to the Book or chapter, the second to the Sūtra or aphorism and the third, within parenthesis, to the annotation. For example, II.18(7) refers to annotation No. 7 in Sūtra 18 of Book II.